CHER HAMPTON

Thrive Through Healing

4 Books in 1 about Inner Child Healing, Setting Boundaries, Codependency & Anxious Attachment Recovery

First edition

This book was professionally typeset on Reedsy.
Find out more at reedsy.com

Contents

BONUS: Your Free Gift

I'm only offering these bonuses for FREE to my readers. This is a way of saying thanks for your purchase. In this gift, you will find a guide with extra tools to start your inner journey and a self-development course.

Healing your Inner Child First Guide

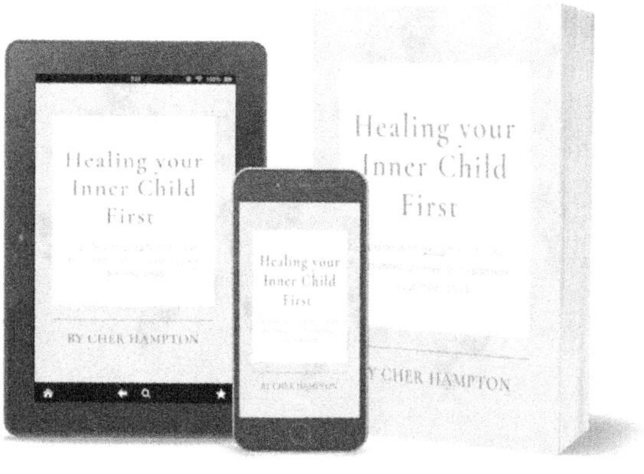

Inside this guide, you'll discover:

1. How to use Journaling in the Healing Process.
2. Questions to Remember Your Inner Child.
3. Space to Write Your Thoughts Down.

4. Questions to Better Understand Your Inner Child's Pain.
5. Motivational Things to Say to Your Inner Child.
6. Positive Affirmations + a 5-Step Method to Make Your Own.
7. An Extra Inner Child Meditation.
8. A Checklist.
9. And More...

The Personality Development Wisdom Course

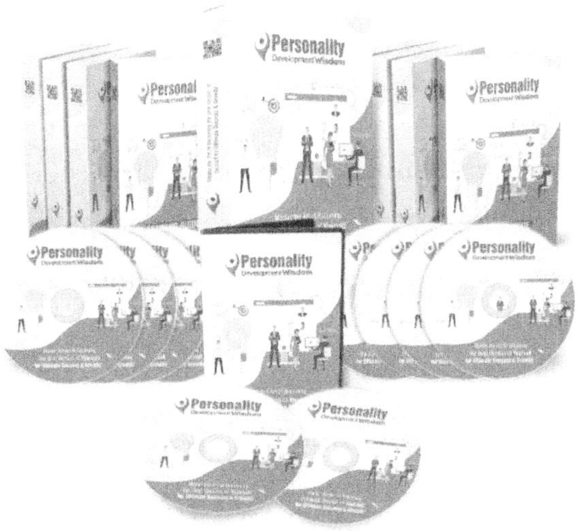

Inside this course, you will find:

1. Personality Development - An Overview
2. How to Transform Yourself into a Better Version
3. How To Improve Your Body Language
4. How to Boost Up Your Self-Confidence, Self-Esteem, and Motivation
5. Best Tips to Overcome Procrastination
6. The Power of Positive Thinking

7. How to Improve Your Workplace Wellness
8. How to Enhance Your Soft skill
9. Learn and Practice the Art of Work-Life Balance
10. How to Deal With Failures
11. How to Manage and Overcome Your Fears
12. Best Ways to Deal With Difficult People
13. Stress and Energy Management
14. How to Have a Productive Day
15. Bonus 1 - Cheat Sheet
16. Bonus 2 - Mind Map
17. Bonus 3 - Top Resource Report
18. Bonus 4 - 10 Extra Articles

To receive these extra **bonuses,** go to: https://booksforbetterlife.com/thrive-through-healing

Or scan the QR code:

About the Author

Meet Cher Hampton, a passionate author, and developmental psychologist whose life journey intertwines intimately with the subjects of her transformative books. Cher's path has been a tapestry of challenges, growth, and the relentless pursuit of healing. Growing up in a complex family dynamic, Cher's personal journey has fueled her dedication to helping others navigate the challenges of their own lives.

From an early age, Cher found herself grappling with intense emotions that often seemed disconnected from the situations at hand. Growing up with a mother diagnosed with bipolar disorder and the loss of a stepfather to suicide at just seven years old, Cher navigated emotional terrain that left lasting imprints. Her resilience carried her through bouts of depression and burnout during her formative years, ultimately inspiring her commitment to foster positive change. These experiences shaped her early maturity and pushed her to confront her own battles with depression and burnout during her teenage years.

Through her personal growth, Cher's determination to heal propelled her toward a path of self-discovery and therapeutic exploration. Over time, she honed her knowledge and skills, pursuing a master's degree in psychology to better understand the complexities of human behavior.

With her profound understanding of the human psyche and extensive background in developmental psychology, Cher can say that the topics in this book affected her and her relationships the most in the past. After tackling these issues, Cher has gained more control over her life and relationships. Now she is a powerful woman who doesn't shy away from challenges and relationships.

Cher's journey has fueled her mission to provide others with tools for healing. Her collection of books delves into the intricate world of inner child healing, overcoming anxious attachment, codependency recovery, and setting boundaries. Her commitment to helping people overcome their challenges and traumas shines through in her work.

Join Cher on a transformative journey toward self-awareness and healing. Through her profound insights and expertise, she invites you to dive into a journey of growth, empowerment, and renewal.

I

Healing Your Inner Child First

Becoming the Best Version of Yourself by Letting Go of the Past, Overcoming Trauma, and Feeling Worthy

Introduction

"The greater a child's terror, and the earlier it is experienced, the harder it becomes to develop a strong and healthy sense of self"

– NATHANIEL BRANDON

Think back to a time when you were having fun with the other kids in your neighborhood. You tumble and fall while racing around on the playground. The other kids make fun of you. You might not recall everything that happened. You could not even recall who was there or your age at the time. But you remember the embarrassment, the tears in your eyes, and the ache of your skinned knee. You can even recall telling yourself, "I'm never going to make a fool of myself like that again."

Although your knee has healed, you are carrying the wounds into adulthood. You are no longer in command. Your inner five-year-old is still in charge, whether you're twenty or fifty years old. Even though taking a risk may benefit you, you can't forget what occurred on the playground—even if you don't remember it.

When we begin the inner child healing journey, we are tapping into a sensitive and impressionable aspect of ourselves. We may be both the 'grown-up' and the 'child,' offering unconditional self-love, compassion, and support.

We are born with a blank slate. As we mature, we learn everything we will take into adulthood, and we do so in two ways. The first is by gaining experience, and the second is by playing. When we play as children, we act out our experiences, ideas, feelings, and dreams. Our imaginations serve as the foundation for how we prepare for life in the actual world.

Adolescence is a period of exploration, but it can also be a time of suffering. As we get older, we begin to have opinions about the world. Those expectations might let us down at times. We have shattered hearts, we have disappointments, and we have aspirations that never come true. Many of us eventually stop playing and let our experiences define who we are and what we desire.

Heal Your Inner Child in the Following Steps

Self-care is being discussed more often than ever before, and for good reason. Healthcare practitioners and therapists alike are discussing techniques for reducing anxiety and making the current moment as serene as possible. But what do you do when your anxieties, pain, and hurt go much deeper than the present events? How can you begin healing when your inner child is crying out for love, acceptance, and comfort?

Learning to confront the past without allowing it to dictate your present and future might be a difficult step to take, but it is doable. Today, we're going to provide six methods you may use to deal with the problem(s) that caused you to lose your innocence, and begin rebuilding the life you deserve.

1. identify the neglect
2. accept the past
3. accommodate your inner child
4. reach out to your inner child
5. embrace your emotions

6. fill the gap by taking action

How to Develop a Meaningful Relationship with Your Inner Child in Two Steps

ONE: Connect with your inner child, starting a discussion with them, and create a connection.

TWO: Begin to truly listen to and learn about your inner child's needs, sorrows, hopes, and dreams, and take measures to make them a reality.

The objective is for you to tune in to how your inner child is doing, to tenderly care for it, and to discover a method to satisfy its needs. Doing so often clarifies what has to change in order for you to go forward.

Furthermore, this internal process frequently softens the resistance and 'stuckness' you are experiencing in your adult life. Some people find that 'reparenting' their inner child is beneficial in this process as well, using the inner child to alleviate stress and inspire optimism and pleasure.

Let's begin here...

To do this, we will first ask your adult self to be a little more open and potentially vulnerable. Bring your inner kid out of hiding and talk about what's going on or what it requires. We must be open to hearing and witnessing their tale, inquiring about his/her life, hopes, aspirations, anxieties, and problems.

We want your inner child to start building trust with your adult self so that it may share freely. We want to know about its expectations, dreams, wishes, as well as its pain, sadness, fears, and worries.

We frequently notice that when the inner child has someone (adult you) who actually cares, slows down, and is there with them, they can calm down and feel the sensations that he/she has had to suppress for years. It's frequently suggested that you perform this work with a qualified therapist who specializes in inner child therapy, childhood emotional neglect, or emotional difficulties since the work can be delicate. A skilled clinician can guide and support your recovery. However, if you can't see a therapist, don't get disheartened. The approaches outlined in this book will allow you to work on yourself and help your inner child.

As you come to know your inner child better, you may find that they need some serious mending. There are several approaches to providing support, love, and healing to one's inner child. They may need to tell you a narrative that they've been keeping hidden for years. Your inner kid could show you the loss and pain it felt years ago but didn't have the tools to process their trauma. He/she might want to demonstrate to you their need for love and attention, and may want you to discover methods to meet those needs in your life before moving on with the goals you've been concentrating on. They may request that you speak up in your relationships since he/she does not want to be ignored like they were as a youngster. It might also be something else. We have no idea what will come up until we begin this procedure.

When the inner child realizes that you are paying attention to them and trying your best to love it and meet its needs, it will frequently be more accessible to you.

It may need greater physical or emotional safety, more attention to how you're taking care of your mind, body, or soul, recovering from previous wounds, creating boundaries in life, or changing who you spend time with. This effort frequently reveals what is genuinely essential. When we deal with the deeper levels of inner child healing, we've observed how many symptoms are alleviated when clients begin to work beyond and through stuck places. We've witnessed clients begin to open their hearts for the first time, allowing love to enter their lives.

For some, completing the deeper work helps them to be present in their parenting so they can connect without the irritation that was previously there. Others begin to show up to work and relationships with confidence, and they begin to ask for what they require more easily. Others find that their worry and dread have subsided significantly, and they can now stand firm on the limits they've been attempting to establish for years.

Now, our inner kid may either be quiet and comfortable (most of the time), or it can act out and make things a little rumbly on the inside: impeding good relationships, organizational abilities, and self-regulation. When it comes to becoming a contributing member of society, or taking steps toward pleasure, our inner child may make or break us.

If you're feeling irritated or trapped in your life, it's likely that your inner child requires some care. Stuck spots might manifest as difficulty at work, in parenting, in finding or maintaining love, in growing relationships, or in creating boundaries.

> ***NOTE:*** *This book will have the best effect when you try to perform all the exercises presented in this book to the best of your ability. Sometimes it can also be good to perform them several times; in the end, listen to what feels right for you.*

Finding and Reconnecting with Your Inner Child

"A grownup is a child with layers on"

— WOODY HARRELSON

This chapter talks about:

- 9 ways to rediscover your inner child
- Root chakra

As per the definition of the inner child by Woody Harrelson, you may ask if your child within is a real person or only a psychological term or hypothesis. There isn't a physical child inside of you, of course (unless you're pregnant). What you must remember is that, while no one can see tangible indications of your child within, it is still real. We evolve, but our minds and bodies retain memories—and occasionally moods and patterns—from the past. The child within might sometimes be the source of how we feel as adults.

You've undoubtedly mentioned your inner kid a few times before. "I'm channeling my inner child," you could declare while leaping off park swings, chasing your roommate across the house with a Nerf pistol, or plunging into the pool while wearing your clothing.

Many people attribute the idea of an inner child to psychiatrist Carl Jung, who identified a child archetype in his writings (Kellend, 2015). He connected this internal child to memories and experiences of innocence, fun, and creativity, as well as optimism for the future.

Other experts define this inner child as a manifestation of not just your kid self, but also your lived experience through all phases of life (Sjöblom et al., 2016). Because early experiences can have a significant impact on your development as an adult, the inner child can be a source of strength.

Recognizing Trauma

The first step toward healing is identifying the impact of our experiences as children because they continue to have an influence on us in adulthood. Trauma has different effects on each individual, which could include loss of sleep or loss of appetite. One is infused with fear after the trauma and this is one of the ways to recognize it. Childhood trauma, and trauma generally, can manifest itself in a variety of ways. Examples of trauma that may affect kids include (but are not limited to):

- neglect or abuse (whether physical or emotional)
- bullying
- natural calamities
- financial upheaval or hardship
- car mishaps
- substance abuse problems in the family
- other mental or physical health problems in the family
- the loss of a loved one
- domestic violence in the family
- being a displaced person
- housing instability

- predictability is lacking
- distancing from caregivers
- isolation

However, when traumatic childhood events influence you, your inner child may continue to bear these scars until you address the root of the pain.

Recovery

If you were instructed as a youngster not to express your emotions, you may have learned to keep them inside. Though this is only one example, emotional suppression may be harmful both emotionally and physically, thus it is critical to treat it. Lower-level traumas, negative sensations and experiences that have lasting influence are common in childhood. Therefore, even if you are the healthiest child, you can do inner child work to resolve lasting traumas.

Furthermore, if the problem is not identified and addressed while you are still a youngster, major and lasting consequences might occur. The following are some frequent issues in adulthood that individuals address or explore when doing inner child work:

- self-sabotage
- self-destructive conduct
- adolescent passive-aggressive conduct
- anger or outbreaks of rage
- suppression or repression of emotions
- attachment insecurity

With this in mind, it's no surprise that working on your inner child may help you live a better, happier, and more confident adult life. It can help you reclaim your power as a result of childhood adversity and become the person you want to be.

9 Ways to Rediscover Your Inner Child

Relive the simple delight and wonder of existence once more.

Despite that we now know that everyone has a child within. We as individuals occasionally forget to embrace the humorous, lighter side of life. Reconnecting with your inner child involves taking life a little less seriously. Allowing oneself time to play, explore, laugh, and observe the world with delight and astonishment is what this connection implies.

Laughing is a Therapy

Do you recall laughing, even giggling, as a youngster since there was nothing to stop you? You didn't have to worry about expenses or waking up early for work. You lived for the present, and what toy you were going to play with next.

Break out in a huge belly laugh if you wish to release your inner kid. The idea is to laugh as if no one is looking and to be unafraid of doing so. There are many things in life that may make you laugh:

- Consider a humorous situation you've been in. If you've just experienced tragedy in your life, try taking advantage of having a good laugh, it may act as a salve.
- One tried-and-true strategy is to keep pretending to laugh until you start laughing naturally. This is a type of treatment that is used in a variety of institutions, so don't dismiss it. Start laughing right now!
- Spend quality time with your friends, colleagues or family members. Sitting and talking with them can turn any situation into a humorous one. Play games like: I Spy, Slug Bug, and other travel competitions with your family or friends.
- Lastly, you can turn to the internet for a good laugh. Put on a comedy

movie or tv show and start laughing your heart out. But remember to not make this an addiction as it may cause negative effects in the future.

Go ahead and be utterly foolish, as the child within connects with your light-hearted and joyful personality. According to the National Library of Medicine, finding opportunities to laugh every day may do wonders for your mental health (Robinson, 2018).

Express Yourself Fully and Honestly

Children appear to express themselves openly via dance, laughter, and play! They also know how to tell it like it is, and may be brutally honest at times!

As you become older, societal standards have a greater influence on your conduct. You may become shy or fearful of expressing yourself. You may speak up less, maybe out of fear of being rejected.

However, your true self deserves to shine! When you don't communicate your actual sentiments, you miss out on important connections and experiences. Learn to talk openly and honestly to re-awaken your inner child. Not everyone will agree with you, and that's fine! When you express yourself, you offer the world your unique perspective, and as a result, attract individuals who actually appreciate you for who you are.

Spend Time with the Kids

Spending more time with children is a great approach to bring out your inner child. Making time to spend with your children, whether you're cracking jokes, running around, or playing games, lets you tap into your inner fun and youthful expression. You will also have the opportunity to share your expertise in order to assist young people in learning and growing. If you don't have children of your own, you might spend time with the children of friends or relatives.

Recognize Your Strengths to Improve Your Inner Peace and Security

Everyone needs to feel safe, especially children. You must build an unbreakable persona that you are confident will protect you. You may do this by being aware of your emotional, physical, and spiritual strengths. Accept that you have obstacles to overcome, and embrace your gift for resilience. If you wish to communicate with your inner child, you must first make them feel protected:

1. Keep an eye out for when you're attempting to modify or deny things that can't be undone. Some individuals interpret warning signs as sentiments such as, "This is unjust, it shouldn't be this way!" or "Why am I here?" Others may experience warning signals in the form of emotions such as rage or irritation.
2. Remember that "it is what it is," and there is nothing you can do about it right now. Depending on the scenario, you may need to repeat this several times each day/hour/minute.
3. Allow yourself to be sad and dissatisfied; these are useful emotions too! Simultaneously, have faith that acceptance will eventually offer you serenity and tranquility.
4. Seek social assistance. Engage in self-care activities to assist you in coping with tough emotions and improving your mood.

Use Your Imagination

Kids like learning via arts and crafts, dance, drawing, singing, and so on. You, too, may bring out your inner kid via creative activity—and reap several health advantages as a result. Creative self-expression aids in the recovery from trauma, the management of emotions, and the promotion of general well-being (Chen, 2020).

Do you need some motivation? There are several adult coloring books available to help you get your creative juices flowing. Start some do-it-yourself projects to decorate your house or business.

Respect Yourself

Perhaps members of your family adored you and showed it frequently. Even so, a tragic occurrence as a youngster may have made you doubt their love for you. If, on the other hand, your caregivers and other key people in your life rarely showed their affection for you, providing your physical requirements but were emotionally aloof, you may have grown up feeling ignored, unwanted, and maybe even unlovable.

How do you teach yourself to embrace your inner child? As you identify and address your childhood needs, such as emotional needs, social requirements, boundaries, the need to relax, and so on, you will likely begin to notice the benefits of this self-care. It might be difficult at times to recognize what you need and offer yourself the love and respect you deserve. If this describes you, a therapist might be able to assist you in recovering from childhood trauma.

Keep Developing Yourself

Adults are more concerned with problem-solving and completing tasks. Children are eager to study and discover the world's many possibilities. Adults grow more into this fixed mindset where they think they know everything and miss the opportunity to learn. Where children have this growth mindset and always want to discover new things. By letting go of the constant drive to correct and control, you may reconnect with your inner child. Instead, have an open mind and look for learning changes every day.

Consult a Therapist

If reaching out to your inner child causes discomfort or difficult emotions, such as loss, traumatic memories, or feelings of helplessness or dread, be sure to obtain support from a competent mental health practitioner. A therapist can provide support and expose you to coping skills that can help you deal with prior trauma and emotions.

Some therapists may have more inner child work experience and training than others. Inquiring about possible therapists' experience with inner child therapy will assist you in finding the proper individual to support your growth and recovery, as this method is based on the premise that mental health problems, relational issues, and other forms of emotional suffering are frequently the result of unresolved pain or suppressed emotions from childhood and/or adolescence.

In therapy, you may learn to 'reparent' your inner child, which will allow you to start addressing and resolving these difficulties.

Clearing Chakra Blockages

Chakra is a Sanskrit word that means "'wheel' and refers to energy points in your body. They are thought to be spinning disks of energy that should remain 'open' and aligned," as they work in relation to "bundles, major organs, and areas of our energetic body that affect our emotional and physical well-being" (Stelter 2016). These wheels are energy places in your body that become blocked when you experience negativity, pain, or illness.

Root Chakra

Energetically, our "Root Chakra Existence Cycle" of seven years, establishes the basis of who we are throughout our first seven years of life. As a result, our fundamental ideas and unconscious behaviors are formed.

Our energy body develops our root chakra (foundation) as well as all of our other chakras during the first seven years of our life. We have a basic human need that we are attempting to fulfill at each age—one, two, three, and so on. When these demands are addressed, the chakra associated with them tends to open. And if a chakra requirement is not supplied, that chakra tends to close down (Howie, 2021).

Meaning

Our body's most primordial and essential energy center, the root chakra, or Muladhara, is located near the base of our spine, or groin area. The energy here is connected with instinct, survival, and safety and regulated by the root chakra, also associated with the color red.

When the root chakra gets tainted as a result of trauma, psychological difficulties such as persistent dread, or psychosomatic suppression and repression, the flow of life is disrupted. Our clogged energy centers frequently cause us ongoing personal, existential, and relational concerns.

The base layer, 1st Chakra of our Unconscious Mind, serves as a hard drive for the ego. This hard drive stores all of our life streams' cellular memories. These memories are not assigned value when they are recorded, and regardless of whether they are perceived as good or harmful, are saved on the root hard drive of every human person. Whether one was a fetus, an infant, or unconscious when the body was subjected to 'abuse,' the incident was stored in one's memory bank, whether it is recallable consciously or not.

Some people will have terrible memories but will have no idea what caused them or where they originated from. Others will be in shock and will have fully shut off these memories as a coping technique. Others have had great success releasing these memories using emotional clearing techniques such as hypnosis or other therapies. Because our autonomic nerve system and autonomic body processes are controlled by our unconscious mind, unhealed memory trauma in these primary areas causes a wide range of physical symptoms and disease.

Healing

The practice of root chakra healing entails the opening, clearing, purifying, maintaining, and strengthening of the root chakra in our bodies. Root chakra therapy employs certain foods, sounds, scents, affirmations, yoga routines, crystals, and other holistic medicines to restore balance to the body-mind unit.

Obtaining Base Security

To restore balance to our root chakra, we must make a concerted effort to break the fallacy of basing one's self-esteem on the appearance or assumption of external conditions. For many of us, the immediate goal is to be psychologically and emotionally free of being harassed, intimidated, and threatened against one's feeling of inner security, stability, foundation, and well-being. It is entirely up to each of us to maintain that relationship. Only you can create faith in that relationship with yourself; no one else can accomplish it for you.

The root chakra, therefore, is the basis of our body's foundation and our form-holding energetic blueprint, which lives as the holographic tree of life. When we carry unresolved and unconscious suffering in our base frequency, it weakens our whole foundation, eroding the roots that hold our personal tree of life at its very base. Without strong, permanent roots for establishing the strong, secure spiritual basis of one's personal tree of life, one's path may fall or be redirected. This is why laying a solid foundation helps to create a balanced root chakra is crucial in laying a spiritual basis that will help to heal your inner child. When one is not spiritually strong in morals and ethics, one is easily influenced, controlled, or possibly hijacked by controlling forces.

To restore balance to our foundation, we must confront negative archetypes and fear thought-forms in order to deliberately work to change them to a higher frequency of love ideas. At this point, you will be directed to the vibrationally matched and appropriate life route in order to complete the needed learning through the highest awareness pathway.

15 Indicators of an Unbalanced Root Chakra

Pay attention to your ideas, feelings, behaviors, and physical sensations within your body to determine whether you require root chakra therapy.

Here are some red flags to keep a watch out for:

1. You have a tendency to obsess over money. For example, you worry that you don't have enough, you have catastrophic thoughts about going poor and homeless, you overwork to alleviate your financial anxiety, you become triggered whenever someone in your family spends too much, you feel you must have complete control over the money in your family, and so on.
2. You are generally distrustful of people (trust issues).
3. You assume that the only person you can rely on is yourself, and you avoid asking people for favors (even when you really need them).
4. You're a workaholic who burns out easily.
5. You don't get along with your family.
6. You have the impression that there is "never enough" to go around and that you must struggle for what you desire.

7. You're afraid of losing control.
8. You are hyper-aware of any potential threat from people or your surroundings.
9. For most of the day, you feel dizzy, uneasy, spacey, and ungrounded.
10. You find it challenging and frightening to be your true self in front of people.
11. You are estranged from other people and nature.
12. You're a hoarder who enjoys 'collecting' a large amount of items, resulting in a small and crowded living space.
13. When you are unhappy or stressed, you binge or stop eating totally.
14. You experience issues with your legs and feet, such as: edema, infection, cramping, and poor circulation.
15. The lower part of your body is where you acquire weight the most (e.g. love handles, thick thighs).

How many of the signs on this list do you recognize?

Do You Have an Excessive or Deficient Root Chakra?

When most people talk about 'blocked' or deficient chakras that hinder energy flow, they're talking about diseased root chakras. But do you realize that your chakras may be excessive—or hyperactive—as well?

So, what is the distinction between a deficient and an overactive root chakra? A weak root chakra is considered docile, whilst an overactive root chakra is considered aggressive.

Here's a rundown:

Deficient chakras are: dead, slow, inactive, blocked, and introverted (not enough energy flows in). As a result, you will be more prone to difficulties like worry, distrust, and withdrawal.

Overactive chakras, on the other hand, are: energetic, agitated, reactive, aggressive, and outwardly directed (too much energy flows in). If your root chakra is overactive, you are prone to hoarding, workaholism, greed, and rage.

Hence, excessiveness compensates for deficiencies, whereas deficiency protects. So the question is, which of them do you have? It is also conceivable to fall someplace in between the two categories.

15 Healing Techniques for the Root Chakra

So, how does a healthy and balanced root chakra feel?

When your root chakra is clean, strong, and harmonious, you will feel anchored and tranquil at first. You will no longer be afraid of money or losing control, but will instead come to trust the divine wisdom of life. Not only will you have more faith in yourself, but you will also feel more intimately connected to others and the environment. When your root chakra is in good condition, it will be simpler to be your real self and connect to the calm that is always there in the present moment. You will let go of the need to battle, guard, and defend, and instead align with the ebb and flow of existence.

Root chakra is also great for healing the inner child as the sacral chakra is totally dedicated to this purpose. This chakra deals with creativity and happiness which is essential for your inner child to thrive. In order to reach out to your inner child, practice the following root chakra exercises:

1. **Repeat the phrase "LAM" to yourself:** This sound corresponds to the vibration of the root chakra. You might also want to listen to binaural beats (a type of music healing therapy that uses alternating sound waves to activate and cleanse all of the chakras). Listening to binaural beats between 7-30 Hz daily will bring a change and help the inner child to heal.

2. **Go for a walk in the woods on a regular basis:** Take conscious notice of your feet's relationship to the soil.
3. **Practice targeted yoga:** Stretch your muscles with the basic yoga poses of child pose, forward bend, mountain pose, squat, and warrior.
4. **Consume grounding foods:** Consider root vegetables such as sweet potatoes, beets, radishes, and others.
5. **Practice mindfulness for 30 seconds:** Make it a habit to pause every day and count your breaths for three counts. This simple exercise will assist you in regaining your footing.
6. **Carry crystals with you and meditate with them:** Use crystals from the root chakra, such as: jasper, hematite, smokey quartz, and carnelian. Black tourmaline is my favorite root chakra gem.
7. **Use aromatherapy smells to cleanse the root chakra:** Sandalwood, vetiver, patchouli, cloves, black pepper, and ginger are some essential oils to try.
8. **Experiment with 'earthing:'** Earthing is the technique of walking on grass or ground to recharge the human energy field.
9. **Sit quietly and envision:** Imagine a crimson ball of light pulsing in your root chakra (your groin area). Consider all of the murky energy dissolving as it comes into contact with the ball of red light.
10. **Set aside time each day to sit outside and connect with nature:** Simply watch what is happening around you: the birds, the breeze, the clouds, the light, and feel your oneness with nature.
11. **Make use of affirmations or mantras:** To change your unconscious thought habits, use mantras or affirmations: "I am grounded," "I am centered and whole," "I trust in the wisdom of life," "I have all I need," "I am safe and secure," "I surrender," and "I am strong, stable, and at peace" are some affirmation/mantra examples.
12. **Drink a grounding tea:** Include root chakra cleansing herbs such as ashwagandha and cloves.
13. **Take a relaxing shower:** Water has the ability to clear sluggish and obstructed energy. Alternatively, take a cleansing bath with mineral

salts like Himalayan pink rock salt.

14. **Look into the source of your anxieties:** Fears arise as a result of your inner beliefs, grudges, and unresolved sorrow. Spend some time in a notebook or with a trusted friend, partner, or therapist, reflecting on the source of your anxieties.
15. **Engage in catharsis:** Every day, engage in catharsis to actively release blocked root chakra energy. You may try dynamic meditation or just leap, kick, punch, yell, or dance your stress away.

Story of Someone Who Has Been Through the Journey

Let's consider for a moment, the story of someone who has previously suffered with a very unbalanced root chakra (Thoughtless Delineation, 2018):

> *I discovered that incorporating greater awareness into my days helped quickly and tremendously. Slowing down, taking more pauses, and connecting with my breath were all basic and straightforward initial steps I took. Following that, I began using the other therapeutic methods, such as: aroma therapy, connecting with nature, and journaling for insight and cathartic release.*
>
> *Childhood trauma may leave an indelible imprint on our minds. These memories might be kept in our bodies, cells, in our very essence. The route to completeness within myself was therefore about providing a safe space for this trauma to be heard and healed.*
>
> *For those, like myself, who have undergone bodily trauma, the energy toll is enormous. It means that the body is never a safe place to be, and the planet is never a secure place to be. It implies that we do not believe we can fall and be caught. It implies submission may evade us, yet the beauty of surrender is that when we do, we get the greatest blessings in life: love, freedom, joy.*

Trauma in the body also means that we are always firing on all cylinders, which can lead to a depletion of resources and energy levels that affect our health on several levels.

I've been fortunate to experience numerous methods of self-knowledge and healing over the years that I've spent learning to own my body and know myself. And this is now influencing the work I share.

My idea is that when we can't figure out why something is the way it is, or why we're stuck in some manner, we turn to the body for solutions. And our body will tell us what is going on.

Many individuals might be in their 30s, 40s, or older, and live very successful lives, but at some level, the terrified kid within them remains frightened. On some level, their bodies are still holding the trauma, and it will have an impact, whether subtle or overt.

Trauma may become such a familiar companion in our body that we may seek out more unpleasant occurrences because the reverse seems incorrect in some way. As a result, many people who come from violent backgrounds may find themselves in similar situations again.

We persist in the pain because we are creatures of habit—familiar equals safe. As a result, the wire tripping persists. However, true comfort comes from teaching the body what is good and healthy.

Key Takeaways

- Don't be afraid of bringing your inner child out as he/she is the one affected. Addressing your inner child will help you to heal.
- Root chakra is the process of healing internally and will help you overcome the trauma. You don't necessarily need to have experienced a traumatic childhood to benefit from this healing—any minor issue

throughout life can also be the reason. No matter what it is, the earlier it is addressed, the better it will be for you.

- The fifteen above mentioned techniques are the guide to healing. If you feel like this is new for you, and you feel overwhelmed, keep reading ahead to trust the process.

Emotional and Psychological Trauma

"The greatest happiness of life is the conviction that we are loved; loved for ourselves, or rather, loved in spite of ourselves"

— VICTOR HUGO

This chapter talks about:

- Effects of trauma in childhood and the risk of future trauma
- Aftermath of emotional and psychological distress

Children whose families and homes do not consistently give regular safety, comfort, and protection may develop coping mechanisms that allow them to live and function on a daily basis. For example, they may be highly sensitive to other people's moods, always monitoring to see what the adults around them are feeling and how they will behave. They may hide their feelings from others, never allowing them to see when they are fearful, sad, or furious. When physical and/or mental threats are constant, these types of learned adaptations make sense. As a child grows older and experiences safe environments and relationships, these adaptations become less useful, and may even be counterproductive, interfering with the ability to live, love, and be free.

What occurs to us in our first ten years of life has an impact on every decade that follows. Our bodies, brains, and personalities are imprinted by our early experiences during this very fast era of growth and development. That is why childhood trauma may have such a profound effect on our mental and physical health and well-being throughout our lives. The definition of childhood trauma varies greatly. Childhood trauma can manifest itself in a variety of ways, including physical or sexual abuse, neglect, unstable or hazardous environment, witnessing violence in the household, and serious illness. Furthermore, children might suffer from relational trauma, which is defined as a break in the primary link with a parent or caregiver. Trauma can also be triggered by events outside the home, ranging from intense bullying to the communal trauma caused by catastrophic events such as a pandemic. What influence can childhood trauma have on an individual's capacity to flourish as they grow older? Here are six ways trauma can appear mentally and physically as children move through adolescence into adulthood.

Trauma and Self-Worth

How we are treated by people closest to us from infancy onwards is critical in forming our perception of ourselves as worthwhile and deserving of love and care. Children who are mistreated or neglected by their primary caregivers learn that they are unlovable. Even loving parents who do not relate with their children may accidentally send this message to them. Furthermore, 'parentification' occurs when parents rely on their children to satisfy their emotional needs, and children learn that their own needs are unimportant. As a result, traumatized youngsters acquire a deep feeling that they are unworthy. They may blame themselves for their treatment, feeling that if they were 'better,' their parents would "love them more." Even if this self-perception is unconscious or semi-conscious, it can be exceedingly difficult to change later in life. An individual may finally realize why their parent(s) acted the way they did, maybe as a result of their own unresolved childhood trauma or a mental or physical disease.

However, awareness alone may not be sufficient to transform the adult child's self-image and feeling of self-worth.

In turn, this fundamental wound, as it is sometimes called, causes a deep well of emotional suffering. As a result, young people who have experienced childhood trauma and the guilt and shame that comes with it are more likely to suffer from anxiety, depression, and maladaptive coping methods such as substance abuse and self-harm.

Relationships and Attachment

It is impossible to emphasize the value of a child's tight bond with a caregiver. Children learn to trust people, manage their emotions, and engage with the environment through interactions with significant attachment figures; they acquire a sense of the world as safe or hazardous, and they start to appreciate their own value as individuals. Children learn that they can't rely on others to aid them when those close interactions are unstable or unpredictable. When a child's primary caregivers exploit and abuse him or her, the youngster internalizes self-hate and comes to believe that the world is a dreadful place.

The majority of abused or neglected children struggle to form a strong, healthy relationship to a caregiver. It has been demonstrated that children who do not develop healthy bonds are more sensitive to stress. They have difficulty managing and expressing their emotions, and they may respond aggressively or improperly in certain situations. Our capacity to have healthy, supportive connections with friends and significant others is dependent on our ability to form such ties in our families. A youngster who has experienced complex trauma may struggle in romantic relationships, friendships, and with authority figures such as teachers or police officers.

Physical Well-Being: Body and Mind

The biology of the body evolves from birth until adolescence. The environment influences normal biological function in certain ways. For instance, when a kid grows up fearful or under persistent or acute stress, the immune system and stress response mechanisms in the body may not develop appropriately. When the kid is later subjected to even moderate amounts of stress in adulthood, these systems may behave as though the individual is under acute stress. When confronted with stressful events, an individual may exhibit strong physiological reactions, such as: fast breathing, heart pounding, or may "shut down" completely. While these reactions are standard biological reactions to stress, they are often out of proportion in the context of typical stress and appear to the outside world as: 'overreacting,' 'unresponsiveness,' or 'disconnection.'

The development of the brain and nervous system can be hampered by stress in the environment. In neglectful situations, a lack of mental stimulation may prevent the brain from growing to its full capacity. Children who have experienced complicated trauma may have persistent or recurring medical issues, such as headaches or stomach aches. Adults with a history of childhood trauma have been found to have more chronic bodily diseases and issues. They may engage in dangerous activities, exacerbating the severity of these illnesses.

Body dysregulation is a common symptom of complexly traumatized adolescents, meaning they either overreact or underreact to sensory inputs. Some may be hypersensitive to noises, scents, touch, or light, for example, or they may be numb in a manner of speaking, to pain, touch, or internal bodily sensations. As a result, individuals may harm themselves without experiencing pain, suffer from physical difficulties without realizing it, or complain of persistent discomfort in numerous body parts for which no physical explanation can be located.

Emotional Reactions

Children who have undergone severe trauma, frequently struggle to: understand, express, and manage their emotions, and may have limited terminology for experiencing such states. They frequently internalize and/or externalize stress reactions, which can lead to considerable melancholy, anxiety, or aggression. Their emotional reactions might be erratic or explosive. Trembling, rage, grief, or avoidance may be displayed by a youngster in response to a reminder of a traumatic experience. Reminders of multiple traumatic incidents may therefore lurk anywhere in everyday surroundings for a youngster with a complicated trauma history. When disturbed, such a youngster may often respond violently, and have difficulties calming down. Because interpersonal traumas are so common, even minimally unpleasant contact with others can function as trauma memories and cause significant emotional reactions.

Children are typically alert and guarded in their dealings with others, and are more prone to view circumstances as stressful or hazardous, having learnt that the world is a terrible place where even loved ones cannot be trusted to protect them. While this defensive stance is beneficial when an individual is being attacked, it becomes troublesome in situations that do not necessitate such ferocious reactions. Many youngsters, on the other hand, learn to "tune out" (emotional numbness) to hazards in their surroundings, leaving them exposed to revictimization.

Difficulty controlling emotions is widespread and occurs even in the absence of partnerships. Many of these youngsters get quickly overwhelmed because they have never learned how to calm themselves down when they are unhappy. In school, for example, they may feel so upset that they abandon even the smallest activities that provide a challenge. Children who have undergone early and strong traumatic incidents are more likely to feel scared all of the time and in a variety of scenarios. They are also more prone to suffer from depression.

Dissociative Symptoms

Dissociation is common in children who have experienced complex trauma. When children are confronted with an overpowering and frightening situation, they may dissociate, or psychologically remove themselves from it. They may feel disconnected from their bodies, floating on the ceiling or elsewhere in the room, witnessing what is occurring to their bodies. They may believe they are in a dream or another altered condition that is not quite real, or that the event is occurring to someone else. Alternatively, individuals may lose all recollections or sense of what occurred to them, resulting in temporal gaps or holes in their personal history. At its most severe, a youngster may cut off or lose contact with numerous parts of his or her life.

Although children do not naturally disassociate intentionally, once they have learned to as a protection strategy, they may dissociate spontaneously in subsequent stressful situations or when confronted with traumatic memories. As a result, dissociation can impair a child's capacity to be completely present in daily activities and drastically disrupt a child's sense of time and continuity, thus having the potential to impair learning, classroom conduct, and social relationships. Others may not always notice when a child is dissociating, and it may appear that the youngster is merely 'pinging,' daydreaming, or not paying attention.

Effects on Cognitive Abilities

When brain function is interrupted, the consequences are far-reaching. Along with the mental and physical health repercussions of childhood trauma outlined above, individuals might also develop cognitive issues—difficulties with memory, logical reasoning, and problem solving. These executive functioning deficits might make it difficult for individuals to establish goals, plan for the future, and achieve success in academic or professional settings. According to research, those who have undergone childhood trauma have a smaller prefrontal cortex, the area of the brain responsible for executive functioning.

Cognitive deficits can be caused by habitual psychological patterns that a child develops as a result of trauma, in addition to brain structure and function. When youngsters are continually exposed to stress, all of their energies are devoted to surviving the stressor. As a result, they have less energy, attention, and interest to devote to learning, developing new abilities, and making sound judgments. Even after the traumatic experience has passed, trauma triggers, and the ongoing struggle to avoid them, divert a child's efforts and attention away from learning new things. As a result, childhood trauma symptoms and PTSD are linked to the following problems in early adulthood and beyond:

- learning disabilities
- memory problems
- language difficulties
- difficulty with organization and planning
- adults are more sensitive to traumatic stress
- a short attention span
- cognitive abilities deteriorate at a faster rate.

Emotional and psychological trauma is produced by very stressful conditions that rob you of your sense of security, leaving you helpless in a dangerous setting. Psychological trauma can leave you with unresolved unpleasant feelings, memories, and anxiety. It can also make you feel numb, distant, and hard to trust others.

Traumatic situations frequently include a threat to one's life or safety, but any circumstance that leaves you feeling overwhelmed and lonely can result in trauma, even if no physical damage is involved. The subjective emotional experience of the event, rather than the objective conditions, determines whether an incident is traumatic. The more terrified and helpless you feel, the more probable it is that you have been traumatized. Below is a list of some traumatic citations that can cause physical and psychological turmoil:

- major and minor incidents, such as an accident, injury, violent attack, losing a loved one, divorce or bullying, can contribute to emotional and psychological stress
- constant and unrelenting stressors, such as living in a high-crime area, suffering a life-threatening illness, or witnessing horrific events on a regular basis, such as, bullying, spousal abuse, or childhood mistreatment
- commonly ignored reasons, such as surgery (particularly in the first three years of life), the unexpected loss of a close relative, the end of an important relationship, or a humiliating or severely disappointing event, especially if someone was intentionally harsh

It might be tough to cope with the trauma of a natural or man-made tragedy, even if you were not personally engaged in the event. In reality, while it's exceedingly improbable that any of us would ever be direct victims of a terrorist attack, aircraft accident, or mass shooting, for example, we're all frequently exposed to awful pictures of those who have been on social media and news outlets. Repeatedly viewing these sights might overload your neural system and cause severe stress. Whatever the origin of your trauma, and whether it occurred years ago or recently, you're encouraged to make therapeutic adjustments and go on with your life.

Trauma in Childhood and the Risk of Future Trauma

While traumatic events may happen to anybody, you're more likely to be traumatized by an incident if you're already under a lot of stress, have recently suffered a string of losses, or have previously been traumatized—especially if the previous trauma occurred when you were a child.

Trauma in childhood can have serious and long-lasting consequences. When childhood trauma is unresolved, the child grows up with a sense of fear and powerlessness, setting the framework for future trauma. Even if your trauma occurred many years ago, there are steps you can take to overcome your pain, regain your emotional balance, and relearn to trust and connect with others.

The effects of a traumatic incident usually last a few days to a few months, gradually dissipating as you absorb the upsetting incident. Even if you're feeling better, you may be bothered by unpleasant recollections or feelings from time to time, especially in reaction to triggers like an anniversary of the occurrence or something that reminds you of the trauma.

Whether a traumatic incident results in death, or not, you must cope with the loss. Grief is the normal reaction to this loss. You, like those who have lost a loved one, must go through a mourning process. The following suggestions can assist you in coping with your sorrow, healing from the trauma, and moving on with your life.

Tip 1: Get going!

Childhood trauma alters your body's natural homeostasis, causing you to become hyper aroused and fearful. These sensations stay embedded within your brain causing it to function in a negative way. Staying idle can worsen the situation especially when you are alone and have nothing to do. Exercise and movement, in addition to burning off adrenaline and creating endorphins, can also assist in restoring your neurological system.

- **On most days, try to exercise for 30 minutes or more.** If it's more convenient, three 10-minute bursts of exercise every day are just as effective. Walking, yoga, jogging, swimming, basketball, or even dancing are examples of rhythmic exercises that utilize both your arms and legs.

- **Include a mindfulness component.** Rather than focusing on your thoughts or distracting yourself while exercising, concentrate on your body and how it feels as you move. Consider the sensation of your feet striking the ground, the rhythm of your breathing, or the sense of wind on your skin. Rock climbing, weight training, boxing, or martial arts can help with this. Remember to focus on your body motions to avoid harm during these sports.

Tip 2: Avoid Isolating Yourself

Isolating oneself after a terrible occurrence may seem like a comfort, but it will only make issues worse. Maintaining relationships and limiting your time alone will help you heal.

- **You are not compelled to talk about the trauma.** Connecting with people does not have to include discussing the trauma. In fact, for some people, this might make matters worse. Feeling involved and welcomed by others provides comfort.
- **Solicit assistance.** While discussing the trauma is not a necessity, it is vital that you have someone with whom you can relate your experiences face-to-face, someone who will listen carefully without judging you. Seek the advice of a trustworthy family member, friend, counselor, or pastor.
- **Even if you don't feel like it, engage in social activities.** Participate in 'normal' activities with other people that have nothing to do with the traumatic incident.
- **Participate in a support group for trauma victims.** Connecting with others who are coping with similar challenges can help you feel less alone, and hearing how others deal with their issues may inspire you to work on your own recovery.
- **Volunteer.** Volunteering, in addition to helping others, may be an excellent method to combat the sense of powerlessness that

frequently accompanies trauma. Helping others might help to remind you of your abilities and restore your sense of power.

Tip 3: Train Your Nervous System to Self-Regulate

It is critical to understand that you can change your arousal system and relax yourself regardless of how anxious, scared, or out of control you feel. It will not only help to alleviate the anxiety associated with trauma, but it will also provide you with a sense of control.

- **Breathing with awareness.** If you're feeling bewildered, confused, or agitated, practicing mindful breathing might help you settle down quickly. Simply take 60 deep breaths, focusing on each 'out' breath.
- **Toning of the voice.** As weird as it may sound, voice tone is an excellent approach to increase social interaction. Sit up straight and make a simple "'mmmm" sound. Adjust the pitch and loudness until you feel a nice vibration in your face.
- **Sensory information.** Is there a certain sight, scent, or flavor that instantly makes you feel calm? Perhaps caressing an animal or listening to music might rapidly calm you down or putting some essential oils on your body? Everyone reacts differently to sensory input, so try out several rapid stress reduction tactics to see what works best for you.
- **Keeping a firm footing.** Sit on a chair to feel more present and grounded. Feel the earth beneath your feet and your back against the chair. Look around you and select six things that include the colors red or blue. Take note of how your breathing becomes deeper and more relaxed.
- **Allow yourself to feel what you need to feel when you need to experience it.** Recognize and embrace your feelings regarding the trauma as they emerge.

Tip 4: Look After Your Health

It's true, having a healthy physique can improve your ability to cope with trauma-related stress.

- **Get lots of rest.** Worry or fear may disrupt your sleep habits after a distressing encounter. A lack of quality sleep, on the other hand, might increase your trauma symptoms and make it more difficult to maintain your emotional equilibrium. Aim for 7 to 9 hours of sleep every night and go to bed and wake up at the same time every day.
- **Stay away from alcohol and drugs.** Their usage can exacerbate your trauma symptoms and heighten feelings of melancholy, anxiety, and isolation.
- **Reduce your tension.** Try relaxing techniques such as meditation, yoga, or deep breathing exercises. Make time for activities that make you happy, such as your favorite pastimes.
- **Consume a well-balanced diet.** Eating modest, well-balanced meals throughout the day will help you maintain your energy and reduce mood fluctuations. To improve your mood, avoid sugary and fried meals and consume enough of omega-3 fats, such as salmon, walnuts, soybeans, and flaxseeds.

A well-balanced diet provides your body with the nutrition it requires to function properly. To receive enough nourishment, the majority of your daily calories should come from:

- fruits
- vegetables
- lean proteins
- legumes
- whole grains

When Should You Seek Professional Trauma Therapy?

It takes time to recover from trauma, and everyone heals at their own speed. However, if you feel that it interferes with your daily life, you may want professional assistance from a trauma specialist. Seek trauma treatment if you are experiencing any of the following circumstances:

- having trouble working at home or at work
- suffering from intense dread, anxiety, or depression
- unable to build strong, rewarding relationships
- experiencing terrible memories, nightmares, or flashbacks
- stay away from anything that reminds you of the trauma
- emotionally numb and alienated from others
- relying on drink or drugs to cope

Working through trauma may be frightening, difficult, and possibly retraumatizing; thus, this healing process is best done with the assistance of an experienced trauma specialist. It may take some time to find the proper therapist. It is critical that the therapist you select has expertise in treating trauma. However, the quality of your relationship with your therapist is just as crucial. Choose a trauma specialist with whom you feel at ease. Find another therapist if you do not feel comfortable, respected, or understood. But keep in mind, at the end of the day, therapists are people as well, trying to help you.

Ask yourself the following questions:

- Did I feel at ease expressing my difficulties with the therapist?
- Did I feel as if the therapist understood what I was saying?
- Were my concerns treated seriously, or were they dismissed?
- Was I handled with kindness and respect?
- Do I think I could come to trust the therapist?

Post Traumatic Stress Disorder

If your symptoms do not improve or worsen, and you are unable to move on from the experience for an extended length of time, you may be suffering from Post Traumatic Stress Disorder (PTSD). While emotional trauma is a normal reaction to a terrible event, it progresses to PTSD when your nervous system becomes 'stuck' and you remain in psychological shock, unable to make sense of what happened or process your feelings.

To recover from psychological and emotional trauma, you must: confront unpleasant sensations and memories, release pent-up "fight-or-flight" energy, learn to manage powerful emotions, and regain your capacity to trust others. In a child's treatment for PTSD, a trauma expert may employ a range of different therapy techniques:

Somatic experience is concerned with physiological sensations rather than ideas and recollections of the traumatic incident. You can release pent-up trauma-related energy through shaking, weeping, and other types of physical release by focusing on what's going on in your body.

Cognitive-behavioral therapy assists you in processing and evaluating your ideas and feelings in the aftermath of a tragedy.

EMDR (Eye Movement Desensitization and Reprocessing) combines cognitive-behavioral therapy aspects with eye movements or other types of rhythmic, left-right stimulation to 'unfreeze' traumatic memories.

Things You Can Do That Help in the Aftermath of Emotional and Psychological Distress?

Regression is a typical reaction to trauma, and there are strategies to assist your inner child to move forward and leave it behind. Firstly, you need to think back to a time when you felt safe before the trauma. Younger children may wet the bed or need a bottle, while older children may be afraid of being alone. If your inner child behaves in this manner, it is critical that you be understanding, patient, and reassuring.

Your inner child believes it is their fault. If you experience major or minor traumas at a young age, you don't know how to recover from it and the inner child takes on the blame. Assure your inner child that he or she is aware that they did not cause the incident.

Some individuals have trouble going to sleep, while others wake up frequently or have disturbing dreams. This is all because your inner child feels alone and all these years of bottling up the feelings keeps him/her on edge. Toss a cuddly animal and a warm blanket into your bed to make yourself comfortable. Make sure to have no screen time at least one hour before you go to bed. Try to do something that you find relaxing, like reading or having a bath.

In the following chapters, we will further discuss how you can break free from negative childhood patterns, different phases in the healing process, and how you can let go of the past.

Key Takeaways

- After experiencing trauma, you may keep thinking about it and asking yourself questions like "why me?" or "what could I have done to get out?" So, just remember that the first step to moving on is accepting that it happened and focusing instead on healing.

- Don't forget to take good care of your health amidst inner child healing. Your food intake is directly linked to this healing so make sure you are eating a balanced diet.
- Your inner child is the one who is wounded, so remember to heal him/her to ultimately heal yourself.

Breaking Free from Negative Childhood Patterns and Reparenting Yourself

"Seeing unhealthy patterns in your family and deciding that those patterns end with you and not be passed down to future generations, is an extremely brave & powerful decision"

— TINY TAT

This chapter talks about:

- Reparenting your inner child to break the cycle of trauma
- What is shadow work? How this practice can help you live a better life

Reparent Your Inner Child to Break the Cycle of Trauma

The following testimonial demonstrates just how deeply entrenched childhood trauma can become in adult life (Pandey, 2021):

> *Finally, the extent of my abhorrent behavior had caught up to me. Seeing my son cowering in the corner with unadulterated fear, fear of being yelled at and beaten, felt like a punch in the gut. My anger issues, and my proclivity to violence and infidelity, resulted in failed*

relationships. My disintegrating marriage, the fear of losing custody of my only child, a child I loved with all my, had finally sunk in. I realized I could not go on like this. I realized I wasn't happy anymore, no matter how hard I tried. It was like I was stuck in an endless loop where similar situations repeated in all the walks of my life. I decided enough was enough. I was going to change this. I was going to dig deeper and give my life a one-eighty degree turn.

The answers to this man's questions lay in his childhood, the family environment he grew up in, the interactions with his parents and peers created the man he had become. Humans are contradictory beings, with both a sophisticated and a basic experience of consciousness. We are a mash-up of every age we've ever been at the same time. We carry the wisdom of our current selves as well as the innocence of our inner kid. People who endured childhood trauma or neglect have scars that have been buried deep inside their subconscious thoughts.

Even persons who grew up in a mostly good atmosphere have the impressions of the terrible experiences they've endured lodged in their mind. Our subconscious mind is created during our youth, particularly between birth to four years of age. It is the time at which we first feel emotions. It is the age when we begin to analyze our emotions, observe our parents' and elders' interactions, learn to set and maintain boundaries, our behavioral patterns, and other nitty-gritty (Pandey, 2021).

Our inner child is a part of ourselves that has been there since we were conceived, through utero and all of the developmental years following when we were young and developing into delicate selves: baby, infant, toddler, young kid, and middle school aged. We all have an inner kid. Your "inner child" is a subconscious part of you that has been gathering up messages long before you were ready to completely grasp what was going on (mentally and emotionally). It contains previous emotions, memories, and beliefs, as well as future aspirations and desires. If you are new to the idea of reparenting your inner child, you may be pondering the following questions:

So, how does this inner child play a role in how we perceive life?

Every person is plagued with troubles in their lives. Some lack the communication skills required for a successful and healthy relationship, others are struggling with harmful habits such as addiction and self-sabotage, and still others are suffering from an identity crisis and lack of self-worth. Everyone suffers from these challenges, which culminate and are expressed in various ways for each individual, but they are all tied to one thing: conditioned behavior performed from childhood.

But why do we need to cure our inner child?

We have a tendency to be protective and defensive about our early experiences. The reason why inner child healing and reparenting are required is rather straightforward. To be immersed in a rich inner world is to experience pure unconditional love from yourself. To become more empathic, caring, and compassionate is to cultivate a strong feeling of self. Most importantly, we must become emotionally robust and conscientious individuals who are aware of our responses and reactions and do not become gluttons for suffering and averse to our own enjoyment. The fact is, as adults, we have a unique chance to recover and intentionally select another behavior, regardless of everything we have gone through in the past.

What does this have to do with our parents? Are they harmful?

No, not always. Our parents, in an ideal world, are two self-actualized individuals who enable their children to be seen and heard as the unique individuals that they are. Because we live in a civilization that does not achieve conscious awareness, the majority of us are born to unaware parents. Our parents are reproducing the same patterns they saw as children and in their own homes. They operate from their own wounded shadow self since they never mastered the skills for constructively processing their emotions or even the understanding of the necessity to process their emotions.

It is critical to remember that our parents behave only on the basis of their own awareness. We can only give what we have practiced receiving. As a result, playing the blame game is futile and can lead to even more strained relationships with our parents and relatives.

So, what is reparenting, exactly?

Reparenting is the act of providing oneself with what you did not receive as a kid, namely all of the emotional understanding, caring, and love that you needed. You deserved unconditional love and support, but you were pushed to think that love and acceptance had to be won by doing specific things. Perhaps you came to view yourself as undeserving of love if you did not behave in a specific manner or meet the expectations of others. Reparenting is our obligation to ourselves to heal this hurt. That is something we owe ourselves.

When is the best moment to repent, and how can we get started?

As soon as you recognize your difficulties and have identified the source. It is doable for everyone. It takes time, dedication, and a great deal of patience. Every day, you will have to show up for yourself. There are no excuses. There are no shortcuts. There are no short-term remedies. However, it will help you to heal, forgive, and go on. A joyful by-product is being able to have happy, loving, and rewarding relationships, friendships, and companionships.

The Four Pillars of Reparenting

The four pillars of reparenting include:

1. discipline
2. joy
3. emotional regulation
4. self-care

Please be advised, some may be more challenging than others, depending on our life experiences.

Discipline is sometimes the most difficult aspect since we naturally seek comfort, and discipline typically has a bad connotation in our thoughts. Some people find it difficult to experience joy because they believe they do not deserve it, that they must earn it.

This is why we must be patient with ourselves and others, because the end result is a life that is extremely satisfying.

So, to begin, here is how to get started:

1. **Breathe.** Keep in mind that reparenting is a process that will likely extend over days, weeks, or months. Doing too much too rapidly might overwhelm you, causing a reversion to our old habits. Pause and take a deep breath if you sense it becoming too intense or uncomfortable. Take it at your own speed—consistent and comfortable.
2. **Make it a habit to maintain your promises to yourself.** Begin small. Every day, make a commitment to yourself and keep it. It may be as simple as drinking 8 glasses of water, listening to a couple of songs, writing a page in your notebook, or meditating for 10 minutes. Anything that doesn't seem excessive to you. Simply avoid making

promises that will take up too much time at first. Anything from a few minutes to a half-hour is OK. If you do this regularly you will see a visible change in terms of reparenting of your inner child.

3. **Believe in someone you can rely on (other than your parents).** Inform the person that you are embarking on this quest. Do not include your parents since it may cause them to feel inadequate as parents. The purpose of reparenting is for you to heal, not for them to feel awful. Inform a friend, partner, or sibling. Any assistance would be greatly appreciated.
4. **Treat yourself.** Consider what you require right now. What can you do to make yourself happy? It may be something as simple as a warm bath, or a massage and spa treatment, or even that snack you crave but don't let yourself enjoy. If you like, you can sunbathe or swim. Alternatively, jump in the puddle while it's pouring rain.
5. **Learn to enjoy yourself.** We will rapidly dismiss the truth that we are showing up for ourselves if we are not recognized, applauded, and seen for the unique individual that we are. It is tough to reparent ourselves. Recognize the bravery required. Take charge of your progress. Celebrate the person you're becoming.

What is Shadow Work? How This Practice Can Help You Live a Better Life

The "shadow self" refers to components of ourselves that have been pushed down into the unconscious—aspects of ourselves about which we feel concerned, humiliated, or frustrated, and hence repress.

The concept of the shadow self is founded on the idea that we metaphorically bury those aspects of our personalities that we are afraid would not be received, accepted, or appreciated by others; hence, we keep them in the 'shadows.' In a nutshell, our shadow selves are the actual versions of ourselves that we fear displaying to the rest of society.

This is the discipline of accepting what has happened to us, and releasing guilt and judgment so that we can be our authentic selves.

Carl Jung, a Swiss psychologist of the twentieth century, devoted his life to researching the human psyche and mind. Among his many contributions to psychoanalysis was the concept of the "shadow self." The inclusion of the word 'shadow' in this statement may appear eerie at first, but this is nothing to be concerned about!

The shadow self frequently presents itself by leading us to be provoked by another person's words or actions, to suffer inner tension and cognitive dissonance, to criticize or lash out at others, or to feel insecure and held back.

Shadow work is the practice of working with our shadow selves to eliminate the negative impact they have on our lives and to integrate the many aspects of ourselves into one whole.

Over the course of a lifetime, we may have pushed small parts of ourselves so far away that we are unaware of what is hidden in our shadow self, perhaps fearing what we may find hidden away. Shadow work is the bringing to light, processing, and re-acceptance of those small parts—piece by piece and one by one—in order to become a whole, entire, and integrated self.

Shadow work is essentially a type of psychoanalysis (as psychoanalysis is at the core of Jungian psychology). Regardless of the terminology chosen, Jung claimed that integrating the segmented versions of the self is a powerful thing (Kellend, 2015).

What Benefits Does Shadow Work Offer?

While shadow work is not always simple, since it is frequently accompanied by the pain of previous rejection, repairing the schism between the aware and shadow selves may be a life-changing experience. "Shadow labor is the way of the heart warrior," according to Jung (Kellend, 2015).

Jung believed that such a procedure may aid in the development of a balanced existence and a sense of harmony within oneself. Feeling whole, rather than fragmented, may give us a new feeling of freedom, allowing us to see life in new ways and experience things we wouldn't or couldn't previously.

Addressing the emotional baggage that has long been buried in our shadows can help us to show up more fully and consciously for our commitments and relationships in life, whether that's being a better spouse, sister, kid, parent, teacher, mentor, friend, or any of the myriad other roles we serve throughout our lives. In an ever-changing and often restrictive environment, shadow work also helps us to feel stronger sensations of power and personal agency.

Shadow work almost assures more authenticity in everything we do by developing us into the most authentic versions of ourselves that we've ever been.

Finally, by accepting and mending the aspects of ourselves that we've assigned to our shadows, we may learn to express those qualities in healthy ways rather than concealing them until they appear in unhealthy, uncontrollable ways (lashing out at others due to anger, or creating a toxic body image and inner dialogue). This acceptance can then bloom into a strong sense of self-love.

Benefits of Shadow Work for Inner Child Healing

It is critical for your mental health and well-being to have a good relationship with the juvenile aspects of your personality.

Inner child shadow work has been linked to a higher sense of safety, love, support, and creativity in people's lives, according to Lule University's research on health throughout one's lifetime (Cotec, 2020).

Shadow work has also been demonstrated to aid in the treatment of relationship problems and depression, and it may be utilized to improve your ability to discover happiness in your life.

Inner child work can assist your healing in the following ways:

- cultivate your creative and free spirit
- stop emotional outbursts (tantrums/outbursts)
- heal toxic shame and guilt, allowing you to experience more love and support in your relationships
- set and maintain firmer limits
- requests should be made without becoming upset or overreacting
- and many more ways!

In essence, completing inner child work and shadow work, will help you to combine diverse components of your personality into a more solid and whole sense of self.

5 Steps to Healing Your Inner Child Through Shadow Work

Healing means connecting with the child who resides inside you by listening to that part of yourself, and assisting it in expressing repressed feelings. Only when you have processed any hurt or trapped memory will you be able to go forward and nurture a healthy inner child.

These five steps can help you mend your inner child:

1. Recognize the trauma or harmful pattern. The purpose of this initial stage is to bring any suppressed components of your personality to the surface. This initial phase is ideal for shadow work.
2. Investigate the source of the trauma. Consider where the trauma triggered and initially manifested itself. Consider your age, where you were, and what was going on.
3. Travel back in time by using your active imagination. If it feels comfortable, attempt to return to the time when the initial trauma occurred. Try to observe with the eyes of a caring adult.
4. Encourage your inner kid. Approach your younger self in your recollection for solace and be a supportive ally to yourself. If no one was there for you back then, you are there for your inner child today.
5. Repeat these steps as many times as you like/need. It may take some time to process these intense feelings from your history. Be patient, and simply show up. You will eventually experience a great deal of healing and a stronger connection with your inner child.

Journal Prompts for Inner Child Shadow Work

Writing prompts are another effective technique for investigating the shadow and the inner child. Set up some time for reflection and writing for this exercise.

When responding to these prompts in a diary or notepad, try to write as quickly as possible. With freestyle writing, you're attempting to enter a flow state, allowing your subconscious to surface. Don't bother about editing or spelling—just write.

Here are some writing prompts:

- Do you think you had a decent childhood? How functional was your

home life while you were growing up?
- What were your favorite childhood activities? If you gave up any in adulthood, what made you decide to stop?
- What do I miss most about being a child?
- What could I do to increase my sense of fun and creativity?

Shadow work is an excellent approach to experiencing inner healing and transformation, and all that is required is self-awareness. Every person on the planet has gone through a terrible phase in their lives that has left them with shadows. The good news is that the entire cosmos is on our side, attempting to help us heal. Every action in the cosmos is geared toward development and expansion.

We are given several opportunities to confront our shadow selves in order to eventually be free of them. It makes no difference how long you stave off your shadow self. It will continue to appear in your reality unless you pay attention to it.

The fragmented self longs to be reunited, and we will be given opportunities to see pieces of ourselves that we have hidden, rejected, denied, and disowned.

The more you recognize and embrace your shadow self, the more embodied you become as a conscious person, and the more control you will have over yourself and your life.

Key Takeaways

- Look out for the impact of trauma on your emotional and physical health.
- No matter what you have been through in childhood, there's no need to get depressed over the past or question, why me? Instead, reparent yourself so you could break free from the vicious cycle of trauma.

- Shadow work brings out the emotions that you have pushed back in order to help you address them and work accordingly. It is essential to follow the methods of shadow work to gain maximum benefits.
- Don't feel lost while reparenting, following the four steps: discipline, joy, emotional regulation and self-care, at your own speed, will help you.
- Though difficult, embrace the journey to help free yourself from the trauma that's holding you back.

Phases of the Healing Process

"Trauma doesn't discriminate and doesn't just happen to "bad" people"

— KRISTIN ANDERSON

This chapter talks about:

- Trauma and recovery stages
- Being your authentic self to win
- The advantages of simply being you
- The personal story of Brené Brown

Trauma and Recovery Stages

These days, we hear a lot about trauma. The news is also rife with horrific events. Trauma does not discriminate and does not only affect 'evil' individuals. Trauma is a human experience that must be understood and treated. But do we truly comprehend the impacts of trauma?

Knowing the phases of trauma might help you heal and feel more in control of what you're going through. Investigate the following steps to become more aware of your recovery process.

Safety and Stabilization

You are likely to retreat as a result of the distressing experience. This retreat process is a form of self-preservation. You are likely to experience rage, guilt, anxiety, and denial during this process. Other emotions may also arise depending on who you are as an individual. It's natural to feel uncomfortable in your own body, in your relationships, and in your surroundings. This stage might span several weeks, months, or even years. This is especially true if the trauma is not processed, acknowledged, and supported throughout therapy.

During the stability and safety stages, begin by assessing your feelings. This is the base to start from because once you find out what you will be working on, it will make the process easier. So, sit back and relax while recalling the trauma. It is easier said than done, but trust the process. This will be the last time you will ever need to recall the trauma, then you will experience the wonders of moving on.

To heal, you must first learn how to manage challenging emotions by developing new coping abilities. Therapists will understand if discussing the trauma is too difficult for you. In this scenario, the therapist may teach you how to settle yourself through mindfulness, yoga, and deep breathing. This period of recuperation should also include the development of new routines.

Mourning and Reminiscence

During this stage, you'll start to come up with your own solutions to the question, "What does it all mean?" This stage of healing is primarily about processing and making sense of the experience. The idea is to create a space where you may reflect on the experience without reliving it. This phase can be completed at your own speed. If you're working with a therapist, they'll continue to prioritize safety and stability. When you are ready, you can lament the losses caused by the traumatic experience. Discuss your feelings. Allow yourself to let go of negative emotions and thoughts. During this period, be kind to yourself. Be patient and empathetic. There is no such thing as a 'correct' time frame.

As mentioned in chapter two, EMDR may also be a useful therapy during this stage. EMDR is a therapy approach that allows you to reflect on a traumatic incident while focusing on bilateral external stimuli. Tapping, buzzing, or eye movements might be the stimulation you need.

Reconnection and Integration

Our sense of ourselves may be distorted following a traumatic occurrence. Because the consequences of the traumatic experience are so severe, it may appear to define us. The final step of trauma rehabilitation assists you in overcoming these consequences so that you can live a full life. You will develop a new sense of self throughout this era. You will also build on positive experiences and start planning for the future. You will have a role in reconnecting with people and redefining important connections.

Taking meaning from pain may be experienced on a smaller scale that is just as powerful. You could opt to live a better lifestyle or change occupations, for example. You empower yourself and others as a result of your efforts. You'll develop new, healthy self-beliefs that will help you to go ahead into your new sense of reality, a reality that is produced by you and that you're motivated to accomplish.

You Are Not Alone: Navigating the Stages of Trauma

Remember that you are never alone in experiencing trauma, even if your reactions and coping techniques differ from those of others. Take the help of a therapist if you need extra help progressing through the phases of trauma. A therapist can help you cope with your trauma in a healthy and helpful way. They can assist you in better understanding yourself and making sense of how you're feeling.

The trauma itself gets ingrained in your past. It no longer defines you, but rather serves as a chapter in your life story. Being able to now fully comprehend the significance of the incident, you are prepared to take action. The goal of this stage is to make use of the traumatic event. For example, you could decide to work with or assist individuals who have been through similar trauma. You may consider publishing a book or giving a public talk on your experience.

Be Your Authentic Self to Win

Still, rather than resorting to external sources, digging within yourself can provide the answers you seek and bring the greatest fulfillment if you ever have the sensation that something is lacking from your life but can't quite put your finger on what it is.

Have you ever been amazed at how a young toddler rushes through life satisfied with no hint of "tone-knowledge?" You were simply yourself when you were younger. You didn't have any other options. Still, when we mature and succumb to the demands imposed by many environments such as education, family, work, or friends, we might sluggishly and unconsciously lose sight of our original tone. Rather, we gradually adapt to what we believe others expect. Finally, we may feel like a fake, a fictitious representation of ourselves that we believe others want to see.

We all put on social masks from time to time. We've all bought into beliefs about what's relevant (and what isn't), and we've all bought into notions of success that aren't ours. They may have originated from our parents, friends, creative organizations, or society as a whole. But we allow these notions to ferment unconsciously in our thoughts, and before long we're crafting a life that conforms to someone else's concept of what a happy life looks like. We're burying our actual passions behind a layer of potential. We lose touch with our true selves. We lose touch with our actual desires and begin to live the life we feel we are meant to or have to live.

Does Being Your True Tone Lead to Loss and Rejection?

Many individuals are concerned that being true to their tone would jeopardize or destroy their security, family, relationships, job, and other vital aspects of their lives. This is simply untrue. When we feel empowered to speak our true tone, rather than losing out, we gain far more than we had ever believed was possible.

What Is Your True Tone?

Your real tone is the "actual you," the person you are after all adaptive masks are removed. Your genuine tone is the person you are when you have a deep inner serenity and awareness. When your values, pretensions, beliefs, words, actions, and public image fit with your specific values, you connect with this state of being. Although it appears to be a straightforward notion, many of us have a difficult time allowing our real tone to take center stage.

How Do You Find Your True Tone?

Consider the following tips when you're ready to investigate and embrace your true tone:

- **Consider a certain force.** A little soul-searching is required to better connect with your real tone. Gather a pen and paper and write a list of the characteristics you admire about yourself. Make another list of the things you like performing and the life consequences that make you happy. What do you enjoy, and why do you enjoy it? This information will be critical in helping you on your journey to finding your unique tone, so take your time assessing your lists.

- **Don't be concerned about what others think.** While it is true that it is easier said than done, you will never be able to be your true tone if you are continually angry over what other people think of you. People-pleasing may appear to be a beneficial attribute, yet pleasing others typically comes at the expense of your own pleasure. Make a vow to quit worrying about being the way other people expect you to be and allow your real tone to show through without making any excuses.

1. *Consider why you care.*
2. *Concentrate on being present in the moment.*
3. *Recognize that most people do not care.*
4. *Practice self-acceptance and love.*
5. *Identify your group of people.*
6. *Recognize that you cannot please everyone.*
7. *Recognize that life is too short.*

- **You should be honored.** The ultimate goal of the journey to becoming your actual tone is to truly appreciate and love oneself. Stop searching for affection and validation from others; no amount of money, love, or renown will fill that gap. If you want to achieve genuine fulfillment in life, you must find and offer yourself love.
- **Accept your fears.** Fear of failing, being judged, disappointing others, or making mistakes is a natural element of human nature, and it may prevent you from being your authentic self. However, the best way to overcome it is to recognize your concerns, appreciate them, and express yourself—go for what you desire. They are, after all, a part of who you are. However, if you're attempting to oppose portions of yourself that you don't like or understand, psychotherapy can assist.

Taking one tiny step at a time is the key to overcoming your worries.

Going too quickly or attempting something too frightening before you're ready might backfire.

However, it is equally critical to keep pushing forward. A reasonable level of anxiousness is OK. Don't wait for your nervousness to go away before taking a step forward, or you'll end up waiting for a change that won't occur on its own.

A fear hierarchy made up of modest steps is the best method to construct an action plan. Here's an example of how one could use exposure therapy to overcome their fear of public speaking one step at a time:

1. Talk to yourself in the mirror.
2. Be sure to hold eye contact as you speak.

This is the tried and true method for confronting and overcoming fear. This provides you an edge in recognizing your worries and then working on them to make them your strength.

The Advantages of Simply Being You

When we don't connect with our inner child, we often try to imitate others. However, when we try to imitate them, we lose sight of our purpose. This section goes into detail about this issue and mentions the exercises to help you be yourself and connect with your inner child. Our culture is obsessed with attaining lofty goals, and some may regard taking the time to concentrate on oneself as self-indulgent. Nonetheless, embodying your real tone might produce significantly smaller rewards than other, more tangible career-focused ambitions. I'm not implying that you stop striving for success; rather, it means shifting your emphasis such that the success you accomplish not only yields tangible benefits, but also provides you with a feeling of purpose that is important and rewarding to you.

It's quite satisfying to be comfortable in your own skin. One of the most significant advantages of adopting your real tone is a sense of fulfillment in life that cannot be obtained in any other manner. Indeed, whether your specific relationships or job are in shambles, finding your real tone may help you soar above it all to feel optimistic about your future. Life counseling may help you stay on track as you integrate your views, values, aspirations, and behavior.

Self-control is Essential

Authenticity necessitates discipline. This refers to the ability to execute your principles despite temptations to forsake them. The world of the moment is saturated with glitz, gaudiness, and an emphasis on material gain. As a result, I recommend adopting the following strategies:

- **Reflection about yourself.** The true you necessitates continual tone-reflection. This talent will place you in a state of perfect harmony, leading you to experience less tension since you aren't concerned with another person's point of view, only your own.
- **Visioning.** When you're truly connected to yourself, you might dream about your future tone. Visioning will allow you to feel excited as your fundamental values assist you in raising the bar. The following visioning exercise can help:

1. *Be sure to sit in a quiet and comfortable place to start visioning.*
2. *Think about your goals instead of the past and plan to achieve them.*
3. *Think how your future self will look once you break free from the past.*

- **Translucency.** The fabric of authenticity is woven via open dialogue. When you are certain of who you are and what you stand for, you walk through life with tone-assurance and a sense of inner value.
- **Harkening that is active.** When you're genuine, you notice little emotional stumbling blocks to your pride, which makes you an

excellent listener. Because you're secure and at ease in your own skin, it's easier now for you to focus on others.

- **Remember:** If we aren't true to ourselves, we are doing the world, not to mention our families, friends, and visitors, a disservice. Maintain your integrity. Accept your natural tone!
- **Focus.** To be successful in business and at home, you must resist urges and focus on the process until it is complete. Your capacity to adopt your real tone improves your ability to ignore distractions. To increase your focus, you can try the following changes:

1. *Exercise to practice patience.*
2. *Eat a healthy diet, preferably with more fats.*
3. *Get a good night's sleep.*
4. *Make a to-do list to achieve smaller milestones.*

In chapter six, we will dive deeper into becoming the best version of yourself by feeling worthy, authentic, and playful.

Personal Story of Brené Brown

Accepting who we are is a journey that begins with honesty, contemplation, and tone-discovery. Keeping in touch with oneself is a life-long journey. Brené Brown shares her personal revelations (Snowise, 2015):

> *I've been there. That pit of confusion where you wonder who the hell you are. Where you wonder if you even actually know yourself at all. I had a moment where I looked in the mirror and stared at myself with almost a foreign level of disconnection. I actually said out loud..."Who am I?" I had lost myself in the chaos and responsibility of modern life. But I was craving to know what made this woman that stood in front of me tick. What did I really want out of life? Standing there staring at myself in the mirror with a feeling of pure confusion was disconcerting to say the least, but those are the exact moments*

that you start to wake up to your authenticity. Without having the courage to ask yourself these questions, and have a willingness to delve into yourself and explore, you can never really be in touch with your authentic self. Authenticity requires that you truly connect and know who you are.

Once you've begun to connect with your inner partner and what truly makes you alive, you must maintain that connection, which requires regular practice and dedication. The current world is hectic, frantic, and noisy. When we don't have that established connection with ourselves, it's easy to get caught up in it and washed away.

Key Takeaways

- Remember that you are not alone in the healing process, so don't put too much pressure on yourself. Following the above mentioned steps will guide you in the process.
- Learning to be authentic might require a lot of guts. When you do, though, you liberate yourself and begin to develop a life that provides you joy and significance. You won't get there overnight, but you can get there.
- Once you have accepted your past and start working on it, no one can stop the change you are about to achieve.

Letting Go of The Past

"Every time your fear is invited up, every time you recognize it and smile at it, your fear will lose some of its strength"

— THICH NHAT HANH

This chapter talks about:

- Letting go of the past
- How to handle fear and anxiety
- Self-apologies: healing shame and guilt with self-forgiveness
- How do I practice self-forgiveness?

Let Go of the Past

Most of us have been subjected to some type of trauma during our lives. We may have had "big trauma" such as abuse, major loss, or a life-threatening incident, but we may have examples of "small trauma" from situations that were not life-threatening but caused emotional anguish and impacted our way of viewing ourselves, other people, and the world.

Childhood trauma of any form may have an impact on our relationships as well as our mental and physical health. The necessity of making meaning of the trauma, regardless of when it occurred or what form it took, cannot be stressed enough.

This is due to the fact that unresolved trauma may haunt us in ways that resolved trauma does not. According to research, when we fail to handle both big and small traumas, we might become imprisoned in our suffering. Our trauma might have unanticipated consequences in our life (Firestone, 2022). It might make us feel worried and triggered for reasons we don't understand at times.

Unresolved trauma occurs when we do not process it immediately after it occurs or when we do not process it at all. Taking a deep dive into our own narrative may thus do a lot of good.

So, what measures can we take to bring our memories to the surface and comprehend our trauma? Here are nine recommendations I make when assisting folks in developing a cohesive story around their experience:

Watch Out for Exaggerations

To begin, we might seek out locations where we have strong emotional ties. Anything from our partner's tone to a baby's cry might set off feelings associated with prior trauma. When we have a heightened emotional reaction that doesn't seem to suit the situation, we should consider whether there is underlying, unresolved trauma affecting us.

Interpersonal neurobiologist, Daniel Siegel, describes a strategy for acquiring insight into our interior state using the acronym SIFT (sensations, images, thoughts, and feelings). First, we can examine any physical symptoms we may be experiencing, such as our heart pounding or our forehead becoming heated. Then, we may evaluate the images that come to mind. This may be anything from a harsh expression on someone's face to a specific piece of wallpaper in a room. We can then focus on any emotions that occur, such as terror, grief, embarrassment, or rage.

Finally, we can make a mental note of any thoughts that arise, such as, *You should get out of here.* In this circumstance, you are not safe (Siegel, n.d.). The sensations, ideas, sentiments, and thoughts evoked may have more to do with the past than with the present. As a result, they provide insight into events or circumstances that may have been distressing to us at a time when we were unable to completely digest the experience.

Immediately Write Out Ten Childhood Traumas You've Endured

Many people who I invite to participate in this exercise begin by stating, "I don't believe I can think of ten traumas that occurred in my early childhood." Others have felt confident in continuing with a considerably larger list. However, starting with ten generally motivates us to expand our brains and memory and delve into situations and events that we may not initially categorize as trauma. These might be "capital T" or "small t" events.

We frequently try to bury or brush over negative things that happened to us, especially if they were terrifying or occurred while we were too young to properly comprehend them. We may never have recounted our own tales about these occurrences, so we don't frequently remember them. As difficult as it may be at first, identifying the events that have influenced us is beneficial. Even things that have had a significant impact on us that we've disregarded or forgotten. Bringing them to light is the first step toward understanding our narrative.

Give it Some Thought

Certain sections of the tale will make little sense to us when we jot down particular occurrences. We may become aware that many portions of our experience remain unsolved or have slipped from our consciousness. We may detect a muddled timeline or memory gaps. Alternatively, we may reconsider a portion of our tale that we previously viewed in one manner but now see in a completely different light.

Many folks I've spoken with blame themselves as youngsters. For example, one lady grew up believing she had murdered her dog when he was hit by a car after she had unintentionally left her back door open.

As we investigate our memories, it is helpful to identify areas where the tale is disjointed and may benefit from greater contemplation.

Use the RAIN Method to Calm Down

Examining our emotions and recollections may be upsetting. When something unpleasant or stressful occurs, psychologists Jack Kornfield and Tara Brach, advocate the RAIN Approach, which consists of the following four steps:

- **Recognize** the trauma or loss. Take time to consider how you're feeling.
- **Allow/Recognize/Accept** whatever powerful feeling is present in the moment. We can recognize that this trauma occurred and that it may not be addressed.
- **Investigate** the experience in relation to your history and present life.
- **Nurturing non-identification** with the experience implies that you should not over-identify with what happened or let it define you. Remember that the recollection isn't occurring to you right now and has nothing to do with who you are.

Collect Information

When we have gaps in our recollection, it might be beneficial to ask others to provide their perspectives. Family members and friends who were present at the time of our trauma may be able to provide us with a more complete knowledge of the event. However, there's the potential for an individual close to the situation to disagree with or dismiss our observations, especially if they're puzzled about an occurrence.

In these instances, it's crucial to realize that what the event meant to us is still significant. It's alright to admit that our experience or personal truth influenced our life if it seems real to us. Even still, the advice of someone we trust can help us piece together items we can't recall or have reservations about.

Feel the Full Extent of What Occurred

When we tell our tale, it is certain to elicit strong emotions. Accept that your feelings are genuine and that they matter rather than trying to justify them away.

Allowing ourselves to completely experience the emotion without judgment or attempts to stop it, is a vital step in processing and overcoming the initial trauma. This will provide us with relief.

Remember that our emotions may be like a wave, rising and falling, finally returning us to a state of peace, but only if we allow them to run their complete course.

Make a Note of it

We may continue to write our tales as they come to the surface. In many circumstances, simply writing about them may be really beneficial. Feelings, ideas, and recollections of any kind are allowed.

We must approach the intricacies of our tale with patience, compassion, and without judgment. It can also be helpful to write down what we believe happened based on our present feelings.

When people begin to do this, their memories frequently come to the surface.

Share Your Experience With Someone

Choose someone you can trust and tell them about your trauma. Others may be able to perceive the issue more objectively and contribute fresh insight. Those close to us frequently have a softer attitude and more sympathy for us than we have for ourselves. This can help us understand what happened and improve our attitude toward ourselves. It can assist us in beginning to confront any long-held negative views we've held about ourselves that have arisen as a result of the traumatic incident.

Construct a Logical Story

After we've begun to identify the traumas that occurred, we might ask, "What's a story that makes sense around that trauma?" Even though the facts themselves are nonsensical, we may begin crafting our story in a coherent fashion in which the events make sense to us.

We might begin to feel less fractured inside when we digest what happened in a cohesive manner. We may come to see how we were innocent in particular situations or how specific events affected us far more than we realized. We may approach our situation with compassion and love, just as we would if a friend told us the same tale.

We can feel more connected when we face and share our narrative in a holistic way. By acquiring crucial insight into our triggers and emotions, we may begin to reclaim the sense of peace that our trauma had previously robbed us of. We may stop blaming ourselves for bad things that have happened to us and start seeing ourselves in a different perspective.

How to Handle Fear and Anxiety

This section discusses what you can do on your own to manage fear and anxiety. There are options, approaches, and techniques available to work on your fear and anxiety that add to the work of professionals. These are critical for persons who have been traumatized or who are experiencing acute dread or anxiety.

Avoid Evasion

The only way to overcome fear is to confront it. Avoiding our concerns simply keeps us from progressing—it makes us uneasy. However, be careful with yourself and just do what seems safe to you! If you sense yourself becoming increasingly panicked, take a pause and look for anything pleasant or reassuring to observe or do. When the feeling passes, you can revisit your phobia, taking breaks as required. If you find it difficult to handle persistent concerns or anxieties on your own, keep in mind that therapists may be quite helpful in working through avoidance methods with you. Working with a therapist to provide a secure setting where you may face your anxiety and recreate your memories is especially crucial if you have suffered trauma.

You can attempt mindfulness meditation if your fear or anxiety is milder. All you have to do is sit quietly and pay attention to the current moment and try to recognize any feelings of dread or worry that occur. Be as inquisitive as you possibly can. Take note of the worry. Take note of how it feels in your body. Take note of any linked ideas. See if you can just observe it as it is; don't get caught up in the tale or try to get rid of or modify it.

And, if necessary, take a pause and focus your attention on something neutral, such as your breath or your hands on your lap. It's worth noting that if you're feeling too upset to be interested, it's best to take a break, open your eyes, and examine what's around you, or go for a short stroll.

Encourage Positivism

Fear encourages us to notice and recall bad occurrences, which confirms our impression that the world is a terrible place. We may attempt to alter that by consciously observing what is positive—the joy we experience when we see someone we care about, the pleasure of a bright day, the beauty in nature, the fun of a trip, the humor in a scenario.

According to Barbara Fredrickson's research, optimism broadens our perspective—we physically have a larger vision, which provides us with more possibilities (Fredrickson, 2014). The more we practice positively, the stronger it becomes, allowing us to operate even in challenging situations.

Look for Significance

Fear has the power to disrupt our perception of the world as we know it. Those who have undergone trauma may have also suffered significant losses, leading them to question the meaning of their existence. Trauma survivors frequently feel guilty about what happened, believing, illogically, that they might have stopped it in some way, and this shame can add to worries about their significance.

However, whether we are suffering from anxiety or trauma, it is critical to re-establish a sense of purpose. An 80-year study of variables that influence lifespan, discovered that those who return to healthy habits after trauma are the ones who can find purpose in the terrible event and rebuild a feeling of security in the world (Delagran, n.d.).

Meaningful Therapy for Healing

Logotherapy, which literally means "healing by meaning," has been shown to be effective in treating people suffering from post-traumatic stress disorder (PTSD).

Part of the success of this treatment stems from just allowing people to speak their stories and feel understood, which aids in the healing process. Another aspect is determining how to put talents and experience, particularly those gained through trauma, to use in a meaningful way. For example, a person who has suffered from PTSD because of childhood trauma, may find purpose in assisting others who have suffered similar trauma.

Seek Assistance

Fear might sometimes make us feel estranged from others. The longevity experiment also discovered that the strength of one's social interactions was a crucial predictor of lifespan among persons who had experienced trauma in their lives (Delagran, n.d.).

This is due to a variety of factors. Friends and relatives can assist us in making an accurate evaluation of the hazard. We are more confident in our ability to deal with problems when we have the support of others. In addition, having a loved one around relaxes us and decreases our fight or flight response.

Embrace the Nature

Being in nature decreases fear and anxiety while increasing pleasant sensations, as evidenced by the emerging area of nature-based treatments. People express their sentiments when they see a scene of natural beauty using terms like peace, beauty, happiness, hope, and aliveness. Being linked to nature not only improves people's mental well-being, but it also lowers blood pressure, heart rate, muscular tension, and the creation of stress hormones—all of which are signs of worry and fear.

So, if you're experiencing sensations of fear or anxiety, go for a walk or run in a park or greenspace. Physical activity will improve your mood in addition to the healing effects of nature.

Self-Compassion Should be Practiced

Many members of racial, sexual, ethnic, and gender minority groups suffer greater levels of dread and anxiety as a result of estrangement and discrimination, which occasionally involves violence, according to research and personal testimonies (Robinson & Segal, 2018). For persons who are facing this sort of chronic threat, self-compassion may be a profoundly therapeutic practice. That's because, in addition to treating oneself as you would a loving friend, self-compassion entails contemplating the shared suffering of others like you.

Face your concerns and anxieties so that they do not become crippling. Determine how you may gain a sense of personal control or mastery over your life. Finally, even if you are plagued with worry, don't neglect other aspects of your life. Even when working towards greater security, it is possible to find happiness in relationships and a sense of purpose.

Consider yourself as a child. Think back to a time when you were feeling vulnerable, when you were being treated harshly, or when you were in emotional distress and needed to be consoled. Take note of any emotions that arise. Some people find it beneficial to look at a photograph of themselves when they were younger. Consider how you would care for that child in a hypothetical situation. What do you think you'd say to him or her? What would you do to comfort this child? Once you answer these questions, you will feel greater relaxation and content in your life.

Self-Apologies: Healing Shame and Guilt with Self-Forgiveness

We often hear how important it is to forgive people who have wronged us, but what about forgiving ourselves? Is it also important? Absolutely. When we injure others, we feel remorse and apologize. However, we frequently punish ourselves for mistakes and create negative self-images as a result. These sensations are accompanied by emotions of shame and guilt. While these sentiments are comparable and can occur concurrently, they are slightly distinct.

Guilt and Shame

Shame and guilt can seem extremely similar in that they both make us feel horrible about ourselves. However, guilt may be defined as being dissatisfied with oneself for breaching an essential internal value or rule of behavior. Feeling guilty can be beneficial since it can lead to good behavioral change. With shame, one may also experience self-dissatisfaction, but no value has been violated. We feel guilty when we feel horrible about anything we did or didn't do. When we are ashamed, we feel horrible about ourselves. When we feel guilty, we must realize that it is OK to make errors. When we feel ashamed, we must understand that it is alright to be ourselves.

Shame refers to feeling bad about a certain feature of your body and then comparing it to others, thus making you feel more judgmental about yourself. Over time, this feeling becomes deeply entrenched within. Thus, when you feel ashamed of your trauma or something you did not do. This affects your adult mindset and behavior.

Shame is harmful because it leads to poor self-esteem (feelings of unworthiness) and behaviors that perpetuate a negative self-image. Shame may lead to self-criticism, blame, neglect, self-destructive actions, self-sabotaging behaviors, the sense that you don't deserve wonderful things, and rage, among other emotions.

Self-Forgiveness

So, how do we lessen our feelings of shame and guilt? Forgiveness of oneself, especially when it comes to humiliation, is key. Self-forgiveness promotes emotional stability and mental tranquility. The more guilt you are able to repair, the more clearly you will be able to see yourself—the good and the troubled. You will be able to identify and acknowledge to yourself and others how you have injured them. Compassion is the cure to embarrassment. Self-compassion works to neutralize guilt and eliminate the poisons that shame creates. Self-forgiveness is an essential component of self-compassion. It relieves the agony produced by shame in our body, mind, and soul, and it aids in the entire healing process.

How Do I Practice Self-Forgiveness?

Self-Understanding

Understanding the events, traumas, and pressures that have led to the formation of harmful thinking patterns in your life can go a long way toward forgiving yourself for the ways you have harmed yourself and/or others. Understanding the reasons behind your coping mechanisms or beliefs might help you avoid blaming yourself for decisions you may or may not have made.

According to research, the long-term impacts of trauma are most visible and noticeable when people are agitated, in unfamiliar settings, or in scenarios that remind them of the circumstances of their trauma. As a result, events might sometimes elicit emotions that we wish we didn't have. Understanding oneself via healthy coping skills, counseling, and support, on the other hand, may significantly increase your ability to forgive and move forward.

Compassion for Oneself and Common Humanity

Kristin Neff, is regarded as a pioneer in the subject of self-compassion. The second key ingredient of self-compassion, according to her conception, is acknowledgment of the universal human experience—or what she refers to as "Common Humanity." She writes in her book, *Self-Compassion*, that "self-compassion recognizes the truth that all human beings are imperfect, that bad decisions and feelings of regret are unavoidable" (Self Apologies, 2021).

We've all committed errors. Knowing this and realizing you are not alone, might help you feel compassion to forgive yourself. Compassion for yourself does not absolve you of responsibility for your actions, but it can liberate you from negative self-talk that keeps you from forgiving yourself, allowing you to respond to the situation with clarity.

When you evaluate your errors, it becomes evident that you did not deliberately choose to do them, and even when you did, the rationale for your actions was tinted by previous traumas. Specific patterns emerged as a result of the guilt you carried, outside situations, and extra pressures. These external influences might include genetics, family history, and living conditions.

"When we begin to see that we are a product of innumerable influences, we don't need to take our 'personal faults' so personally," Kristin Neff states in *Self-Compassion* (Self Apologies, 2021). We might be less judgemental of ourselves and others when we recognize the complicated web of conditions in which we are all enmeshed. A thorough awareness of interconnection enables us to feel compassion for the reality that we're doing the best we can with the hand life has dealt us (Self Apologies, 2021).

Having to Earn Your Forgiveness

If you are having difficulty engaging in self-forgiveness, be open and inquire with yourself. "Why wouldn't I want to forgive myself?" you might ask. If you say, "I don't deserve it" that's your shame speaking. If you still believe you don't deserve forgiveness, you may believe you must earn it.

What steps do you take to earn forgiveness? Be honest about what you believe you require forgiveness for and what you believe you have done, as this may help you to alter some negative ideas and be more compassionate and forgiving of yourself.

Write a letter to the person who you want to forgive (in this case yourself). In this letter you'll write about what you want to forgive yourself for and why. After it is written, you will burn it, and leave it behind.

Your Inner Child and Soft Boundaries

Assume you grew up believing you were unloved. As a result, whether consciously or subconsciously, you will spend your entire life yearning for love, thinking: *I need to be a nice girl or a good guy; and in order to feel loved, I must not ever say no.* And so you wind up giving and giving to the point of contempt because saying no is something you find really difficult to do.

Your Inner Child and Rigid Boundaries

Assume you grew up witnessing your mother or father struggle to say no, and you saw what this lack of boundaries caused them, or perhaps to both of you. So, as a youngster, you make a promise to yourself that you will never allow anyone to get too close to you and that you will never let your guard down. From that perspective, you create hard boundaries, believing that you must protect yourself by erecting those walls, and that if you don't, you will suffer in the same way that others close to you have suffered.

The reason that limits are set in both situations is because they are ego-based reactions. Because of a painful event, the ego protects you by establishing these limits. It ultimately backfires.

So, what steps can you take to remedy the desire to set rigid boundaries?

Step 1: Let Go of Your Grip on the Agony

There is a need to defend oneself if the ego is involved. Because your inner child did not feel secure and was injured, the ego made agreements and limits to help your inner child feel comfortable. If you let go of your grief, you will behave and react from a place of neutrality rather than anguish. To let go of agony:

- ***Write.*** Writing is a therapy for almost all of the issues out there. So make sure to write it all out so there is nothing holding you back.
- ***Grow your creativity.*** Drawing, knitting, painting, dancing, photography, music, ceramics, or any other hobby that you like is acceptable. This practice is comparable to journal writing in that it allows for the discharge of emotions.
- ***Divert your attention to something else.*** Our emotional condition can become overpowering and difficult to regulate at times. This is when having a diversion might help you cope. A diversion might be as easy as watching a movie or going out for coffee with a buddy.
- ***Exercise.*** Physical activity is an important component of mind-body wellbeing. Movement can help our unpleasant emotions get unstuck, allowing us to process and release them.
- ***Eliminate unhealthy thinking patterns.*** Learn to recognize harmful habits of thought, such as rumination or negative thinking, and

attempt to change such patterns. This is a frequent cognitive-behavioral method used to treat stress, as well as depression and trauma. For example, if you see yourself indulging in negative thinking or obsessing on a traumatic scenario, utilize self-talk to break the cycle. You might tell yourself, "I will get through this," "I am strong," or "I am bold."

Step 2– Act From a Place of Loving Neutrality

Once you've let go of the fear and given yourself what you need, you'll be in a better position to see and comprehend that other people have their own things going on as well—their own filters and viewpoints through which they see and live. They, too, frequently behave or respond depending on their own experiences. With that in mind, act, respond, and make decisions from a neutral, loving place.

This neutrality becomes simpler to maintain as you have a better understanding of others' point of view. When you approach the world and those around you with loving neutrality, no matter what life throws at you, you help bring clarity and healing to all involved, including yourself. There will be no need for hard boundaries.

Step 3– Positively Express Yourself

Even if you're dealing with a challenging or unfavorable situation, it's necessary to express yourself. But you must do so in a productive and respectful manner.

Don't be scared to stand up for yourself and confront those who question you and/or your rights. You may even allow yourself to get irritated! But remember to keep your emotions under check and to be courteous at all times.

Key Takeaways

- Childhood trauma may have an impact on our adult relationships as well as our mental and physical health.
- Trauma remains unresolved if we do not face it.
- Creating an unified story entails admitting our mistakes, sharing our stories, and feeling the agony of our trauma.
- Use stress-reduction practices like mindfulness, meditation, or cardiovascular exercise to help you relax.
- Refocus your attention on the pleasant emotions you experience on a regular basis.
- Work to discover your life's meaning and purpose.

Feeling Worthy, Authentic, and Playful: Becoming Your Best Self

"It takes a very long time to become young"

— PABLO PICASSO

This chapter talks about:

- 8 easy ways to release your inner child's creativity
- Inner child vs. inner critic: a creative fight
- Reparent your inner child to improve your self-esteem and live a happier life
- Parenting with intention
- 5 ways to live your best life

8 Easy Ways to Release Your Inner Child's Creativity

The joy of childhood play is an excellent source of inspiration for adult creativity.

Do You Need a Creative Outlet?

Perhaps your day job entails arranging Excel sheets as your most creative task. Perhaps being creative is your day job, and you're exhausted by the continual need to come up with new ideas.

Whether you're a full-time creative or don't have a creative bone in your body, having a creative outlet aside from your day-to-day work is important.

Why is Having a Creative Outlet so Important?

We have an intrinsic drive to express ourselves as humans. We require a means to express our feelings and experiences, which allows us to deal with our everyday lives and comprehend the world around us. Simply discussing our difficulties isn't enough. We require a creative retreat to assist us in connecting with ourselves on a deeper level.

Furthermore, there are scientific studies that corroborate the multiple benefits of creativity. It can help reduce stress and anxiety, enhance physical and mental health, and increase IQ (Chen, 2020; Robinson, 2021). Fortunately, there are several methods for releasing your creativity. And you don't have to be Picasso or Mozart to benefit. In fact, you probably already know how to perform a number of activities since you did them as a youngster.

Here are some ideas for making time for yourself and maintaining a creative outlet.

Things to consider while looking for a creative outlet:

- **Have a sense of humor.** As adults, we are often too focused on attaining positive outcomes. We'll quit a creative project if we don't excel at it quickly. Allow yourself to be surprised when it comes to finding a creative expression. Consider when you were a child and doodled or played make-believe. Attempt to channel that sense of enjoyment and enjoy the process.

- **Have some structure.** Is it possible to have fun while following the rules? Yes! Structure and regularity will really assist you in connecting with your creative side. There's a reason why writers are overwhelmed by the blank page: the sensation of possibilities may be overpowering.

1. *Try setting up a regular day and time to engage in creative pursuits, whatever they may be.*
2. *If you're just getting started with creative writing, try keeping a word prompt diary. Instead of feeling obligated to create anything from scratch, you may utilize the word prompt as a jumping-off point for brainstorming ideas.*

Suggestions to Be Creative

- **Adult coloring books** - For good reason, adult coloring books are a popular creative activity. Coloring has been shown in studies to reduce stress and anxiety. Coloring enables you to get out of your thoughts and concentrate on the subject at hand. We spend so much of our adult lives problem-solving, evaluating, and juggling job and home life. Coloring allows our minds to rest and be inspired by the colors on a page, taking a break from all of the thinking and fretting.
- **Watercolors** - You may get started straight away by purchasing inexpensive paints and brushes. Smooth paint brush strokes and a soothing palette of water colors are so pleasant and relaxing.
- **Dance class** - Getting in touch with your physical side is the best way to get out of your thoughts. Try a salsa or flamenco class, or any other activity that allows you to express yourself through dance. Because it helps you to connect with your physical body, a dance class might

be especially beneficial if your profession demands you to write and communicate all day.

- **Make a collage** - Create a physical Pinterest board by gathering periodicals and catalogs and clipping out any image that speaks to you. Maybe you'll make a vision or inspiration board – go with your gut and see what you come up with. These graphics may be glued to a paper or pinned to a corkboard.
- **Build with Legos** - Legos, like adult coloring books, are making a resurgence as adult sets. Allow your imagination to soar as you construct vast universes one brick at a time.
- **Cook a dinner** - Being creative does not require you to learn a new instrument or write a poem. In fact, when you're inspired by ingredients and flavors, creating a meal can be a creative endeavor. Furthermore, the physical sensations of cutting, dicing, and stirring are guaranteed to be a terrific stress reliever, and the ingestion of flavors and fragrances will alert the senses, making you more susceptible to creative thoughts.
- **Playing instruments** - Playing instruments is beneficial to your health and creativity. They might help you relax and enter a meditative state, and learning different instruments is a great way to relieve tension! If you've grown weary of crunching statistics or staring at text all day, take an instrument lesson or simply get a bongo to pound on at home while listening to music.
- **Solve riddles** - If music and dancing aren't your thing, perhaps board games and puzzles are. Make some tea and get out a puzzle. And by fitting the puzzle pieces together, you might just be able to see the greater picture–not just on the board, but also in your own life!

Remember that the simpler the creative activity, the better. Consider the things you enjoyed as a youngster, the pure thrill of doing something enjoyable that engages your imagination is what childhood enjoyment is all about.

We hope you discover a creative outlet that is both soothing and pleasant, whether you're building a collage or coloring in a book.

Inner Child vs. Inner Critic: A Creative Fight

Adults mourn their childhood's pure curiosity, and artists attempt to recover their lost childish inventiveness. The creative process might feel like a never-ending conflict between an inner child and an inner critic. Can this creative conflict be resolved in favor of creative balance?

Getting Older

Being a youngster is synonymous with being inquisitive. It seems as though children ask 107 questions each hour. However, as we become older, we begin to accumulate factual information, practical shortcuts, and mental models to help us make faster judgments. In a society that values speed as a metric of performance, we seek the shortest road to our objectives. We place so much emphasis on understanding *how* quickly we can arrive at a desired end that we neglect to pause and ask *why* along the way.

And when we do ask ourselves questions, we are frequently motivated by self-doubt. Is my labor sufficient? What will the public think? Our inner critic is trained by a learning system that emphasizes getting the right answer and outperforming others on prescribed assignments. Listening to our inner critic may lead to conformist work rather than superior creative work.

While the inner child has typically been employed in psychology to represent an unconscious archetype pointing to unresolved childhood events, it may be welcomed to help us better balance our creativity. In his book, *Psychotherapy for the Soul*, psychologist Stephen Diamond asks, "Has your adult self spent time with your inner child today?" (Diamond,

2008).

Retraining the Inner Critic

We frequently discuss silencing our inner critic. Connecting with your inner child and releasing your youthful creativity does not mean we need to quiet our inner critic. Instead, it's about retraining how the inner critic interacts with the inner child: unlearning self-doubt, pointless competitiveness, and dread of failure.

As with many unfavorable emotional experiences, accepting the voice within might help us better comprehend it. Turning self-criticism into self-reflection may boost your creativity by allowing you to go deeper into your own mind and confront your ideas and feelings in a healthy manner. We disarm the inner critic with love rather than violence.

So, how do you go about doing so? Positive self-talk is a simple technique for transforming self-criticism into self-reflection. For instance, positive self-talk appears to assist athletes enhance both their performance and their mental condition. A meta-analysis of 32 studies on the subject backs up these claims (Diamond, 2008).

There are easy steps you may take to make room for positive self-talk:

- **Create your own fun.** Integrate playfulness into your creative work as a discipline. Talk yourself into doing new things, let go of the aim, and surround yourself with people who are fun to be around.
- **Accept JOMO (Joy of Missing Out)**. It's fine to forgo an adult event in order to spend time with your inner kid at home. Do you want to sketch, write poems, or learn how to 3D print instead of going out for drinks with your coworkers? Proceed with caution. Feel the thrill of missing out.
- **Inquire why**. Don't allow your lack of apparent expertise keep

you from asking questions. Continue to ask why, as if you were a child. Train your inner critic to convert self-doubt into exploratory inquiries.

Over time, your inner critic transforms into your inner coach. Instead of it being a paralyzing fight that stifles your creative process, it propels your personal progress. *What would others think?* becomes instead, *Who could provide me constructive feedback?* and *Does it feel good enough?* based upon societal criteria, we ask ourselves, *Does it feel pleasant?* based on our own feeling of play and curiosity.

"It is never too late to have a good childhood," Tom Robbins wrote. It is never too late to make amends. Kill your inner critic with love so that it becomes your inner coach, and embrace your inner child's fun and curiosity to boost your creativity. Your inner dialogues will be a lot more joyful, and this will be reflected in your life and job (Diamond, 2008).

Heal Your Inner Child to Improve Your Self-Esteem and Live a Happier Life!

As mentioned before, reparenting is an effective method for healing childhood emotional traumas. In essence, you become the parent you lacked as a child. And, by providing to yourself what you did not receive as a child, you are liberated from the past.

This is also critical for developing self-esteem and mending emotional traumas from the past. As a consequence, you will be able to have good relationships and live a happy life.

Childhood Adversity

Sometimes parents fail to offer the psychological, emotional, and physical support necessary for a child's healthy growth. Adults who are stuck in their prior trauma might be dominated by their wounded inner child indefinitely.

And this may lead to bad adult decisions, particularly when it comes to relationships and creating appropriate boundaries. Because you were unable to build a strong sense of self as a youngster, emotional or physical abuse will have an impact on your future judgment. As a consequence, you may be unsure of how to establish healthy limits with others. Regrettably, this may lead to a lot of heartache, stress, and drama later in life.

Hurting Words

If you're harboring childhood scars as an adult, there are very genuine and, sadly, frequent causes for this. Your parents may have tried to teach and protect you, but they may have really done the opposite. The following are some of the most typical ways that children's feelings are rejected or minimized:

- You were made to feel bad for expressing your feelings.
- You were yelled at.
- You were penalized for attempting to speak out or express your uniqueness.
- You were humiliated by your parents or other family members.
- You were subjected to criticism or verbal assaults.
- You were raised to believe that you were responsible for your parents' unhappiness.
- You were dragged into grownup topics and discussions.
- You were taught that having your own ideas is unacceptable.
- You did not get proper physical attention, such as hugs, kisses, or

cuddles.

- Your emotions were not validated or given any weight.
- You were physically disciplined with spankings, slaps, pinches, and other forms of corporal punishment.

So, if you were unwanted as a child or were mentally/physically mistreated or neglected, you most likely have poor self-esteem since you never learned how to connect with yourself.

Then vs. Now

You might be asking yourself why this is so significant. Some people are still unknowingly affected or governed by their unconscious inner child. This is because they lack a true connection to themselves.

As a result, they are unable to attract good partnerships into their life. Childhood trauma causes these harmful and self-destructive behavioral habits.

It also explains why you can be apprehensive, fearful, or insecure. That, however, is not your fault. How else could you feel when you were a youngster and never had adequate safety or mental shelter? And it is for this reason that you must now reparent your inner child in order to mend your life and make good changes!

Taking a Look Outside Yourself

Unfortunately, when your parents do not affirm you or teach you the value of your feelings, you are trained to believe the same. You can't care for yourself or establish self-esteem if you don't appreciate your own feelings. As a result, you evolve into adulthood without knowing you have a self to care for.

When you don't have enough self-confidence, you're taught to ignore your feelings in order to please others. So you search outside of yourself for everything you should be offering to yourself: love, approval, self-esteem, validation. Only when things go really terrible, or you've reached your emotional rock bottom, will you begin to look inside because there's nowhere else to turn.

Parenting with Intention

You can heal your inner child no matter what has happened to you. So, try these activities to accept and strengthen your inner child and become a joyful, healthy adult.

Identify Your Inner Child

When you are hurt as a kid, it is all too common for you to become codependent. This implies that you seek recognition, validation, and affection from sources other than yourself. As a result, the world may become perplexing, if not frightening.

- Maintain an open mind.
- Seek advice from someone younger, most often a child.
- Try going over your childhood recollections, both happy and sad. It can help to make a timeline and write these moments down.
- As a child, take pleasure in the simple things.
- Speak with your inner kid.

Make Use of the Present Moment

You may ground yourself in the present moment by living in the now, not stressing about the future or focusing on the past. Every minute of the day is a new chance to be unconditionally loving, caring, and kind to yourself. And this is just what your inner kid requires to grow and thrive.

You may be the attentive parent you wished you had as a child by taking care of yourself.

Self-Care

Self-care is a powerful method for connecting with your inner self. This is a profoundly restorative activity that has the potential to transform the path of your life. Nobody understands what you require better than you.

So, ask yourself, *What brings me joy?* Then do whatever it is that brings you joy. Instead of looking outside of yourself, change your attention and learn to rely on yourself! Consider yourself to be a tiny child. Then, acknowledge your inner being, which is constantly with you. Speak with her (or him). Find out exactly what they require from you.

You are the only one who has the ability to cure your wounds. So, offer your inner child what you wished for as a youngster but did not get. Throughout the day, check in with yourself frequently, by exploring, *How do I feel about this emotion/situation/event?* And then cultivate those emotions.

Recognize Your Inner Child's Requirements

Based on our unique experiences, we all have distinct demands. As a result, everyone's reparenting experience will be unique. This means setting limits, making time for yourself, and being gentle with yourself during the process.

Reparenting is "simply self care," according to Dr. LePera, creator of the "Holistic Psychologist" website. In other words, the idea of reparenting your inner child is predicated on the assumption that you are capable of meeting your own needs. "It's making choices every day in your own best interest." She continues, "It is about becoming conscious of your habits and actions, particularly why you do what you do" (Estrada, 2019).

Parental Reflection

When you are young, the adults who raise you, teach you about yourself. This occurs as a result of parental mirroring.

"Parental mirroring" is defined as a caregiver's ability to precisely reflect a child's expressed thoughts and feelings. And the child's perception of acceptance and validity will be enhanced as a result of this affirmation that he or she has been heard.

As a result, in order to reparent your inner child, you must first supply him/her with what she needed to hear as a youngster. Here are a few major examples of words of healing that your inner child needs to hear:

- I adore you.
- I understand.
- You are flawless and complete.
- You did not deserve it.
- That must have been a really tough situation for you.
- I'm very sorry for what happened to you.
- You are astute.
- You gave it your all.

Visualization of the Inner Child

The following practice can be utilized to heal your inner child:

- Take a seat or lie down in a comfortable, peaceful location.
- Pay attention to your breathing.
- Take slow, deep breaths in and softly exhale. If you notice any stiffness in your body, concentrate on it and breathe into it.

- Exhale to let go of the stress. Continue to take slow, deep breaths in and out.
- Allow your mind to relax and simply accept whatever feelings occur.
- When old hurtful emotions come to the surface, pause and take several deep breaths.
- Imagine a brilliant light streaming through your body, bringing you back to a state of tranquility.

Repeat this practice as soon as you feel responsive and ready.

Love as a Healer

The most powerful healing force in the universe is love. And love has the power to heal even the most profound childhood traumas and grief.

You can choose to consider different ideas and make new decisions when in peaceful contemplation. You will cultivate loving feelings of forgiveness and compassion as you reparent your inner child. This will offer up new avenues for you to cultivate better, happier connections.

True maturity is dependent on recognizing, embracing, and accepting responsibility for loving and raising one's own inner child. And only you have the ability to make positive changes by reconnecting with yourself, increasing your self-esteem, and your confidence. This is an efficient and healthful method to begin making great changes right away!

5 Ways to Live Your Best Life

In the midst of a pandemic that has undeniably aged us all, the urge to embrace our inner child is all the more pressing. We may learn a lot from youngsters, such as their curious, fearless, and carefree attitude toward life. With bills to pay, money to save, errands to do, and a life full of rules and obligations, it's all too easy to lose sight of our curiosity for life and excitement for each day.

That doesn't mean we can't restore those characteristics. Getting in touch with your inner kid is a terrific approach to de-stress and rediscover the creativity and vigor that you had as a youngster and that you still have deep within.

"We get caught up in the grown-up trap and forget to have fun; embracing your inner child can reconnect you with the contentment and simplicity you once experienced as a child," says Nicky Taylor, co-author of the book, *Be More Kid* (Meyerowitz, 2020).

As we get older, we believe that grownups have all of the answers; but what if the reverse is true? What if, in order to live a meaningful and satisfying life, we need to unlearn the harmful behaviors we've picked up as adults and embrace our inner child?

"We've all had the resources within us all along, not only to help us through difficult times, but to thrive," Nicky says. "We just need to unlearn detrimental adult tendencies and 'be more childlike'" (Meyerowitz, 2020).

So, here are five methods to embrace your inner kid, based upon Nicky Taylor, Mark Taylor, and Ed James' principles (Meyerowitz, 2020):

Re-establish Connection with Lost Dreams

Children think they can be anything they want - they have no doubts that restrict them, and adults around them encourage them to believe everything is possible. As we get older, our goals and prospects vanish and are replaced with "have to's" and "must do's." Those same individuals who previously encouraged our aspirations, now tell us that we need to find something practical to do that pays well or our dreams won't come true.

Get in touch with your childhood dreams. What were they? What was significant to you about the things you used to fantasize about? How could you do something similar as an adult? Why not take classes if you once aspired to be a ballerina? Write those dreams down for yourself and place them somewhere you can be reminded of them.

Rekindle your unflinching faith in yourself and your abilities. Surround yourself with those who believe in you, completely.

The Art and Science of Thinking

Children think in a very simple manner. It never occurs to them that something may go wrong. Obstacles are just non-existent. If you explain why they can't accomplish something, they will tell you all of the ways they can!

Adults, on the other hand, believe their own reasons for not trying something, and if they do push through fears, they frequently wind up feeling guilty or visualizing everything that could go wrong, which ruins their enjoyment of a pursuit. Retrain your mind to concentrate on everything that is going well. To accomplish this, think of something particular that is coming up, and spend some time picturing what the scenario looks like after it has ended. What are you going to see, hear, feel, and think to yourself?

Remember that pleasant image every time you think about that incident—this is the only version you need to envision. Take note of how cheerful and calm you now feel about that occasion, perhaps even a bit eager, like a child might. Once you know how, it's simple to embrace your inner child!

Be Constant

Consider how persistent a youngster is when he or she wants something. They will keep repeating their request until they obtain what they want, no matter how obnoxious it is!

As adults, we may only ask for something once, and if our request is ignored or we do not receive the desired result, we may feel unable to ask again. You don't have to go to such lengths as a child, but if something is essential to you, use that childlike desire to make it happen. Look for an alternative way, put yourself in the shoes of the other person, and discover a win-win situation that benefits both of you. It's your life, you owe it to yourself to live it to the fullest.

Play a lot

Kids are extremely imaginative and can transform almost any situation into a game. They like having fun and easily invite their new best buddy over for a sleepover, despite the fact that they have just recently met them.

Adults, on the other hand, will perform the chores they dislike, miserably, rather than finding a way to enjoy them—even putting off doing the ones that they do enjoy as a result. Find innovative methods to make things you don't like into a game or a competition; you'll be surprised at how fast you can do them when they're enjoyable.

As we age, making new acquaintances can become a significant challenge, and those who are overly pleasant are even considered suspect! Everywhere you go, take advantage of the opportunity to meet new individuals. Simply be yourself and take in the friendliness for what it is. You'd be astonished at how many intriguing stories folks have to share (It would be advisable to wait a little longer before inviting them over for a sleepover!).

Contentment Overhead of Happiness

Kids discover satisfaction in the present moment, getting immersed in what they are doing or will do next. They don't consider anything else. Adults search for happiness outside of themselves or believe they will be happy in the future when circumstances change, such as when they have more money or can retire. As a result, they lose out entirely on the opportunity to be present in the moment.

Maintain complete focus on what you're doing right now. Enjoy the sensation of being in the now rather than waiting to go somewhere else. Instead, simply enjoy the ride that is life.

Key Takeaways

- Creativity is the key to letting the inner child express themself. There are different techniques to be creative from coloring to building with legos. Make sure to try a variety of creative ideas to help your inner kid.
- Your inner child is still a part of you, so they have a right to live a fulfilling life. Working on the above mentioned techniques will help you achieve the goal.
- Recovery from trauma happens in stages, if you feel like it is coming back again, don't lose hope. Keep the practice going.

Extra Healing Practices

"Healing is an art.
It takes time.
It takes practice.
It takes love."

— MAZA DOHTA

This chapter talks about:

- A letter to my inner child
- Your inner child's message to you
- The mindfulness energy
- A healing meditation for your inner child

Your inner kid is no longer estranged or lost. However, they still require some healing in order to let go of the past and accept the future. He/she is now grateful to you since you recognized them after all these years, just when they believed they were alone. This chapter outlines additional healing procedures that will be helpful in the healing process.

A Letter to My Inner Child

Your inner child is that part of you, the 'original' self, that still views and responds to the world through the eyes of a child who is innocent (and occasionally hurt).

It's about bringing the fragments of your history into the light of day so you can see what has yet to be resolved—where you have yet to be seen and heard. It's facing your limits and making a peace offering to the pieces of yourself that you've never forgiven. The versions of you who are still bound by past fear, treading water and unable to go on. It's a method to bring softness to your stress, to breathe into your heart's neglected chambers. It's about re-orienting yourself in light of your totality by piecing together your fractured self like a puzzle.

It boils down to becoming a mom to the pieces of yourself that were left behind when the rest of you developed. It's you, lavishing yourself with the love, attention, and approval you never had. It's not an easy job, sorting through the belongings you've been dragging about for far too long. Your recovery is complicated because you are human, and all humans are complicated.

Inner child work may be quite therapeutic if you allow yourself to be receptive to it. You could have a breakdown and then have a breakthrough. You may suddenly realize that the sensitive region behind your right shoulder blade is where the trauma settled when your father died.

Even what you've educated your mind to forget, your body remembers. Fear is stored in the muscles, humiliation in the cells, and sadness in the bones.

Your heart, too, recalls everything. You only need to be quiet enough to hear the facts you've been hiding from yourself, and it's enlightening when you do.

Whatever you've gone through, this letter may be exactly what your younger self requires.

You are the one speaking to your innermost self when you read this. You're speaking to the part of yourself that has been damaged, starved, abused, abandoned, ashamed, left out, and left behind: your inner child.

You're paying attention. You're hearing them. You are present in every facet and season of oneself. Allow yourself plenty of time. Read this letter as though it were your own, because it is yours:

> *Hello there,*
>
> *Firstly, I ask for your apology for ignoring you for all these years. In my defense, I was scared of approaching you after the incident and locked you away. With time, I grew to be the best version of me but little did I know that my every decision had an impact on you. Please forgive me for approaching this late, but, better late than never, right?*
>
> *You felt isolated and misunderstood for many years. You felt that no matter how hard you tried, you were never good enough. Everything seemed to be your fault. I'm writing to affirm your sentiments and let you know you're not alone.*
>
> *Today is the day we confront your suffering, or, more accurately, our pain, and cut off the old roots.*
>
> *You did an excellent job of concealing yourself. I now see that this caused you to bottle up all of your feelings and become the person you are today. But don't be afraid to express yourself since today is*

the day we make a difference.

You are not insane, overly emotional, or too sensitive. Those that told you that, were simply emotionally immature themselves and did not completely comprehend your situation. Please accept that it is not your fault. Your emotions are valid, and you have the right to express them. You needed to defend yourself, and you were doing your best with what you had. I appreciate you for that. You don't have to conceal yourself any longer. You don't have anything to prove.

I know how many times you've suppressed your needs for fear of being condemned for expressing them. I know how many times you've kept your rage disguised when you felt you weren't being treated fairly. And I know how much sorrow that has caused you. You don't have to hang on to this humiliation, disappointment, and anguish any longer. You are not required to hold yourself together anymore.

It's about time to let it go...

I am here for all the re-assurance. I will keep sending the positivity your way so you can heal. You are worthy of being told "I love you." And I am here to make sure that you keep hearing it.

I hope you find the strength inside yourself to remember that your value is not determined by the thoughts and judgments of others, and that you do not need to satisfy anybody in order to be appreciated and adored. I hope you learn to always love and respect yourself even though you were never taught how. I hope you'll now consider yourself a priority in this cruel world.

It's all right to let go.

You're no longer in danger. I'm here to help you, with new information and better tools.

You're still here, and I'm grateful for that. When you point out the locations that still ache, I learn more about what you require. You educate me to pay attention with every sensation of guilt, anxiety, or envy.

I apologize for the things you wish you could have handled better or learned sooner. Please forgive me. Thank you very much. I adore you.

You may forget it from time to time, but you are always loved.

You have always been sufficient.

I haven't always noticed you, but now I do.

I haven't always listened to you, but I am listening now.

Thank you for your courage. When you had so much to cope with, you continued smiling and being friendly. Even when you were in pain, you made people feel seen and heard.

I hope your heart remains open even when you are not treated with kindness. I love you.

Your Inner Child's Message to You

Our minds have the ability to entirely alter our perception of a situation. It contains receptors that are associated with certain types of feelings and are only activated when we experience emotions. Similarly, as children, we retained a feeling of surprise, awe, and innocence in our brains. It never lets us grow old and keeps the spark of excitement alive within us. It keeps us interested in new things, seeking joy, and inspiring astonishment in the world around us. This positivity, however, is out of reach to our inner child who has experienced trauma as a youngster. Instead, feelings of dread, worry, loneliness, or uncertainty dominate their outlook, which then may appear in our thoughts, behaviors, and decisions as adults. When our inner child takes hold in stressful situations and drives us in the incorrect direction based on those sensations, it may wreak havoc on our life.

Those who were traumatized and harmed as children are not the only ones who may have felt unsafe as a youngster. In reality, most people can certainly reflect back on pleasant childhoods and identify areas where their needs were not addressed. There is no such thing as the 'ideal' parent. It's the most difficult duty anybody has, and most parents do their best with the information, education, and maturity they possess. Recognizing where our parents fell short in making us feel secure, isn't a process of assigning blame, rather it's a way for us to become aware of the sensations their lack of protection has caused. A kid may feel unsafe in a variety of ways, including: physical or emotional abuse or neglect, a lack of positive reinforcement, a lack of space for emotional expression, feeling criticism or humiliation, being forced to succeed at a high level, or growing up too fast, to name a few.

Your inner child grows up with you. They grow angrier and more furious with you because you continue to ignore it. Working directly with this part of you (and any other parts within it) may help you to: heal trauma, stop dysfunctional habits, connect with your essence and personal truth, meet your needs, experience joy, and live according to your internal compass, among other benefits. There are several approaches to working with the inner child. One such approach is, allowing your inner child to also send you a letter as though he or she has journeyed across time.

This type of practice can aid in the connection between you and your inner child. As youngsters, there was no open discussion with our parents, and we were often misunderstood. Before we can acknowledge our inner child, we must first understand one of the reasons they "act out" through us—they feel unheard. Examine your upbringing carefully to identify times when your inner child felt unheard or insecure. Connect with them to reassure them that they are protected and provide them a safe space to vent their unpleasant emotions.

Begin drafting the letter to your inner child. Remember, it's almost like talking to yourself, so take it easy. Don't worry about the sentence structure or using difficult words. Be simple. Make sure you are sitting in a comfortable place away from any distractions. Begin brainstorming the feelings you recognize on a sheet of paper. This is only the starting point. From here on out, all of your questions/statements will be based on the core reasons you've identified. Begin by acting as though your inner child is a stranger to you, and you want to learn more about him or her and become friends with them. "Hello, how are you?" is a good place to start. "It's been a long time, and I hope everything is going well with you." These inquiries will sway your inner child's affection towards you and minimize their anger.

Ask your inner child if he or she prefers talking or writing. If they want to write, begin by writing about the event you want to address or the reason you feel led down a different road. If they prefer to converse, stand in front of the mirror and look yourself in the eyes to address the inner child. Don't be afraid or think you're crazy, this is the most effective technique to get your subconscious to listen to you.

Don't be harsh on your inner child and don't place any demands on him/her. Instead, let them speak for themselves and develop a shared foundation of understanding, because all meaningful dialogue is born from mutual understanding. Allow your inner child to voice his or her concerns openly, but you may ask specific questions such as, "Where did it start?" "How has life changed for you?" "How come you didn't reach out to me?" Questions like these can help you better grasp the issue and may lead to a greater knowledge of your inner child. Never forget that your inner child is also full of love and life. They may be furious at first, he/she will soon see the wonderful side of it.

Our inner child needs love and reassurance, just like any other human being. Using reassuring words like, "I will protect you," "I am here for you," and "I have got your back" will calm him/her. It will soothe the negative feelings and create the feelings of safety they previously lacked. This can be further accomplished through guided meditations or visualizations, which are amazing in aiding us to envision ourselves sitting next to our inner child, giving us the ability to imagine hugging and consoling them. You can also indulge your inner child by playing the way they want to, go to a park or amusement park, watch a movie you loved as a child, color, or do any other activity they'd enjoy.

Here is a sample of the letter you can look to for guidance:

> *Hello there Adult,*
>
> *It's great to hear from you after such a long time. After all this time, I had given up on the possibility of reconnecting with you and having a heart-to-heart. Growing up brought you many difficulties, which drove you away from me. You're probably in need of a rest and someone to chat to. It amazes me how you seek affection from other people when I am right here. I know you're worried that I've been injured and transformed as a result of that traumatic experience. But you have to believe me when I say that it was just the wrong moment, not the wrong life. I, too, need to appreciate the beauty of life rather than reliving the pain over and over again. I'M OVER IT! You locked me up after the event and continued on with your life, while I was hidden away here, imprisoned. SET ME FREE. Make a*

> *difference in your life. Reunite with me to realize your true potential and conquer the world. I'm hoping to get some attention from you before I shut myself away for good.*

Practice this exercise of reaching out to your inner child to sort things out. Once you have done it, you will feel content with life. Always remember, you and your inner child will become friends now, so you can reach out for him/her in case of any obstacles. You are now teammates.

The Mindfulness Energy

To repair your inner child, you must first cultivate and nourish your attention so that you can awaken yourself to the truth of your pain, which you would otherwise want to escape. If you choose to pay attention, there are clear warning signs of greater suffering: you've become engrossed in your pain, recounting and retelling your story to anyone who will listen, as though you are competing—my misery is greater than yours. Without realizing it, you are keeping your sorrow alive by courting it.

Continually courting our suffering is an unpleasant romance, as we could find ourselves in a codependent relationship that must be acknowledged by its actual name: addiction. We get physiologically and emotionally entangled in our pain to the point where we cannot live without it, even if it is ruining our well-being. Yes, we clutch for momentary insights—this is suffering—but only when they arise to the surface of our awareness. The buried sorrow, on the other hand, has a way of gaining speed and energy until it suddenly erupts in its entirety—the tiny serpent has grown into a monster. Our mental condition is now infected with an addiction to misery. We react to every sight of sorrow with such destructive emotion that we reinforce the reasons and situations that caused the misery to begin with. As a result, we keep shooting ourselves in the foot—again and again.

Mindfulness is thought to have started some 2500 years ago in ancient eastern and Buddhist philosophy. Jon Kabat-Zinn popularized the notion of mindfulness in the Western world. Kabat-Zinn initially found awareness while practicing Zen Buddhist meditation with Zen Buddhist meditation masters, Philip Kapleau, and Korean Zen Master, Seung Sahn Haengwon. Kabat-Zinn secularized historical Buddhist mindfulness principles by detaching them from Buddhist cultural, religious, and ideological factors and orienting them to the "Western mind" and culture, resulting in the development of the first formalized Mindfulness-Based Intervention (MBI), known as Mindfulness-Based Stress Reduction (MBSR) (Kabat-Zinn, 2003).

The store of consciousness, also known as root consciousness, is the foundation of human awareness. In Western psychology, this is referred to as "the unconscious mind." It is the repository for all of our prior experiences. Store awareness is capable of learning and processing information.

Our minds are frequently absent from our bodies. Sometimes we go through our everyday routines without even thinking about it. We can do a lot with only store consciousness, and mind consciousness can think of a thousand more things. For example, while we drive across the city, our mental consciousness may not be thinking about driving at all, yet we can still arrive at our destination without getting lost or in an accident. That is our store consciousness at work. Awareness is analogous to a home, with the basement representing our store consciousness and the living room representing our mind consciousness. Mental formations such as rage, grief, or joy exist in the store of awareness as seeds. We have seeds of wrath, despair, prejudice, and fear, mindfulness, compassion, understanding, and so on. Store awareness is composed of all of the seeds, and is also the soil that sustains them. The seeds remain until we hear, see, read, or think of anything that reaches a seed, causing us to feel anger, joy, or sadness. In our living room, a seed is sprouting and blossoming on the level of mental consciousness. We no longer refer to it as a seed, but rather as a mental creation.

When someone touches the seed of anger by saying or doing anything that irritates us, that seed of anger rises to the surface and manifests in mind consciousness as the mental formation of rage. My hand is a biological structure. My rage is a mental construct. Seed varieties can appear as mental forms. One of them is anger. Anger is referred to as a seed in store awareness. It's referred to as a mental formation in mind consciousness.

The first thing we may do when a seed, like the seed of anger, rises up in our living room and emerges as a mental formation, is to touch the seed of mindfulness and ask it to come up as well. In the living room, we now have two mental forms. This is angry mindfulness. Mindfulness is always focused on something. Mindfulness of breathing occurs when we breathe thoughtfully. When we walk attentively, we are practicing walking awareness. When we eat consciously, we are practicing mindfulness of eating. So, in this scenario, mindfulness is rage mindfulness. Mindfulness acknowledges and accepts rage.

This technique is founded on the nonduality insight that anger is not an adversary. Both awareness and anger are aspects of us. Mindfulness exists not to repress or combat anger, but to notice and manage it—much like a big brother assisting a younger sibling. As a result, the energy of awareness recognizes and gently embraces the energy of rage.

When we need the energy of mindfulness, we just tap that seed with our thoughtful breathing or mindful walking, give a smile, and then we'll have the energy to undertake the job of identifying, welcoming, and, in time, profoundly transforming. Whatever we are doing, whether it is cooking, sweeping, washing, strolling, or being aware of our breathing, we may continue to produce mindfulness energy, and the seed of mindfulness in us will grow strong. The seed of focus is contained within the seed of awareness. We may free ourselves from ailments by using these two powers.

The Mind Requires Circulation

Toxins are known to exist in human bodies, and build up in our blood if it does not circulate properly. Toxins must be expelled from our bodies in order for us to be healthy. When the blood flows properly, the kidneys and liver can fulfill their jobs of eliminating pollutants. Massage, for example, can be used to improve blood circulation.

Our awareness, too, may be in poor circulation. We may be carrying a poison in our awareness in the form of anguish, agony, sadness, or despair. This is referred to as an interior knot or structure. The technique of massaging our consciousness involves embracing our grief and sadness with the energy of mindfulness. When our blood does not flow properly, our organs are unable to work effectively, and we become ill. When our psyche does not flow properly, our mind becomes unwell. Mindfulness boosts and speeds up circulation throughout pain blockages.

Taking Over the Living Room

Because our blockages of pain, sadness, rage, and despair have grown large and want our attention, they always try to come up into our mental consciousness, into our living room. They want to come out, but we don't want these unwanted visitors since they're terrible to look at. As a result, we attempt to obstruct their path. We'd like them to sleep in the basement. We don't want to confront them, so we fill the living room with other people. We do all we can to keep our living room occupied whenever we have ten or fifteen minutes to spare. We dial a friend's number. We take out a book. We switch on the television. We go for a drive. We are hoping that if the living room is occupied, these nasty thought formations will not arise.

However, all mental forms must circulate. If we don't allow them to surface, they cause poor circulation in our brain, and symptoms of mental illness and sadness begin to show in our mind and body. Doctors often prescribe medicine for physical symptoms, yet might occasionally ignore our internal structures, exacerbating our illness.

Taking Down Obstacles

If we can learn to face our knots of anguish, we may gradually allow them to grow up into our living room. We start to learn how to embrace and change them with the energy of awareness. When we remove the barrier between the basement and the living room, blocks of anguish will emerge, and we will have to be prepared to endure a period of suffering. Our inner child may have a lot of dread and wrath pent up from spending so much time in the basement. There is unfortunately no way around it.

That is why mindfulness practice is so vital. It is really uncomfortable to have these seeds sprout if attention is not paid. But if we know how to produce the energy of awareness, it's incredibly therapeutic to encourage and accept it every day. Mindfulness is a powerful energy source that can detect, welcome, and care for these negative energies. Maybe these seeds don't want to sprout at first because there's too much fear and distrust, so we'll have to encourage them a little. After some time of being embraced, a powerful feeling will return to the basement, inevitably forming a seed again, but this time it will be weaker than before.

Every moment you bathe your internal forms in mindfulness, the barriers of suffering within you dissolve. So, every day, give your wrath, despair, and dread a thoughtful wash. After a few days or weeks of bringing them up regularly and then assisting them to go back down, you build proper circulation in your psyche.

The Purpose of Mindfulness

Mindfulness' primary purpose is to take pause at any time and become aware of the child within us. All we have to do when we first see the wounded youngster is to be aware of him or her and say hello. That's it. Perhaps this child is depressed. If we observe this, we might simply take a deep breath in and tell ourselves, "I realize that grief has manifested in me. Hello, my pity. I will take good care of you," and exhale.

The second role of mindfulness is to accept our inner child after we have identified him or her. This is a really enjoyable practice. Rather than fighting our feelings, we are taking care of ourselves. Concentration is an ally that mindfulness brings with her. The initial few minutes of tenderly identifying and nurturing our inner child will provide some solace. The painful feelings will remain, but we will not suffer as greatly.

The third role of mindfulness, after acknowledging and welcoming our inner child, is to calm and ease our painful emotions. By gently cradling this infant, we may soothe our tough feelings and begin to feel at peace. We will be able to see the origins of these mental constructions when we welcome our powerful emotions with mindfulness and attention. We'll be able to pinpoint the source of our pain. Our suffering will be alleviated if we can recognize the source of the problem. As a result, mindfulness acknowledges, embraces, and relieves.

The energy of mindfulness includes both the energy of concentration and the energy of insight. Concentration allows us to focus on only one subject at a time. The energy of staring gets more powerful with focus, and enlightenment is attainable. Insight has the ability to liberate us at all times. If we can maintain our attention, enlightenment will surely follow. Therefore, the energy of mindfulness allows us to examine ourselves deeply and obtain the understanding we require for transformation.

A Healing Meditation for Your Inner Child

The following meditation will assist in healing from early childhood trauma. Utilize this meditation on a daily basis because it creates a gentle place for the body, heart, and mind to recall. As you will continue to develop and grow in self-love, it will provide a living place of inclusion and compassion for childhood memories and all past experiences.

Make Use of Your Love and Support Resources

Thich Nhat Hanh once reminded us that we can build a good fire with pieces of straw or paper. The straw bits that assist us in developing loving-kindness energy are our resources for, "cooking up love" (Rowe Ward & Ward, 2021).

People, places, pets, activities, and lovely memories that soften our hearts and nurture our appreciation, love, and compassion, are all resources that help us grow self-love. Take a few minutes in your practice to thoroughly recollect such a resource. Make it come to life by engaging your senses.

We are thankful to the intelligent and caring therapists, body healers, and shamans who have assisted us on our journey of transformation and healing. A somatic and trauma-informed therapist may be an invaluable support person for individuals on a spiritual journey. For example, a puppy is a great resource to open hearts. Imagine his weight on your lap and the feel of his fur against your hand. Now imagine his bouncy, jaunty step and smiles. You will feel your body relax when you think about the puppy.

Pay Attention to Your Body

Once we have experienced the good sensations of being in touch with our resources, we pay attention to our body. The body is the initial basis of awareness. We love ourselves by being connected to our bodies and acknowledging the marvel that is our bodies.

Find a spot where you can slow down without being distracted, so you can be aware of your body and breathing with some ease. Practice setting your posture thoroughly so that your breath is easy and you can genuinely be present.

Scan your body from head to toe, paying focused attention to your entire body with care. Invite your body to soften and relax, nestling onto your cushion or chair. According to Thich Nhat Hanh, this is how we maintain our appointments with life. He further suggests, "we halt, we relax, we rest, we heal, and we evolve" (Hanh, 2022). Sending this loving, attentive energy to your body is an act of self-love.

Show Your Inner Child Love

Then, silently, offer yourself these guided meditation words:

- I'm breathing in, and I'm aware that I'm doing so.
- I know I'm breathing out, so I pay close attention to the out-breath.
- As I take a deep breath, I am aware of my entire body, in the present moment.
- As I exhale, I am aware of my entire body, in the present moment.
- When I take a deep breath, I imagine myself as a five-year-old child, frail and defenseless.
- As I exhale, I smile to myself as if I were a five-year-old child.

As a follow-up, you can start a conversation with your inner child, if you would like to proceed a bit further. This meditation has assisted us in seeing ourselves as children and seeing the very genuine fragility of being human. We typically undervalue our resilience and strength, as well as our fragility and susceptibility. They are not distinct. In actuality, our fragility contains tremendous power and strength. While it may not be easy at first, being in touch with vulnerability offers a great opportunity to connect with life and our own goodness. The hidden divine child inside can be healed and strengthened as a result.

Key Takeaways

- Healing takes time so don't get frustrated if the things don't work out in the initial days of your practice. Keep the exercises going and you will soon see the change.
- Your inner child will heal and reach out to you through these techniques.
- Listening to your inner child's feelings and allowing yourself to experience them rather than pushing them away might help you understand and validate the anguish you've felt.
- Mindfulness can help you heal your inner child as your practice will focus all your energy into its rightful place.

Conclusion

"The wound is not my fault. But the healing is my responsibility"

— MARIANNE WILLIAMSON

Our inner child is a part of ourselves, which lives within us. They have been there since we were conceived, through utero and all of the developmental years that followed. The inner child frequently remembers both positive and negative childhood events, such as anxieties, traumas, neglect, or profound loss. When we begin to investigate our inner environment, we might begin to see internal patterns that have left us with subconscious "bread crumb trails." Our inner child is always interacting with us...

All we have to do now is learn to listen.

Now, our inner child may either be quiet and comfortable, or they can act out and make things a little rumbly on the inside—impeding good relationships, organizational abilities, and self-regulation.

When it comes to becoming a productive member of society, or taking steps toward pleasure, our inner child may make or break us.

If you're feeling irritated or trapped in your life, it's likely that your inner child requires some care. Stuck spots might manifest as difficulty at work, in parenting, in finding or maintaining love, in growing relationships, or in creating boundaries.

We were all children once, and those children are still alive and well today. Many of them have gone into hiding—waiting for someone to notice their anguish.

They'll be ready to appreciate every moment, carefree and light, once it happens. They want to be able to express themselves. They need to feel protected and loved in order to do so. When they are unable to, it is frequently due to unresolved childhood trauma. These are the bitter memories from your past that you have learned to ignore. In regular life, you might not see them. But it doesn't mean they aren't present.

Unfortunately, your inner child may try to ruin your adult experience by attempting to cope with their unresolved difficulties. However, you can help them to heal by reparenting yourself. This entails offering your inner child the loving presence and self-compassion you wished you had as a child.

What does it mean to reparent your inner child? Reparenting is an effective strategy for mending emotional scars from childhood. In essence, you take on the role of the parent you lacked as a child, emancipating your inner child from the past by providing for yourself what you did not receive as a child.

This is crucial for the development of self-esteem and the healing of emotional wounds from the past. As a result, you will be able to maintain positive connections and live a happy life. You may begin satisfying your developmental requirements yourself after you've become aware of the ways you weren't getting them fulfilled in childhood. Being your own excellent parent is what this entails.

Journaling, writing a letter to your inner child, and drawing, are just a few ways to feel connected with your inner child. Once you build the bridge and feel a connection, you can reparent your inner child as per your wants and needs.

How to Rediscover Your Inner Child?

Most of us have scars from our childhood that need to be healed. Connecting with our inner child may aid in this process, regardless of the amount of trauma our inner child has experienced. Childhood scars can manifest in a variety of ways in our adult lives.

The following are the six ways to rediscover your inner child:

1. identify the neglect
2. accept the past
3. accommodate your inner child
4. reach out to your inner child
5. embrace your emotions
6. fill the gap by taking action

Inner child work has several advantages. It might be especially beneficial for people who experienced general dysfunction, neglect, physical abuse, or sexual abuse as youngsters. Inner child work can assist people in processing trauma by recognizing and resolving the underlying causes of any ongoing psychological scars that interfere with their capacity to function as adults. The following are some of the advantages of inner-child work:

- increased living quality
- relief from depression
- enhanced reactions that are situationally appropriate
- better performance integration of ego states

- improved interpersonal interactions
- increased vitality
- a regained sense of childlike awe
- enhanced emotional control and maturity
- higher levels of genuineness
- a holistic sense of self

We saw the world through a completely different lens as children. As a result, many of the things we believe never wounded us as children, may still have left lasting impressions. This is why it's critical to avoid making assumptions about your inner child.

Through inner child therapy, you may learn to grieve, heal, and resolve whichever causes of trauma you've been knowingly or unknowingly hanging on to for years through your inner child. The practices mentioned within this book, such as: writing a letter to your inner child, a healing meditation for your inner child, five ways to live your best life, having mindful energy, and clearing your root chakra blockages, are some examples of the techniques that will help your inner child to heal!

II

Overcoming Anxious Attachment

A 3-step Healing Journey to Emotional Freedom, Finding Love and Security, and Building Healthy Relationships

Introduction

"A securely attached child will store an internal working model of a responsive, loving, reliable care-giver, and of a self that is worthy of love and attention and will bring these assumptions to bear on all other relationships."

— JEREMY HOLMES

We all desire to feel loved and appreciated by others. This is because when we are in the company of those who love us, our basic human need for safety is fulfilled. However, as comforting as feeling loved can be, it is also a terrifying experience for those who have developed anxious attachment.

Nobody chooses to be anxiously attached to people. If it were a choice, perhaps everybody would have gone with secure attachment. However, our attachment styles are created from the early relationships we formed in life, particularly the mother-child relationship.

An adult who both desires and fears love was once a child who received hot and cold parenting. One minute their parent was emotionally present and affectionate, then the next minute they were dismissive and withdrawn. Since survival was on the line, the child had to learn how to cope with these inconsistencies, and that is how they developed anxious attachment.

You have picked up this book because to some degree, you have been exposed to someone or perhaps have lived with anxious attachment for all of your life. You may be able to relate to the experience of receiving hot and cold treatment from your parent and growing up feeling insecure about who you are and where your place is in the world.

During moments in your childhood when you needed love the most, you could not find it. The unspoken message that you internalized was *Love is complicated*. Little did you know how much the attachment formed with your parent, and all of the harmful beliefs and coping mechanisms you adopted back then, would reinforce the same relational patterns in future relationships.

The purpose of this book is to take a deep dive into the anxious attachment style, which is explained in the attachment theory discovered by psychologists John Bowlby and Mary Ainsworth (Bretherton, 1992). This type of attachment is a result of inconsistent parenting patterns that cause a child to develop a deep sense of rejection and suffer with a low self-esteem.

Not only will we explore the origins and causes of anxious attachment, but we will also look at how it can affect relationship building and cultivating a strong sense of self as an adult. The takeaway message from this book should be that anxious attachment can be healed through introspection, reparenting, and discovering your sense of self-worth.

How to Use This Book

This book is your guide to healing anxious attachment and developing a deeper appreciation for yourself. The book is divided into three parts, namely:

Part 1: Recognizing Anxious Attachment
Part 2: Confronting Anxious Attachment

Part 3: Reconnecting With Yourself

The final chapter will include exercises, meditations, and journal prompts to help you practice the various strategies discussed throughout the book.

Please note that due to the nature of the subject, some examples included in the book may be triggering for sensitive readers.

The Four Attachment Styles

Step 1: Recognizing Anxious Attachment

"Some of us wonder if we can feel secure without being abandoned and some of us wonder if we can feel secure without being overwhelmed. Some of us a little of both."

— ALLYSON DINNEEN

This chapter talks about:

- How the parent-child bond is formed
- The origins of attachment theory and how attachment styles develop
- How to identify your attachment style

The Bond That Begins in the Womb

The unspoken bond between a mother and her child begins in the womb. Even though the fetus cannot see its mother, it can respond to touch and emotions. If you read birth stories, you will hear of mothers who bond with their unborn children by massaging their bellies, singing, or reading children's books. To show that they are paying attention, the children might respond by kicking back or changing positions.

Research has also shown that children begin to intuitively pick up on their parents' emotions while inside the womb. When a mother is upset, for example, the child's heart rate can double.

This doesn't usually have a negative effect on the child when the negative emotions felt by the mother happen once in a while. However, if the mother is in severe distress for a good portion of her pregnancy, the constant stress felt by the child can impact their personality and continued development outside the womb (Sorgen, n.d.).

The reason why it is important to speak about life inside the womb is because that is where the mother-child bond begins. Being able to lovingly respond to the nudges of the unborn child and create a safe environment for them to grow is the first sign or evidence of love and what the child can look forward to outside the womb.

Babies can see, feel, taste, hear, and think before birth. The question for mothers is: *What thoughts, emotions, or memories about your connection will the newborn come into the world with?*

Attachment Outside the Womb

An attachment is an emotional connection between two people that is seen by the way they interact with each other. Newborns form attachments with their birth parents or caregivers who provide for their needs.

It is important to make a distinction between attachment and genuine love since these terms tend to be used interchangeably. The main point to emphasize is that children form attachments with their caregivers out of necessity. Since they cannot survive in the world without being fed, burped, changed, or put to sleep, the care they receive from their primary caregivers creates a strong connection—regardless of the presence of affection and nurturing.

Love is a feeling that is formed separately.

There are some parents who develop love for their newborns and others who don't. When an attachment is formed without love, taking care of the child becomes no more than a duty. The parent knows they are responsible for raising their child, but they don't have any genuine feelings of love that inspire them to be selflessly devoted to parenting.

A sign of a healthy attachment is the presence of love, and an unhealthy attachment the absence of it. One way that we can identify the presence of love between parents and children is to see if the parents are "moved" by their children. In other words, do they respond timeously and appropriately to the children's needs?

Relationship researcher Dr. John Gottman believes that in healthy and loving relationships, both parties will respond favorably to each other's bids for connection. He goes on to describe a bid as "an attempt to get attention, affection, or acceptance" (Eanes, 2016).

For older children, the question "Will you play with me?" is a direct bid to connect, which can be answered with a yes or no (i.e. accepting or declining the bid). But for newborns and toddlers who are not able to verbalize their bids, crying, smiling, or making eye contact are ways in which they attempt to connect with their parents. There are three ways parents can respond to these bids:

- turning toward the child and responding to the bid
- turning away from the child and dismissing the bid
- turning against the child and showing no response or action at all

For example, a toddler who is visibly upset might crawl up to their mother and signal to be picked up. This signal is a bid to connect and receive their mother's affection and reassurance. In response, the mother can respond in three ways:

1. **Turning toward:** Mirror the child's facial expressions, pick them up, and offer a warm hug.
2. **Turning away:** Give the child a puzzled look and tell them to stop crying.
3. **Turning against:** Avoid eye contact with the child and continue to work on the task they were busy with.

Circling back to the connection between love and attachment, parents who turn toward their children and respond to their bids make them feel loved and nurtured. However, those who turn away from or against their children can make them feel unloved and insecure. Note that it takes numerous missed opportunities to connect to make children feel unloved. In other words, there must be a pattern or habit of ignoring children's bids to create an unhealthy attachment.

Attachment Theory

Whenever the topic of attachment is brought up, you will hear the mention of attachment theory. In the field of psychology, attachment theory is often used to explain the emotional bonds between people, particularly the bond between a mother and child.

John Bowlby was the first psychologist to write on attachments. In his work, he described them as psychological connectedness between human beings (Bowlby, 1969). Bowlby wanted to understand why children would become anxious or distressed when separated from their parents. He learned that separation anxiety was caused by distinct behavioral patterns.

A year later, a second psychologist, Mary Ainsworth, expanded on Bowlby's work in a famous study that explored the effects of early attachment on children's behaviors. The participants were mothers with children between 12 to 18 months old. They were given the instruction to leave their babies in a room for a brief moment, before reuniting. Based on the results of the study, Ainsworth identified three attachment styles: secure, ambivalent-insecure, and avoidant-insecure (Ainsworth & Bell, 1970). A few years later, two researchers, Main and Solomon, wrote a chapter about a fourth attachment style they called disorganized-insecure, in a book titled *Affective Development in Infancy* (Brazelton & Yogman, 1986).

There have been countless studies undertaken to support and explain how these four attachment styles impact relationship building later in life. Below is a brief introduction to each attachment style and some of their characteristics.

Secure Attachment

Secure attachment occurs when caregivers are able to respond and validate their children's needs. This enables children to confidently express their thoughts and feelings and develop a stable identity. The hallmark of secure attachment is emotional availability and providing children with positive reinforcement. Other signs of secure attachment include:

- good emotional regulation
- high self-esteem
- easily trusting others
- effective communication skills
- the ability to set healthy boundaries
- the ability to self-reflect in relationships

In adulthood: While secure attachment is the ideal style of attachment in any relationship, it isn't perfect. For instance, those who have secure attachments can experience relationship struggles like anybody else.

However, the difference is that they are more psychologically equipped to handle the highs and lows of relationships.

Ambivalent-Insecure Attachment

Ambivalence-insecure attachment, also known as anxious attachment, occurs when children receive inconsistent parenting. This creates a push and pull dynamic between caregivers and their children, which causes children to feel insecure. Some of the consequences of developing this type of attachment are forming an unstable identity, developing a fear of rejection or abandonment, or seeking constant reassurance from others. Other signs of ambivalent-insecure attachment that can manifest include:

- sensitive to real or perceived rejection/criticism
- developing clingy or needy tendencies
- low self-esteem
- difficulty trusting others
- feeling unworthy of love

In adulthood: What makes this style of attachment interesting is how it creates an intense desire and fear of affection and intimacy. On the one hand, someone might yearn for their romantic partner's embrace, but once they have it, they might feel smothered or deeply unsettled. The familiar push and pull dynamic learned from the earlier relationship with their parents informs their ability to give and receive love later on.

Avoidant-Insecure Attachment

Avoidant-insecure attachment, also known as avoidant-dismissive attachment, occurs when caregivers have been absent or neglectful during their children's upbringing. Instead of feeling insecure about affection or intimacy (as with the ambivalent-insecure attachment), children grow up being fearful or dismissive of them. The pain of emotionally unavailable parents can be harbored by children until adulthood. Some of the signs of this style of attachment include:

- pattern of avoiding physical or emotional intimacy
- unconsciously sabotaging romantic or platonic relationships
- fear of expressing strong emotions
- feeling threatened by people who want to connect
- developing a fear of commitment

In adulthood: Some mistakenly believe that people with this style of attachment are incapable of giving or receiving love. The truth is that they don't have "love issues" but rather trust issues. It is their chronic mistrust of others that makes them reject any signs of intimacy or connection. Working through these trust issues can significantly improve their relationships.

Disorganized-Insecure Attachment

Disorganized-insecure attachment occurs when children develop an unstable relationship with their caregivers due to being exposed to abuse, trauma, alcoholism, or mental illness. For instance, a child raised by an alcoholic parent may have had to assume the parental role and mature ahead of time, in order to take care of their younger siblings or the household. Having this type of parent-child relationship confuses the child and causes both symptoms of anxious and avoidant attachment. The child may also experience:

- fear of rejection
- high levels of anxiety
- unstable sense of self
- poor emotional regulation

In adulthood: In most cases, people who develop this style of attachment were exposed to early childhood trauma, either at the hands of their parents or with their parents' knowledge. They may experience similar outcomes as those with anxious or avoidant attachment styles and may also be vulnerable to mental illness like substance abuse disorder, mood disorders, or eating disorders.

Can You Heal From Your Attachment Style?

Children who aren't able to form secure attachments with their caregivers develop psychological wounds. They may be able to forget the memories of being neglected by their parents, but the pain of that emotional disconnect is very much alive in their subconscious minds.

The big question is: Can adults heal from the early attachments formed with their parents? The answer is yes; however, there is a lot of inner work required to recognize and process childhood psychological wounds. The purpose of this book is to focus on identifying and healing anxious attachment, which is possible through applying a variety of interventions, including psychotherapy, making healthy lifestyle choices, and embracing spirituality.

Quiz: Discover Your Attachment Style

You may or may not have an idea about which attachment style you fall under. This quiz is a fun activity to familiarize you with each style of attachment.

The tables present four styles of attachment. Go through each table and consider how much you agree with the statements. Place a tick inside the appropriate column, then tally your score after completing the table. The table with the highest score will likely represent the style of attachment you resonate with most.

Table 2: Ambivalent-Insecure Attachment				
Statement	**Disagree**	**Sometimes Agree**	**Mostly Agree**	**Strongly Agree**
I am constantly longing for someone or something that I cannot have.	0	1	2	3
I tend to be over-accommodating or over-apologize in relationships to keep the connection stable.	0	1	2	3
I tend to lose myself in relationships because of being overly focused on others.	0	1	2	3
I struggle to say "no" to others or set healthy boundaries.	0	1	2	3
I tend to second-guess myself and wish I had done or said things differently.	0	1	2	3
I secretly harbor resentment when I give more than I receive.	0	1	2	3
I try to avoid being alone because it makes me feel hurt, stressed, or abandoned.	0	1	2	3
I have a chronic fear of being abandoned by my romantic partner.	0	1	2	3
As much as I love to be around my romantic partner, I sometimes pick fights to test the strength of the relationship.	0	1	2	3
I unconsciously take on the mannerisms and personality traits of my romantic partner.	0	1	2	3
Section Total:				

Table 1: Secure Attachment				
Statement	**Disagree**	**Sometimes Agree**	**Mostly Agree**	**Strongly Agree**
I feel at ease in my relationships most of the time.	0	1	2	3
I am comfortable being alone just as much as I enjoy being with others.	0	1	2	3
When I get into conflict with others, I am able to self-reflect and apologize if I was in the wrong.	0	1	2	3
I believe that, in general, human beings are naturally good hearted.	0	1	2	3
I honor commitments made with other people most of the time.	0	1	2	3
I seek to fulfill the needs of my loved ones, and I am confident expressing my own needs.	0	1	2	3
I am protective over my loved ones and seek to maintain physical and emotional safety in our relationships.	0	1	2	3
I have a positive perception of the people that matter most to me.	0	1	2	3
I enjoy physical touch and intimacy with my partner.	0	1	2	3
I take my partner's boundaries seriously.	0	1	2	3
Section Total:				

Table 4: Disorganized-Insecure Attachment				
Statement	**Disagree**	**Sometimes Agree**	**Mostly Agree**	**Strongly Agree**
When I develop a strong emotional connection with others, I feel a sense of fear.	0	1	2	3
When I am faced with problems, I tend to freeze and feel hopeless.	0	1	2	3
I get startled easily, especially when others approach me unexpectedly.	0	1	2	3
Friends and family often express that I am controlling.	0	1	2	3
I tend to expect the worst to happen in my relationships.	0	1	2	3
I struggle to feel safe and relaxed in romantic relationships.	0	1	2	3
I have difficulty remembering past memories related to my attachment issues.	0	1	2	3
Even though I desire closeness, I struggle to make the effort to get to know people.	0	1	2	3
I fail to protect myself when faced with threatening situations.	0	1	2	3
Since I tend to freeze or disconnect when feeling stressed, I prefer simple and clear communication.	0	1	2	3
Section Total:				

Table 3: Avoidant-Insecure Attachment				
Statement	**Disagree**	**Sometimes Agree**	**Mostly Agree**	**Strongly Agree**
When others request to spend time with me, I feel inexplicably stressed.	0	1	2	3
I tend to downplay the importance of close relationships in my life.	0	1	2	3
I struggle to ask for help from others. I believe in being self-reliant.	0	1	2	3
I feel a sense of relief in not needing other people.	0	1	2	3
I need to have plenty of time and space to myself in relationships.	0	1	2	3
Sometimes I prefer to have casual sex than a fully committed relationship.	0	1	2	3
I feel less anxious in relationships with animals or things like work or hobbies.	0	1	2	3
I dislike many forms of intimacy like holding hands or making eye contact.	0	1	2	3
I tend to rationalize my emotions instead of feeling them.	0	1	2	3
I feel a sense of freedom when I break up with a romantic partner, which is followed by depressive emotions.	0	1	2	3
Section Total:				

Key Takeaways

- The parent-child bond begins in the womb through the mother's responsiveness to her unborn child.
- Psychologists John Bowlby and Mary Ainsworth are attributed for

creating what we know today as the attachment theory. The theory seeks to explain the various emotional bonds children can form with their caregivers.

- Every child develops an attachment to their parents out of the need to survive, but this doesn't always mean that the attachment is healthy.
- From an early age, children make bids for affection by seeking their mother's attention. Genuine love between a parent and child is formed when the mother is willing and enthusiastic about responding to bids.

How Attachment Styles Affect Relationships

Step 1: Recognizing Anxious Attachment

"The key to finding a mate who can fulfill those needs is to first fully acknowledge your need for intimacy, availability, and security in a relationship—and to believe that they are legitimate."

— AMIR LEVINE & RACHEL S.F. HELLER

This chapter talks about:

- How attachment styles affect different areas of your life
- The barriers that anxious, avoidant, and disorganized attachment create with communication, empathy, intimacy, and stress management

Everyday Interactions With Different Attachment Styles

Jane has a secure attachment style. She was raised by emotionally available parents, who offered a predictable and structured environment with regular positive reinforcement. Growing up, Jane didn't have difficulty building and maintaining friendships. However, she also didn't feel obliged to keep friendships that were no longer mutually beneficial. Her openness to express needs and wants allowed her to communicate healthy boundaries and hold others accountable to them. In the face of rejection or invalidation, she was able to set limits, issue consequences, and quickly restabilize herself.

Timothy has an ambivalent-insecure attachment style. He was raised by a single mother who worked two jobs and often left the role of parenting to different babysitters. There is no doubt that Timothy was dearly loved by his mother, but he often yearned for her attention and affection.

Since his emotional needs were neglected as a child, he grew up seeking relationships that will fill that inner void. Once attached to an individual, he would become clingy and codependent. At the back of his mind, he feared losing close relationships because his identity was wrapped up in them. He often wondered how he would survive without the people he cared about most.

Mariah has an avoidant-insecure attachment style. She was raised in a traditional and strict household by parents who were ex-military officers. Her parents were not affectionate or emotionally expressive; they showed love by providing a safe and predictable lifestyle, as well as rewarding good behaviors.

Growing up, Mariah struggled to share her thoughts and feelings openly with her parents, out of fear of being judged or misunderstood. This pattern continued into adulthood and caused communication and intimacy problems in her relationships. While she desired love and closeness, she was very uncomfortable with it, and often preferred shallow and less intense connections.

Sonia has a disorganized-insecure attachment style. She was raised in a dysfunctional home environment where substance abuse was rampant with both parents. Growing up, Sonia never developed a healthy bond with her parents. She learned to protect herself by creating two different personas; one that was hard and emotionless and another that was authentic and trusting.

In adult relationships, these two personas often appeared together and created confusion and drama. People often didn't know "which Sonia" they were going to get whenever they interacted with her. Sonia felt the same frustration not being able to let go of her defensiveness and seek closeness. She believed that perhaps there were underlying mental health problems that were also keeping her from establishing a healthy sense of self.

Your attachment style begins with your early caregivers, but ultimately affects platonic, romantic, and professional relationships you will form later in life. Before starting the process of healing your attachment style, it is important to consider the various ways it can impact the quality of your relationships. What follows are five aspects of relationships that are influenced by attachment styles.

Communication

Communication skills are an essential part of human development. Without being able to clearly communicate what you are thinking and feeling to others, you won't be able to meet your needs.

Being a good communicator isn't based on simply talking. If that was the case, then there wouldn't be such a thing as misunderstandings. In order for talking to be effective, your messages must be expressed with clarity and honesty. Unfortunately, your attachment style can get in the way of how you talk and get your messages across to others.

For instance, secure types are known to be straightforward communicators. They may not always express themselves appropriately, but they are able to reflect on their thoughts and emotions and share them with others. This ability enables them to set boundaries, notify others when boundaries have been broken, and negotiate a positive way forward.

Anxious types spend more time attempting to figure out what others are thinking and feeling, which makes them detached from their own thoughts and feelings. It is common for them to be confused about what they want, and this delays their needs being met. Since anxious types are also prone to be people-pleasers, they are likely to say whatever they believe others want to hear, rather than openly stating their opinions—especially when they believe stating their opinions can lead to conflict or judgment.

Avoidant-insecure types can easily be triggered by what others think and feel. They will typically be dismissive of others when they are told something that they don't approve of. Dismissive behavior may include yelling, using threatening language, or giving the silent treatment. Since avoidant-insecure types are sensitive to negative emotions, they may also find it difficult to accept when they have been hurt by others. It is easier for them to suppress their emotions and simply ignore or move away from the wrongdoer.

Disorganized types tend to adopt the same communication behaviors as anxious and avoidant-insecure people. However, what is particularly unique about this type is that they tend to crave connection but become equally stressed in close relationships. They may find it difficult to express their needs, even when it is in their best interest to (e.g. when their basic human needs are in jeopardy).

Empathy

Empathy is a personality trait that describes the ability to show compassion for other people's experiences. It seeks to help you understand what others may be thinking or feeling and the emotional impact of their circumstances.

Generally speaking, human beings are not born empathetic. This trait is usually taught through interactions with caregivers. For example, from a young age, parents can teach empathy by creating an emotionally safe space for their children to express their thoughts and feelings at home and using validating language as part of everyday communication.

A 2012 study found that attachment styles could predict whether or not people were inclined to be empathetic. The study invited 260 nursing students, both male and female, and they were asked to fill out the Interpersonal Reactivity Index (IRI) and the Attachment Style Questionnaire (ASQ). The results from the study showed that students with secure attachment had a positive correlation with empathy, while students with insecure attachment styles (including both ambivalent-insecure and avoidant-insecure attachment) had a negative correlation with empathy (Khodabakhsh, 2012).

Note that findings like these don't suggest that those with insecure attachment styles cannot be empathetic; however, they may struggle to display empathy due to being low in openness. Moreover, it is worth considering that since people with insecure attachment styles struggled to form safe and close bonds with caregivers at a young age, they are more likely to shy away from getting too close to others. Seeing other people express negative emotions could also be something that makes them feel uncomfortable.

Another interesting aspect of empathy is compassion, which is the act of being kind and supportive of others. In order to show compassion, one must first be compassionate to themselves, which means being good at responding to one's own needs. Since those with insecure attachment styles tend to develop a pattern of repressing their needs, self-care is an area that is typically lacking in their lives. This makes it harder for them to respond to the needs of others.

While ambivalent-insecure types can pour from an empty cup and overextend themselves to others, this shouldn't be seen as an example of compassion. If we study the intentions of their seemingly selfless giving, we will see that ambivalent-insecure types extend themselves to others from a place of fear, rather than love (e.g. fear of ruining their reputation or losing a loved one). Avoidant-insecure types, on the other hand, won't attempt to win the favor of others. Their feelings of inner emptiness drive their flighty and dismissive behaviors.

Intimacy

Intimacy can be described as a feeling of closeness, sometimes sexual in nature, within interpersonal relationships. Building healthy intimacy takes time and a great deal of trust. However, the reward of this is that you can feel safe and free to express yourself in relationships.

Those with secure attachment are often raised in loving and child-friendly environments that allow them to feel safe expressing their needs and wants and making bids for affection to their caregivers. Knowing that they can trust their caregivers to behave consistently, regardless of how they might feel toward them, creates a powerful bond. It also boosts their self-confidence and cultivates a healthy sense of self-worth. As adults, securely attached people will display low levels of anxiety and avoidance in relationships. They are also less likely to use sex as a way to "buy" affection or boost their self-esteem.

The other attachment styles (i.e. ambivalent-insecure, avoidant-insecure, and disorganized-insecure) are also capable of developing intimacy, but the difference is that it tends to look and feel unhealthy. A pop culture term that describes this type of unhealthy intimacy is "toxic love."

Those with ambivalent-insecure attachment crave healthy intimacy but are also deathly afraid of it. They are the type of people who will fantasize about being in loving and committed romantic relationships, but they will unconsciously sabotage their unions through codependent behaviors or distrusting their partners. What makes them behave in this way?

As children, their experience of love was hot and cold. They could never fully relax in the parent-child relationship because unexpectedly, the bond would be tested. For instance, their parents would pull away, become emotionally abusive, or become preoccupied with something or someone they deemed more important. A parent who was a workaholic could have spent more time at work than home, or one who was in a codependent romantic relationship could have prioritized their partner over their child.

In adult relationships, ambivalent-insecure types tend to obsess about closeness and worry excessively about whether their relationships will last. This can make them self-conscious, jealous, and codependent. Moreover, they often struggle to trust others fully, which affects their ability to form healthy intimacy. What they believe to be "true love" could in some cases be neediness or dependency.

Avoidant-insecure people treat intimacy differently. They do not fantasize about closeness, nor do they desire that kind of bond with others. The idea of being vulnerable and allowing others to know them on a deeper level is off putting. The reason they behave in this way can also be traced back to the parent-child relationship. As children, avoidant types were not shown open displays of affection and nurturing, such as being comforted with hugs, kissed on the cheek, or told "I love you." For this reason, they grew up being weary of relationships that require emotional investment.

In adult relationships, avoidant types prefer casual sexual encounters and easy-going shallow connections over long-term commitment. They tend to view partners who seek intimacy as being overly needy and demanding too much out of them. Additionally, they may fear their sense of independence being threatened when sharing space or being too close to others. Similar to anxious types, they can also sabotage relationships by giving into their fears.

Lastly, people with disorganized-insecure attachment tend to reflect anxious and avoidant tendencies when getting close to others. These behaviors are caused by a low self-esteem and a sense of unworthiness to being loved. Similar to avoidant types, they prefer to have shallow friendships or casual sexual encounters instead of being in deeply committed relationships.

Stress Management

Research has shown how early childhood attachment impacts the body's physiological and psychological response to stress (Munger, n.d.). The stress response, also known as "fight flight freeze mode," is a trigger that is activated whenever the brain perceives threats. There are usually three primal responses or reactions that ensue: attack, run away, or freeze.

However, when we study attachment theory, we can see the various ways that people react in stressful situations, such as:

- how one perceives stress in challenging situations
- how one reacts at the moment, as well as how one recovers from a stressful situation

- the effect that friends and family have on helping one cope with stress
- the various coping strategies that one uses to adapt to ongoing stressful situations

Secure types, for example, cope with stress by proactively looking for solutions, leaning on loved ones, or taking a different perspective. These coping strategies reduce feelings of fear and panic and encourage logical thinking. Of course, this doesn't mean that people with secure attachment don't overreact. Just like any human being, they can sometimes react negatively to stress or unforeseen events. Nevertheless, their overreaction is short-lived due to their solutions-based approach to stress management. Typical phrases that a secure person might say when feeling stressed are "I'm so disappointed, but I will get through this" or "I am feeling overwhelmed. I need to speak with someone."

Ambivalent-insecure types almost anticipate stressful events, even when there are no signs of threats in their environment. In fact, many anxious people will create worst-case scenarios in their minds to justify their anxious feelings. For example, when they notice that a loved one's cell phone has been off the entire morning, they might assume they are in danger. This scenario can feel so real in their minds that it triggers a panic and interferes with their productivity.

Calm or stable situations often feel "too good to be true" for someone with ambivalent-insecure attachment. In relationships, this can sometimes translate as feeling anxious in harmonious relationships and more relaxed in the presence of drama. Another characteristic of anxiously attached people is that they struggle to bounce back after coming out of a stressful situation. Intense fears may linger in their bodies for weeks and months after the event took place. Nevertheless, this doesn't stop them from connecting with people, as they continue to crave safety and intimacy. Typical phrases that an ambivalent-insecure person might say when feeling stressed are "Why does this always happen?" or "I can't trust anyone."

Avoidant-insecure types have a very detached and clinical way of dealing with stress. On the surface, you would think that they are unaffected by what happens around them—but this is just a facade. Avoidant people feel the full effects of stress, similar to anyone else, but they choose to cope by minimizing or denying the impact. They act as though the stressful event is not a big deal and that perhaps everyone around them is overreacting to the stress. Deep down, they feel a heavy burden to solve the problem or maintain a strong self-image, in order to be seen as being in control.

When dealing with stress in interpersonal relationships, avoidant-insecure people are prone to shutting down, dismissing other people's feelings, or showing little empathy. While this may come across as callous, it is simply their way of self-regulating. Since the avoidant person has a lot of bottled emotions trapped inside of them, they are always fearful of being triggered and stepping out of character. Typical phrases they might say when feeling stressed are "I have this under control," or "Why are you making a big deal out of this?"

Disorganized-insecure types are more likely to feel confused than angry during times of stress. They might appear dazed, mentally dissociated, or withdrawn from what is happening around them. Due to their traumatic history, they have learned to "check out" or hide inside their shell whenever things feel too intense. They will also internalize the strong emotions they feel toward others or their life situation. Out of all the attachment types, these individuals are more prone to obsessions, like working a lot or eating excessively, or substance abuse problems, which occur as a result of not addressing their issues.

Key Takeaways

- Whether or not you are aware of it, your everyday interactions are influenced by your attachment style. This can stretch as far as to how you enjoy sexual intimacy.
- The benefit of learning more about your attachment style is that you can anticipate your responses to certain behaviors or events and mindfully adjust your reactions.

A Deep Dive Into Ambivalent-Insecure Attachment

Step 1: Recognizing Anxious Attachment

"Imagine how much unnecessary anxiety we create when we live under the impression that our relationships should feel amazing all the time and that perfect happiness is an attainable goal!"

— SHEVA RAJEE

This chapter talks about:

- How ambivalence-insecure attachment develops
- Common signs of ambivalence-insecure attachment in relationships
- Some of the harmful habits that are practiced whenever attachment anxiety is triggered

How Does Ambivalent-Insecure Attachment Occur?

It's normal to be cautious when getting to know someone. After all, you aren't sure what type of person they are or how much you can trust them. However, these feelings subside the more information you learn about the individual and the deeper your connection grows.

The difference with people who have anxious attachment is that they never fully get comfortable around others, even when the connection has moved beyond surface level. The reason why we call this type of attachment "ambivalent" is because it is characterized by having "mixed feelings" or embracing contradictory ideas about others. In general, the contradiction occurs over feeling love and fear toward others—an experience that the anxious person had repeatedly when they were growing up.

An ambivalent-insecure attachment develops from early childhood when a child learns that they cannot rely on receiving consistent nurturing from their parents. Due to a variety of factors, their parents are unable to be emotionally available and responsive to their needs. This creates insecurity around the capacity to trust others and receive unconditional love. As adults, they can demonstrate a deep fear of rejection and abandonment in their relationships.

Many people assume that anxious children were never loved by their parents. However, this isn't always the case. It's possible that an anxious child was loved so much by their parents, to the extent of being overprotected. Perhaps you have encountered parents who are hypervigilant about their child's environment, where they go, what they eat, and who they hang around with.

Their desire to protect their child often causes them to invalidate the child's physical and emotional needs. This kind of "helicopter parenting" isn't necessarily inconsistent, but it can teach the child to associate closeness with controlling behavior. Later on in life, they might have mixed feelings about intimacy because they associate it with losing their sense of self.

Another example of loving children too much but invalidating their needs is a child raised by parents who are overly invested in their careers. They may undeniably love their child very much and view their work habits as a sacrifice to give their child the best possible life, yet being physically or emotionally absent creates an unstable and inconsistent connection with the child.

The role of caregiving may be assigned to nannies, schoolteachers, grandparents, or unfairly passed back to the child. This is made worse when nannies are constantly changed or the child is frequently moved from one school to another (or sent to boarding school at a young age). The child learns to fear making strong and lasting bonds because they can suddenly be taken away.

Signs of Ambivalent-Insecure Attachment

Researchers have found that not every anxious attachment looks the same. When looking for the signs of ambivalent-insecure attachment, we should remember that it exists on a spectrum. For instance, an individual can be ambivalent passive, ambivalent resistant, or lie somewhere in between those extremes.

Ambivalent resistant individuals tend to become visibly upset or withdrawn when they perceive a sense of rejection or abandonment. As children, they may have cried uncontrollably when being left by their parents. They may also engage in positive or negative attention-seeking behaviors to seek the approval of others or "win back" the affection of lovers. However, when others become emotionally available again, they may show their disapproval by being moody, withdrawing, or becoming angry.

On the other end of the spectrum, ambivalent passive individuals appear calm, cool, and collected on the surface, which might cause others to believe they are secure and unbothered about the perceived sense of rejection or abandonment. Instead of showing signs of anxiety, they typically internalize their emotions and downplay their own needs. Like other anxious people, they crave consistent and unconditional love but doubt that it is possible.

Both types of anxious people will, however, experience the same symptoms, which may include:

- **Clinginess:** An anxious person displays neediness in relationships, such as requiring constant reassurance about your partner's commitment, wanting constant communication with loved ones throughout the day (i.e. texting and calling religiously), and requiring regular support and check-ins.
- **Overwhelmed with emotional connections:** Ironically, those with anxious attachment can quickly become overwhelmed when relationships get too intense, as much as they are clingy. Since they are not used to being in consistent relationships where they are shown respect and love, they may develop a push and pull behavioral pattern.
- **Feel anxious in relationships:** A person with ambivalent-insecure attachment may be confident and secure in other areas of their life but get easily triggered in close relationships. Small behaviors can raise fears of rejection and abandonment, such as a friend making an ambiguous comment.
- **Unpredictability:** Due to an anxious person's deep-seated trust issues, they find it difficult to see relationships lasting in the long-term. As a result, they don't do well in relationships with unpredictable or impulsive people because they trigger fears of abandonment.
- **Seeking validation:** An anxious person seeks constant reassurance from others to prove that their relationship is solid, that their connection is genuine, and that they are acceptable. Low self-esteem is one of the challenges that anxious people are faced with, regardless of how smart, attractive, or successful they are. When they are invalidated, they can become angry, withdrawn, or try even harder.

It may seem that anxious people are constantly looking for problems in a stable relationship, but what they are actually seeking is emotional safety. Remember, anxiety is the main driving force behind these unhealthy relational patterns, thus when an anxious person feels emotionally safe, they are able to manage their triggers.

It is therefore crucial for these individuals to learn about the different attachment styles and be mindful of the people they choose to connect with. Secure people bring out the best in them, while avoidant-insecure people bring out the worst in them. However, due to the behaviors of anxious people, they are more likely to attract avoidants, who confirm their fears of rejection and abandonment.

Harmful Habits to Avoid When Attachment Anxiety Is Triggered

The reason it can be so difficult to heal anxious attachment is due to the neurological changes made to the brain at an early age. Researchers have found that children with ambivalent-insecure attachment have a larger amygdala, which is the part of the brain that detects threats. As such, they tend to be more hyper-aware and prone to stress and anxiety than children with secure attachment. It also means that they can become easily triggered by threats that are unreal or blown out of proportion.

If you are prone to feeling anxious and vulnerable in relationships, it is important to carefully consider your actions. Of course, your first instinct may be to overreact and get as far away from the perceived danger. But what has been the outcome of taking this action over the years? Has it helped or harmed your relationships?

The following are a few more harmful habits that are likely to occur when your attachment anxiety is triggered. As you go through each habit, ask yourself: What have been the outcomes of taking these actions over the years?

Being Too Available and Consequently Abandoning Yourself

When you begin to feel insecure in a relationship, due to real or perceived signs of rejection or abandonment, you may start to become increasingly needy and self-sacrificing. Investing so much energy in maintaining the relationship means less time spent on taking care of yourself. Signs that you are abandoning yourself include double-texting or being the one to always initiate conversations, stalking the person on social media, or dedicating all of your weekends to being with them.

Compromising Your Beliefs and Values to Make the Other Person Happy

Have you ever found yourself silently cringing when one of your values is violated, but you pretend as though it isn't such a big deal because you don't want to upset the other person? This pattern tends to show up in codependent relationships, where you merge identities and adopt the same values and interests as your partner. In the long run, this can lead to the loss of individuality and weak boundaries.

Self-Sabotage Instead of Self-Awareness

In many cases, when you feel anxious in relationships, old childhood trauma is triggered. In that moment, you can "black out" and time travel back to the past. How you react is dependent on how you reacted as a child whenever you felt neglected. For instance, you might withdraw without saying a word to your friend or partner because that is how you coped with these strong feelings when you were younger. You may also turn to other forms of self-sabotage that you picked up later in life, such as binge drinking, starting an affair, self-harm, or working extreme hours.

Negative Self-Talk

You may have a habit of internalizing your hurt feelings and subsequently blaming yourself for the inconsistencies in a relationship. For example, if you don't hear back from a colleague after a certain number of days, you might assume that you have offended them. The pattern of self-blame leads to negative self-talk, where you constantly criticize yourself for not living up to others' standards or not being able to maintain a relationship. Due to the negative self-talk, you may even fear entering new relationships because of not wanting to replay the negative thoughts in your mind.

Fantasizing About Being Saved

The inconsistencies in love that you experienced early in life may create fantasies about finding true love or being rescued by someone who understands and accepts you. These fantasies aren't necessarily bad, as long as they aren't projected onto people. For example, projecting the fantasy of a soulmate onto a new romantic partner can lead to neediness and people-pleasing behavior. In exchange for your devotion, you expect them to live up to your dream of an ideal partner. When they don't live up to this fantasy—and instead show you that they are only human—you can feel a sense of betrayal and become distrustful of them.

Most of the time, you may not be aware of these habits. But if you take the time to reflect on your current or past relationship patterns, you will see the same triggers and reactions playing out. It's important not to judge yourself for reacting unfavorably when you are triggered, but instead seek to learn more about what unmet needs are being revealed in those moments.

Key Takeaways

- Ambivalent-insecure attachment style develops as a result of inconsistent parenting. A child learns very early on that they cannot trust their parents to be emotionally available and responsive all of the time.
- There are two ways ambivalent-insecure attachment can manifest: an individual can either be ambivalent resistant (lashing out when their needs aren't met) or ambivalent passive (suppressing unmet needs and pretending as though they are unaffected).
- Common signs of an anxious attachment in relationships include clinginess, seeking validation, feeling anxious with unpredictability, and pushing people away when the emotional connection starts to deepen.
- Since anxiety is one of the main markers of anxious attachment, it is important to recognize how you react whenever your anxiety is triggered. Being aware of your reactions can help you find alternative coping strategies that allow you to manage anxiety in more positive ways.

Different Ways to Regulate Your Nervous System

Step 2: Confronting Anxious Attachment

"When you are feeling emotional, it is helpful to remind yourself, as a self-regulating measure, 'The past is not here. This is the present.'"

— SHELLEY KLAMMER

This chapter talks about:

- How the stress response is triggered in the brain and physiological signs to look out for
- Different relaxation techniques to regulate your nervous system and return to a calm and balanced state of mind
- How to create your own stress management toolkit, including a crisis management plan and weekly relaxation practice

Recognizing When You Are Triggered

When your sense of security is threatened in a relationship, for whatever possible reason, you become triggered. The word "trigger" is popular in psychology and pop culture, and it seeks to explain an experience where an individual has a strong emotional reaction to something or someone that reminds them of a past traumatic event.

Author of *It's Not Always Depression,* Hilary Jacobs Hendel mentions how triggers activate the "three brains," namely the thinking, emotional, and body brain (Hendel, 2018). When you are triggered, the three brains respond as follows:

- The thinking brain says, "This situation looks awfully familiar to what I have experienced before."
- The emotional brain says, "I feel anxious, therefore I must be in trouble!"
- The body brain says, "My heart is racing faster, I find it difficult to breathe. Run as fast as you can from this situation!"

None of the three brains take a moment to understand what is actually happening in the present moment or choose to see the situation from a fresh perspective. They react based on existing patterns of thinking and behavior.

In other words, if you have always withdrawn yourself from others when you sense rejection, your three brains will encourage you to follow the same behavior. This reveals something very important about triggers: They exist because of unresolved past trauma.

Due to the fact that you are unconsciously carrying emotional wounds from stressful or abusive past relationships, everyday encounters with people make you feel vulnerable. You are more likely to be triggered by a text, call, or snarky remark—even when these events aren't offensive—because of the trauma-based information that informs your thoughts, emotions, and behaviors.

Understanding your anxious attachment style can come in handy when seeking to learn more about your relationship triggers. It enables you to look at the different kinds of interactions or experiences that bring up feelings of anxiety. For instance, you might discover that your attachment anxiety is caused by external and internal relationship triggers.

External relationship triggers arise from your interpersonal relationships with close friends and family, coworkers, romantic partners, and other members of your community. You might be triggered by the words, phrases, tones of voice, body gestures, facial expressions, or attitudes displayed by others. For example, a friend who has the tendency of not checking up on you can be a source of trigger, so can a romantic partner who shows a lack of empathy.

What's worth remembering about external relationship triggers is that you cannot blame another individual for the emotional distress you experience. The only thing you can hold them accountable for are their actions or misjudgments, but the strong reaction that develops inside of you has more to do with your attachment issues than the individual's behavior. This is why when you express feeling hurt by someone's actions, you are advised to use "I" statements to show ownership of your emotional experience.

Another type of trigger you might experience are internal relationship triggers. These tend to arise from within and are based on troublesome thoughts or unpleasant emotions. Examples include negative self-talk, limiting self-beliefs, anxiety, loneliness, and depression. When you experience a thought or emotion that reminds you of a time when you were most vulnerable, full of self-doubt or anger, or felt confused, your brain assumes that the same incident is taking place again and you react with the same coping mechanisms as before.

Your reactions may be alarming to those around you because they don't understand how the current situation justifies the extreme emotional reaction. They may see your behavior as being exaggerated, dramatic, or impulsive because it doesn't match reality. The truth of the matter is that they are correct but that doesn't mean what you are experiencing isn't valid. If they aren't familiar with your attachment style, they won't be able to empathize with your behaviors and see that you have mentally regressed to the little boy or girl who felt anxious and unsafe.

Both external and internal triggers will continue to feature in your life until you get behind them and heal the parts of you that are still wounded. Nevertheless, recognizing triggers is winning half of the battle. When you are aware of your reactions to various triggering situations, you have the power to choose a favorable response.

How to Calm Your Nervous System

When your attachment anxiety is triggered, you can feel lost and helpless. The initial thought might be "Here we go again!" before a wave of anxiety floods your body. The first step of healing from anxious attachment is acknowledging that relationships are stressful for you. As much as you would like to open up to others and sustain long-term mutually beneficial relationships, this won't be easy for you.

Acknowledging that you find relationships stressful helps you anticipate flare ups of anxiety in everyday encounters, rather than being shocked by them. You anticipate that your brain will ring alarm bells for trivial mistakes that others make, almost like a whining child who cries out when feeling the slightest discomfort. Try not to judge yourself for being so sensitive to offense or sudden changes in relationships; simply acknowledge that due to your upbringing, you are constantly on high alert.

Besides acknowledgment, another important step to take is to learn about the natural stress response and the process that is carried out whenever your brain senses potential threats. The following is a brief summary of the interaction between the brain, nervous system, and the rest of your body. Note that this interaction happens within seconds, and you won't always be aware of it.

- Your eyes or ears send information to a part of your brain known as the amygdala. The amygdala is responsible for emotionally processing the information, such as interpreting whether a situation is safe or unsafe.
- When danger is perceived, the amygdala sends a distress signal to another part of your brain known as the hypothalamus. The hypothalamus is responsible for ringing the alarm bells and notifying the rest of the body of a possible threat. This communication happens through the autonomic nervous system.
- The autonomic nervous system controls a host of body functions, like breathing, heart rate, and blood pressure. Since its job is so large, it is divided into two parts: the sympathetic and parasympathetic nervous system.
- The sympathetic nervous system sends stress signals throughout the body and activates the fight-flight-freeze response. When it is engaged, you may notice your heart rate accelerating, breath shortening, blood pressure rising, etc.
- The parasympathetic nervous system is responsible for regulating and reducing stress signals until the body returns to a resting state. It is usually engaged after the perceived threat is removed, but if you are familiar with relaxation techniques, you can switch it on.

What is "natural" for your brain and body when you experience attachment anxiety is to send distress signals to the sympathetic nervous system and begin a chain of physiological reactions to stress. What is less common is becoming aware of what is happening and immediately activating the parasympathetic nervous system, so you can regulate the stress response and remain grounded.

There are a number of different relaxation techniques that you can turn to whenever you sense a trigger or notice physiological signs of being stressed. Here are just a few of these techniques, which you can practice in the comfort of your home. After going through the techniques, create your own stress management toolkit, including a crisis management plan and weekly relaxation practice (more instructions to follow).

Breathing Exercises

"Just breathe" sounds like a straightforward instruction, but when you are anxious and your heart rate and breathing are irregular, it can be difficult to remember how to "just breathe."

Research has shown that breathing not only sustains life but can also activate your parasympathetic nervous system, which sends signals to your brain that the perceived threat no longer exists (Sinclair, 2021). Taking slower and deeper breaths also allows more oxygen to the brain, which can leave you feeling calm.

So, how do you just breathe? One of the most common and effective breathing exercises taught in therapy is diaphragmatic breathing, or belly breathing. The aim is to lengthen each breath as much as possible and slowly release.

Patients are usually told to direct their breaths to their stomachs, rather than staying at the chest area, to ensure they take fuller breaths. Follow these steps to practice diaphragmatic breathing:

1. Lie down on a bed with your face looking toward the ceiling and legs slightly apart. Take a few normal breaths to get comfortable in this position.
2. Place your left hand on your chest and your right hand on your belly. For the rest of the exercise, ensure that your left hand remains

completely still. Only your right hand should move up and down.

3. When you are ready, inhale slowly through your nose and stretch your breath until it reaches your belly. A good way to tell if you are doing the movement correctly is to watch your stomach rise.
4. Hold the breath for a brief moment, then slowly exhale out of your mouth, until there is no more air left inside of you. Once again, you will know that you are doing the movement correctly by watching your stomach fall back down.
5. Continue taking slow and full breaths for another five minutes.

Diaphragmatic breathing is not the only exercise that can help you regulate your breathing. Another effective exercise is known as box breathing. The aim of box breathing is to teach you how to take control of your breathing and gradually bring your heart and breathing rate back to a resting state. The following are the instructions to perform box breathing:

1. Inhale through your nose for five slow and consistent counts.
2. Hold your breath for another five slow and consistent counts.
3. Exhale out of your mouth for five slow and consistent counts.
4. Hold your breath for another five slow and consistent counts.
5. If five counts is uncomfortable for you, feel free to drop the count to four or three.
6. Continue practicing this breathing pattern multiple times.

The magic of breathing exercises is how they simultaneously relax the mind and body. The final breathing exercise that will be presented to you seeks to strengthen the mind-body connection by making mental suggestions. It is known as focused breathing.

The aim of focused breathing is to think of a positive word, mental or emotional state, or mantra that you can bring to mind whenever you inhale. Imagine that you were filling your body with an abundance of this particular experience. As you exhale, imagine that you are ridding your body of the opposite, negative experience that you may be exposed to.

For example, after having a call with your parent, you feel a sudden emergence of frustration. This would be the negative experience you want to get rid of. But what could be the positive experience you desire in its place? Maybe you would like to feel peace whenever you speak to your parent, or maybe you need a mantra that reminds you that you cannot change or control other people.

The next step is to close your eyes, take a deep breath in, and imagine you were taking in an abundance of peace. Hold your breath for a brief moment, then as you exhale, imagine you were releasing the pent up frustration. Continue doing this until you feel a noticeable difference in your mood.

Mindfulness Exercises

Mindfulness is a relaxation technique that is borrowed and has been adapted from the Buddhist tradition. Being mindful involves focusing on present experiences, whether it be sounds, sights, smells, thoughts, or feelings.

The reason mindfulness is so effective in calming the nervous system is due to how it reduces mind wandering. Remember, attachment anxiety is triggered by the recollection of past traumatic experiences in intimate relationships.

When you are able to refocus on the present moment, you will notice that the fears of rejection or abandonment become less intense or believable. Moreover, you are able to correctly perceive what is taking place, without mentally regressing to the past.

There are many different kinds of mindfulness exercises you can practice embracing the present moment. One of them is to complete a simple mindfulness meditation.

With your eyes closed, the aim is to acknowledge thoughts passing through your mind, without unpacking them or forming opinions about them. After acknowledging each thought, you take a deep breath and let it go. You can follow this script to complete a mindfulness meditation:

> *Find a quiet spot at home or in the office. Put your phone on silent and set a timer for 5 minutes. Get yourself in a comfortable position where your body is relaxed and muscles disengaged. Close your eyes and complete a short box breathing exercise.*
>
> *When you are ready, take a deep breath and listen for any incoming thoughts. Your mind may be buzzing with thoughts like a busy highway, or it may be calm like a suburban street on a Sunday afternoon. Take a few moments to observe the activity without participating in it.*
>
> *Categorize each thought by its size. Notice how many large, medium, and small thoughts are circulating in your mind. Choose whichever thoughts you want to acknowledge. Perhaps during this session, you only want to acknowledge small thoughts, but in another session you may be willing to acknowledge larger thoughts.*
>
> *Once you have chosen the category of thoughts to acknowledge, focus on a single thought within that category. Make this thought the sole focus of your mind. Be careful not to identify with or attach yourself to the thought. Just look at it, accept the message it has to share with you, then let it go.*
>
> *For example, a fear-based thought may want to alert you about*

somebody's unfavorable behavior. Acknowledge and accept the message, then let the thought go. Continue doing this until there are no more thoughts left in that specific category or until the timer goes off.

Another great mindfulness exercise is the body scan. This is an awareness exercise that can improve your sensory perceptiveness, which is the ability to recognize the different sensations you are feeling in your body.

This kind of awareness can help you detect the physical signs of stress or emotional triggers before they get bigger and become overwhelming.

The traditional way of completing a body scan requires you to lie down on a bed (similar position as diaphragmatic breathing) and take your time moving from one muscle group to the next, looking for any physical or emotional discomfort.

To identify emotional discomfort, it might help to close your eyes and visualize the specific muscle group in your mind and see if there are any thoughts or emotions that arise.

An alternative way to practice the body scan is to match a body sensation with a feeling. For this, you don't need to lie down, but the exercise works best when you are resting. Take your right hand and place it on an area of your body where you sense physical or emotional discomfort. Thereafter, mention what you are sensing and what feeling it brings up.

For example, you may sense physical discomfort around your chest area. You can proceed by taking your right hand and placing it on your chest. Then you can say a simple phrase like "My chest is tight. I feel anxious."

This level of awareness can immediately bring some sort of relief because you are able to gain control of your experience and choose how to react moving forward.

Grounding Exercises

Grounding is an effective relaxation technique, especially for countering anxiety and panic attacks. The aim of grounding is to "connect to earth" or snap back to reality.

Grounding exercises put the power back in your hands by giving you control of the moment. You are able to disengage from negative self-talk or overthinking, empty your mind, and interact with your surroundings.

Some people refer to grounding exercises as positive distractions, and this is true. Essentially, you are distracting yourself from the ongoing chitter-chatter in the mind by focusing on something emotionally neutral, like counting the objects in a room. This can give your body enough time to de-stress and return to a normal resting state.

There are various types of grounding exercises you can experiment with. All of them seek to reconnect you with your surroundings. The first is known as the "5-4-3-2-1 exercise." The challenge is to activate your five senses, scan your environment, and identify:

- 5 things you can see with your eyes
- 4 things you can smell with your nose
- 3 things you can touch with your hands
- 2 things you can hear with your ears
- 1 thing you can taste with your tongue

If you like, you can walk around the room and physically point or grab the items. Adding some movement to the exercise further brings you into the present moment.

Another great grounding exercise is to deliberately adjust your body temperature by exposing yourself to colder temperatures. This triggers a shock in your body and activates the parasympathetic nervous system. Simple ways to do this are running your hands under cold tap water, taking a cold shower or swim, suckling on an ice cube, or placing a cold cloth on your forehead.

Furthermore, you can ground yourself by completing a reorienting exercise. This involves reminding yourself, out loud, what date it is, where you are, what is taking place, etc. For example, when you are triggered at the office you can say to yourself:

"My name is Ashley. I am 32 years old. The date today is May 3rd. The year is 2023. The time is 12 noon. I am in the office boardroom trying to calm myself down. In a few minutes I will stand up and take my lunch. I am having a sandwich and soda for lunch."

Reorienting yourself prevents mental regression, which is common when your attachment anxiety is triggered. It sends a message to your brain that you are not having the same childhood experience. You are older now, in a different place, having a completely new experience.

Examples of a few more positive distractions to ground yourself include:

- Count from 0 to 10 then from 10 to 0, slowly. If your mind wanders, start the counting again.
- Count how many letters are in the phrase "I am safe and in control," or any other phrase you can think of.
- Try to recall whose birthday is this month. Or whose birthday is coming up. What date is their birthday?
- Recite the lyrics to your favorite positive song.
- Recite the alphabet backward.
- Recall the recipe to make your favorite meal.

- Call a friend who puts a smile on your face.
- Read a page from a daily devotional.
- Say a silent prayer.
- Complete 10 jumping jacks and 10 squats.

Visualization Exercises

Visualization is about seeing things in your mind that haven't yet materialized. This requires tapping into your imagination and envisioning a future-based outcome. Since the brain doesn't understand the concept of time (i.e. past, present, future), it assumes that what you are visualizing is taking place in the present moment.

In therapy, visualization exercises are used to make positive mental suggestions that, with enough repetition, can positively affect your mood and overall sense of well-being. When you sense a trigger coming along, for example, you can close your eyes and visualize a peaceful setting. Not only can this serve as a positive distraction, but it can also suggest to your brain that you are safe and calm.

There are some who discount visualization exercises, citing that it is merely "wishful thinking." But study the lives of top-performing athletes or successful entrepreneurs, and you will notice how mental rehearsals (i.e. visualization) are an important part of planning, decision-making, and executing goals.

There are many ways to practice visualization; some are conventional, and others will push you outside of your comfort zone. A conventional visualization exercise is creating a vision or mood board, which is a tool used to constantly remind you of the life or relationship goals you are striving for.

All you need to create a vision or mood board is a large piece of cardboard paper, a few magazine images and word cut outs, and craft supplies. If you wish to create a digital board, you can download an app like Corkulous or Dream Vision Board App. Place your board somewhere accessible so that you can look at it on a regular basis.

Another conventional exercise is to create index cards. These cards also serve as a positive reminder of your goals. The aim is to read over your cards once a day, preferably in the morning, or whenever you are feeling overwhelmed.

On about 10–20 flashcards, write down goals for your relationships. You can include goals like being a good listener, holding emotional space for someone, or taking deep breaths when feeling attacked. Under each goal, write a short description of what that might look like in real life. Every day, shuffle your cards and go through as many as you like. Pause after reading each goal and reflect on the progress you are making in that area.

Now for some unconventional visualization exercises! You have probably heard of positive affirmations before but perhaps haven't practiced them because you don't like the sound of your voice or maybe don't think they work.

Positive affirmations are affirmative statements that suggest certain thoughts and feelings to the subconscious mind. Since the work happens on a subconscious level, you might assume the statements aren't working. But the truth is that each time you recite affirmative statements to yourself, you are dismantling old thinking patterns and building new ones.

Whether you repeat the positive affirmations in front of a mirror or on the car ride to work, what matters is that you say them out loud. Hearing yourself speak positively is part of the reprogramming. Essentially, you are convincing your brain to adopt a positive truth.

The basic structure of a positive affirmation is to start with "I" and structure the sentence in present tense, as though what you are affirming about yourself is already happening. For example, you might say

- I show up as my authentic self in relationships.
- I am an asset to my friends and family.
- I am open to accepting people who are different from me.
- I am patient with myself and others.
- I am calm during conflict.

What makes positive affirmations effective is personalizing them for the specific areas of your relationship you struggle with, such as trusting others, feeling relaxed, or expressing your feelings. Your affirmations need to make sense to you and target your anxiety triggers.

Another unconventional visualization exercise is exposing yourself to the desired experiences you hope to achieve. In practical terms, getting exposure requires you to step outside of your comfort zone and immerse yourself in a new environment.

For example, if you would like to adopt a secure attachment in your romantic relationship, getting exposure would entail hanging around couples who have a secure attachment or watching videos of people talking about secure attachment.

This could also mean avoiding online content or couples that promote or exhibit insecure attachments or unhealthy patterns of behavior. The more you saturate your world with people or content that encourage strictly secure attachment, the more "normal" it will be for you to behave in secure ways in your romantic relationship.

Stress Management Toolkit

Now that you have gone through the different types of relaxation exercises to regulate your nervous system, it is time to put together your own stress management toolkit. The toolkit will consist of your selection of exercises to practice whenever you are feeling overwhelmed.

To create your toolkit, start by writing down a list of common anxiety triggers you experience in everyday life. For example, a trigger at home might be receiving the silent treatment from your partner and a trigger at work might be being spoken to harshly by your boss.

For each trigger, find at least one relaxation exercise you can practice whenever it arises. Write them down on the lines provided.

Next, think about the situations that you fear most in relationships, such as being rejected, criticized, verbally attacked, or alienated by your group of friends. Write them down.

For each situation, find at least one relaxation exercise that can help you cope whenever the fear is triggered. For example, what can you do when you start to feel alienated or pushed out of your friendship group? Note that the fear can be triggered even when there isn't a real threat.

Part of managing stress involves making relaxation a daily practice. Think about the types of stressors you deal with on a daily basis, such as parenting, dealing with a toxic boss, taking care of an ill parent, etc.

Create a daily relaxation routine, either morning or evening routine, which can help to alleviate stress and anxiety. Your routine should have a minimum of three exercises. Feel free to include other calming exercises that were not included in this chapter.

Commit to your morning or evening relaxation routine for three consecutive days and journal about your experience.

Key Takeaways

- When the brain detects a perceived threat, it sends warning signals to the autonomic nervous system, which activates the sympathetic nervous system. This leads to a chain of physiological changes to the body, including increased heart and breathing rate.
- Eventually, when the threat subsides, the parasympathetic nervous system will be activated, which brings the heart and breathing rate back to normal and induces a state of calm.
- When you understand how the nervous system works, you can manage the stress response and control your mental and physical state. The relaxation exercises mentioned in this chapter are effective in reversing the effects of stress and calming the mind and body.

Daily practice of these exercises can help you respond to signs of stress from the onset and maintain a sense of balance.

Prepare for a Paradigm Shift

Step 2: Confronting Anxious Attachment

"We speak about losing our minds as if it is a bad thing. I say, lose your mind. Do it purposefully. Find out who you really are beyond your thoughts and beliefs. Lose your mind, find your soul."

— VIRONIKA TUGALEVA

This chapter talks about:

- The nature of limiting beliefs and how to tell when you are ready to let them go
- The five steps to complete the CBT cognitive restructuring technique and replace limiting beliefs

Outgrowing Your Attachment Style

One of the things worth emphasizing time again is the importance of not judging yourself for having developed anxious attachment.

Judgment implies that how you have approached relationships for the past decades has been wrong, shameful, or unacceptable. However, the story around how you developed your anxious attachment is more complicated than that.

Your attachment style developed out of survival, not a deliberate choice. If you could have chosen, you would have gone with a secure attachment. After all, which child doesn't crave unconditional love and acceptance from their parents? But unfortunately, due to various life circumstances, your parents weren't emotionally available for you, and you were left with no other choice than to adapt and find ways to cope.

Back when you were a child, withdrawing to your room, faking happiness, or seeking approval from others was what worked. Of course, in hindsight, you can see how harmful these coping strategies were (and continue to be) but in your younger years they created a sense of safety.

Now that you are much older, and maybe have kids of your own, you desire to respond to your attachment anxiety differently-using coping strategies that don't sabotage your relationships.

Everybody reaches a stage in their lives where they feel unsatisfied with their current belief system and wish to update how they perceive the world and others. This drive for change can be triggered by personal growth, forgiving a wrongdoer (or receiving an apology from a wrongdoer), making positive new connections, or having a life-altering spiritual experience.

Due to the changes in your life, you start to ask questions about your childhood, relationships with your parents, or about your personality traits. Living under the old belief system, carrying out the old routines, or maintaining dysfunctional relationships becomes increasingly uncomfortable.

If you are at this stage, it is no coincidence that you are reading a book about how to overcome anxious attachment. In your attempts to understand yourself better, you have often wondered why relationships are so stressful and difficult for you.

In many healing journeys, the first step is always acknowledgment. Acknowledging what is not working out creates enough openness to dig deeper and find relief for your pain. Now that you are beginning to acknowledge that your anxious attachment isn't bringing fulfillment in your relationships, you can start to look deeper and understand the beliefs that are holding you back.

Limiting Beliefs That Sabotage Your Relationships

There is a quote by Deepak Chopra that says, "The less you open your heart to others, the more your heart suffers" (Vishnu, 2015). Some might challenge this argument and state the opposite, that the less you open your heart, the less suffering you will experience.

You can test this second argument by reflecting back on your life. Grab a pen and two sheets of paper and write two diary entries as though you had time traveled to two periods of your life: A period when your heart was open and you were able to give and receive love, and a period when your heart was closed and you could not give or receive love. Your diary entry can include typical thoughts, emotions, beliefs, and behaviors you exhibited during both periods.

Now that you have completed the exercise, what can you say about Chopra's quote? Would you side with him and agree that closing your heart brings on suffering or would you say that closing your heart prevents suffering?

Exercises like these, often referred to as cognitive restructuring or reappraisal, are extremely important when you are gearing toward making lifestyle changes. They allow you to pause, think about your beliefs, weigh the pros and cons, and arrive at your own conclusions about whether they are helpful or harmful to your understanding of people and life in general.

When you were a child, you didn't have the psychological tools to critically think about and challenge your beliefs. You simply saw behavior taking place around you and came up with a simple explanation of what was happening. For example, a little child often cries when their parents drop them off at school because in their minds they believe that is the last time they will see their parents.

Of course, this isn't what is actually taking place because within a few hours, their parents will return to pick them up. But in the absence of reflecting and challenging their belief, they are left with a painful wound of separation. Now imagine that the same child faced multiple traumas during their childhood, which caused them to come up with multiple beliefs that were not "fact-checked" or challenged. How differently might they perceive the world around them due to holding onto these beliefs?

Unchecked and unchallenged beliefs continue with you into adulthood and affect your relationships in many ways, such as triggering attachment anxiety. The earlier you identify them and go through the process of cognitive restructuring or reappraisal, the sooner you can decide to keep or discard them.

Here are examples of limiting beliefs that are common among people with anxious attachment:

- **"I'm broken."**

In the previous chapter we spoke about the power of positive affirmations and how they seek to reprogram subconscious thought patterns. The belief "I'm broken" is a negative affirmation that confirms a feeling or state of brokenness.

When you repeatedly tell yourself that something is wrong with you, you subconsciously validate dysfunctional patterns of behavior. After all, if something is truly wrong with you, then it makes sense why you cannot maintain healthy and mutually beneficial relationships, right?

You might be saying to yourself, "Well, what if I actually feel broken, is it so wrong to believe that?" The answer is no, it is not wrong to feel broken-what's wrong is identifying with brokenness. There is a difference between saying "I feel broken" and "I am broken." The latter makes it more difficult to challenge the belief because that is who you are.

- **"No one will ever love me again."**

It is common when coming out of a good relationship to believe that you won't ever find another partner who can love you the same. This belief only sounds true because you can only compare your ex-partner to past partners. But since you cannot travel to the future, there is no way of knowing if your previous good relationship was indeed your last.

What's also worth noting about this belief is the extreme exaggeration, also known as catastrophizing. This is a harmful thinking habit that causes you to make the worst possible conclusion, which most times doesn't match reality. There are so many logical errors with the belief that it cannot be conceivably true. Nonetheless, your mind is inclined to believe that it's true because of the constant reinforcement.

- **"I don't bring any value to relationships."**

One of the side effects of having low self-esteem is thinking that there is nothing good that you have to offer others. Overtime, this belief becomes a self-fulfilling prophecy because if you don't believe you have anything worthwhile to share, you are less likely to reveal your strengths in relationships. You won't see the point of trying to get to know people, revealing your nurturing side, or serving others.

Furthermore, when people believe they bring no value, many times they are referring to extrinsic value, which is the value given to someone by society based on status, power, acceptable standards (i.e. beauty), or materialistic possession (i.e. how much money you have).

Evaluating your worth based on extrinsic value is like gambling with your self-esteem. For example, when you're in a committed relationship, you feel valuable, but the moment you break up, you feel worthless because singleness is looked down upon. Perhaps when you have a lot of disposable money to spend on your partner, you feel valuable, but the moment you can't afford to shower them with gifts, you feel worthless because of the pressure to protect and provide (often experienced by men in the dating world).

Instead it is better to evaluate your sense of self-worth based on intrinsic value, which is the value you determine for yourself based on unique character traits, skills and talents, personal achievements, and the positive impact you make in the lives of others. Intrinsic value doesn't rise or drop when your external circumstances change. It remains consistent whether you've reached a successful point in your life or are still working toward it.

Moreover, your intrinsic value isn't decreased when others fail to recognize your strengths and uniqueness. This can also free you from constantly seeking validation from others or blaming yourself for others' actions.

- **"Knowing myself, I'll find a way to sabotage this new relationship."**

Another self-fulfilling prophecy is believing that what has happened in the past will happen again.

There is some level of truth to this belief but only in certain contexts. For example, the past repeats itself if the same patterns are followed. If your pattern is to pull back whenever a relationship starts to get intense, then that is what will continue to happen. The past will also repeat itself when the environment stays the same. For example, if you continue to surround yourself or maintain relationships that are invalidating, lack boundaries, and fail to respond to your needs, then there isn't much fulfillment you can expect to receive from your relationships.

Take the time to think about the reasons you sabotage relationships. What informs that behavior? Is there a harmful pattern that you continue to follow, or are you part of an unsupportive and unhealthy environment? Take accountability where it is due and make the necessary changes.

- **"It's dangerous to be vulnerable."**

Children who develop anxious attachment learn not to trust those closest to them. Later on in life, they may struggle to be vulnerable with others because of deep trust issues.

As a child, it might have felt safest to shut down your emotions and put on a tough exterior, but that could've also led to feelings of loneliness and depression. The truth is vulnerability isn't dangerous. It is the gateway to unconditional love and intimacy. Only by choosing to be vulnerable can a person experience what it means to be known and accepted by someone else.

The danger is opening up to the wrong people who don't have your best interests at heart. Having core values and knowing your personal boundaries can help you keep the wrong people at a distance, while remaining open to those who genuinely care about you.

Making a Paradigm Shift

A paradigm shift is a term that was coined by physicist Thomas Kuhn and explained in his book *The Structure of Scientific Revolutions* (MasterClass, 2022). From a scientific point of view, a paradigm shift refers to a change that occurs when a scientific activity contradicts previous belief that experts found to be indisputable. As a result, a new "paradigm" or belief replaces the old.

In modern psychology, a paradigm shift can refer to the process of challenging existing beliefs that previously seemed indisputable and replacing them with newer beliefs that match your current worldview. These shifts don't happen regularly since they involve questioning the status quo of your life. Even then, it is still difficult to confront beliefs that have played a major role in how you see yourself and interact with others.

Nonetheless, making a paradigm shift can be liberating. The best way to explain the benefit of a paradigm shift is making an analogy with tight jeans. Have you ever had a favorite pair of jeans that became too tight after years? At some point, those tight jeans fit you like a glove, but with time—and generous helpings of candy and desserts—they become uncomfortable to wear.

From the outside, nobody knew how pressed you felt in those jeans because they looked perfectly normal, but since you were aware of the body changes that had taken place and how the jeans were supposed to feel, you preferred to end your misery and buy a new pair.

When current beliefs become limiting, they start to feel constricting and uncomfortable. In the past you may have been able to justify the beliefs and even support why you felt that way, but with time and change that is no longer how you feel. Making a paradigm shift can help you rethink ideas, thoughts, and memories that have gone unchallenged for many years. Doing this allows you to audit your belief system and replace those beliefs that are no longer appropriate or aligned to your evolved worldview.

Signs You Are Ready for a Paradigm Shift

As you grow and encounter new experiences, your mind expands with new information. You can now look at the same life circumstances from multiple perspectives and challenge ideas that you previously didn't have the knowledge to oppose.

There are a few signs you can look out for that show you are ready for a paradigm shift. These include:

1. You feel disconnected from your current norms and routines.
The first sign that you are ready for a paradigm shift is that you no longer find satisfaction in the everyday norms and routines. Life may start to feel like a drag, and you don't have the same energy and passion for your work, health, and relationships.

2. You feel a void that cannot be filled.
It is also common to sense an inner void or emptiness that doesn't seem to go away, regardless of how you might fill it. Another way of saying this is that you feel stuck and can't move your life forward. Deep down, you know that something is wrong but don't exactly know what the issue might be.

3. You expect more from your relationships.
You are ready for a paradigm shift when you start to expect more from your relationships. Unpleasant behaviors that you previously allowed become increasingly intolerable for you. You may even be more aware of boundary violations than you were before, which can lead to avoidant

behaviors or confrontations.

4. You start to question your past narratives.

When you are ready for a paradigm shift, your past becomes a fascination or obsession. You start to ask yourself questions about the way you were raised, the traumas you experienced, and why things had to turn out the way they did. The big questions are about getting as close as possible to understanding the truth about your life and breaking free from disempowering ideas and beliefs.

5. Your outlook on the world is changing.

Life looks different when you are in survival mode compared to when you are venturing on a journey of healing. The difference is the way in which you perceive the world. When you are about to embark on a paradigm shift, you may look at the world with openness and greater self-awareness. Instead of maintaining high walls that prevent others from getting close, you approach new experiences with curiosity.

Five Steps to Challenge and Replace Limiting Beliefs

If you are ready for a paradigm shift and can attest to experiencing one or more of the signs mentioned in the previous section, then you can proceed by embarking on the process of cognitive restructuring. As mentioned earlier, cognitive restructuring is a psychological technique based on the principles of cognitive behavioral therapy (CBT), which can help you challenge and replace limiting beliefs.

The aim of cognitive restructuring is to create enough distance between you and your thoughts, emotions, and beliefs, so that you can examine them objectively. Therefore, as you follow the five steps of cognitive restructuring outlined next, avoid identifying with your thoughts, emotions, and beliefs. Imagine that you were an observer looking into your situation and assessing it from an unbiased viewpoint.

Step 1: Describe the Situation

In general, beliefs aren't triggered out of nowhere. There is usually a situation in question that triggers a particular limiting belief. For the purpose of this exercise, recall a recent relationship situation that triggered attachment anxiety. It could have been an altercation with a coworker, misunderstanding with your partner, or actions taken by your family members, etc.

In the space provided, describe what happened. Mention the actions that were taken by all parties involved. Avoid making any assumptions.

Step 2: Express How You Felt

Now that the details are out of the way, share your emotional experience. Describe how you felt before, during, and after the situation. Strictly mention your own emotional experience and how you were impacted. Use "I" statements to show ownership of your emotions. For example, "I felt disrespected because he refused to listen to me."

Step 3: Identify Your Limiting Beliefs

In CBT, patients learn that their emotions, thoughts, and behaviors are related. For instance, feeling an intense emotion can trigger an unwanted thought or belief, which causes you to take certain actions or reinforce behavioral patterns.

Therefore, in this step, identify the limiting beliefs that flooded your mind while you were processing your emotions. For example, if you were anxious, what bad thing did you expect to happen? Or if you felt disrespected, how did you see yourself in that moment? Look for the "negative meaning" that you ascribed to the situation taking place.

Step 4: Challenge Your Limiting Beliefs

This step is the most critical because it is when the paradigm shift occurs. For all this time, you have allowed the limiting beliefs to go unchecked and unchallenged. It may not have been an issue for you until now. Without being biased, you have an opportunity to look at the belief from all angles, weigh the pros and cons, and assess whether you believe it to be true.

The goal of challenging your limiting beliefs isn't to assume that they are wrong simply because they sound negative. You must provide your brain with enough substantial proof (e.g. factual evidence) to show that your belief is inaccurate. With enough evidence, it will be easier to ignore the belief whenever it appears in your mind or to replace it with a more convincing one.

There are different ways to challenge beliefs. The first is to write down a list of reasons why you feel that way. Afterward, go through each reason and write down whether it is a fact or opinion. Count how many of the reasons are facts versus opinions. If there are more facts than opinions, it means that there is substantial evidence to prove the belief is true. However, if many of the reasons are opinions, then the belief needs to undergo further questioning.

Another way is to reflect on where the belief originated. Try to recall the earliest memory of embracing the belief. How old were you? What was happening? How did you feel at the time? Some beliefs emerge out of childhood trauma and pain. During this time, they seem helpful because they bring instant comfort or shed light on a situation. But overtime, they can be limiting and cause you to adopt an inaccurate understanding of what actually happened.

You might also find that some limiting beliefs were borrowed from other people. For example, if you were raised by a parent who had low self-esteem, you might have adopted similar beliefs about yourself. Or if your parent had particularly negative beliefs about love, intimacy, or relationships, you might find that you have adopted some of those beliefs too.

The final way of challenging limiting beliefs is to ask yourself objective questions concerning them. In psychology this is known as Socratic questioning, named after Socrates, who developed a method of getting to answers by asking questions. A few objective questions that you can ask concerning your limiting beliefs are

- Is there another way of looking at this?
- Does this belief match reality?

- Are you being fair to yourself?
- Are you basing this belief on new or old information?
- Is the belief based on how you feel or what you know?
- Does this belief show an unrealistic standard you might be holding onto?
- What would happen if you continued to look at life this way?
- Would someone else draw the same conclusion? Would they look at things differently?

Be mindful of the urge to defend the belief. This is common and expected during a paradigm shift. Remember, at a point in time, this belief made you feel safe or helped you make sense of life. A part of you still feels indebted to the belief, and you may feel the need to defend it.

When this urge arises, pause from the exercise and take a few deep breaths. Bring your awareness to the urge and rate its intensity. Take a few more deep breaths and rate the intensity again until you no longer feel its presence. You can then return to the exercise.

Step 5: Make a Decision

After challenging your limiting beliefs, you have a choice to make. If there was substantial factual evidence found, you can reasonably assume that the belief is accurate, which means it matches reality. Perhaps it seems limiting because it has negative undertones, but since life can be difficult sometimes, it is normal to be critical.

If you find that the negative undertones bother you, consider rephrasing the belief in a positive way. For example, instead of believing that "Not everyone has good intentions for me," which is a true statement, you can believe that "Everyone has a different colored heart." The core message is the same, but the updated version has less negative undertones.

In contrast, you may find little to no factual evidence to substantiate your limiting belief. In this case, you are safe to assume that it is inaccurate and doesn't match reality. The best way forward is to replace the belief with one that is fair and balanced.

For example, instead of believing that "I can't sustain healthy relationships," which is found to be a false statement, you can believe that "I sometimes let my anxiety get in the way of building strong relationships." The updated version can be proven true with facts, yet it still provides you with enough room to change your behavioral patterns.

After making a decision, go a step further and create an action plan on how you can respond better to similar situations that might trigger the same limiting beliefs. For instance, what exercises or actions can you take to remind you of the new and updated beliefs? Do you need to step aside and practice positive affirmations? Pull out a note from your pocket or read an encouraging quote or passage from your phone? Have the relevant tools ready and on hand because you never know when the limiting belief may be triggered.

Key Takeaways

- It isn't helpful to look at limiting beliefs as being good or bad because at some point in your life they were important for survival. Instead you might look at them as being helpful or harmful for the current life stage you find yourself in.
- Paradigm shifts don't happen every day. They usually occur when maintaining the status quo becomes too uncomfortable. We can describe a paradigm shift as questioning beliefs that were previously seen to be true and replacing them with those that align with your current worldview.
- The best way to facilitate a paradigm shift is to undergo a process known as cognitive restructuring, which is the ability to evaluate and challenge existing thought patterns. The aim of this process is to find

enough evidence for or against a belief so that a positive replacement can be found and reinforced.

Heal Your Inner Child

Step 2: Confronting Anxious Attachment

"She held herself until the sobs of the child inside subsided entirely. I love you, she told herself. It will all be okay."

— H. RAVEN ROSE

This chapter talks about:

- An introduction into inner child therapy
- Signs of a wounded inner child and the importance of inner child healing
- Steps to heal the inner child and begin the lifelong process of reparenting

Who Is the Inner Child?

In psychology, there is a concept known as inner child therapy, which describes a type of healing intervention that involves reconnecting with younger versions of yourself. The inner child is symbolic of the child version of you that exists in memories. Many believe that the age of your inner child is determined by the age when your emotional development was hindered, such as when a traumatic event occurred and you could no longer experience the world the same.

Inner child therapy allows you to have conversations with this metaphoric child, learn more about your early childhood development, and perhaps piece together the puzzle about your life. Inner child therapy can also be a great way to discover who you are, what your interests are, what you deeply care about, and what makes you so unique. Your most authentic qualities, talents, and aspirations were displayed more strongly when you were an uninhibited child, before you were conditioned to think and behave a certain way.

The idea of an inner child may sound quite childish to some people. They might perceive the concept of reconnecting to a younger self as a sign of not letting go of the past. But what is an adult if not a grown-up child? The truth of the matter is that you are a collection of "selves" that have adapted to the different stages of life and evolved to who you are today. Your inner child has played a big role in shaping the individual you are today—and he or she will continue to influence how you integrate the past with your present and future.

When you fail to establish a relationship with younger versions of yourself, you are unable to access wisdom about who you truly are and the source of the pain you are carrying. Don't be fooled into thinking just because the inner child is a much younger version of you that it is naive. Remember, that little boy or girl survived 100% of the highs and lows you experienced as a kid. Not only are they incredibly resilient, but they also have a wealth of life experience to teach you.

Author Tara Bianca, who wrote the book *The Flower of Heaven*, has a quote that says, "Children are closest to God. They reveal creation. They are the embodiment of love and connection" (Goodreads, n.d.). That childlike innocence, purity, youth, and openness that you naturally displayed as a child is what kept you going when everything around you seemed unstable.

It is unfortunate that with the passing of time, these qualities are lost or forgotten because they are what facilitate healing. The purpose of inner child therapy is to recapture those golden moments of childhood, find closure from past hurts, and commit to a lifelong journey of nurturing the inner child.

Taking a Closer Look at Inner Child Healing

Inner child healing is another interesting concept. The aim is to address unprocessed emotional wounds through communicating and responding to the unmet needs of the inner child. Once again, the assumption is that the inner child holds the answers about what exactly happened many years ago and what steps need to be taken in order to get closure and heal.

Another goal for inner child healing is to address current behavioral and relationship issues, which may be causing conflict in your life. The assumption made here is that these unwanted patterns are a result of a wounded inner child who seeks attention through projection.

For example, when you are misunderstood by a colleague, the wounded inner child might be triggered to believe that you are being disrespected, which could be a familiar emotion the child grew up experiencing. Thus, you may respond to the situation with an overly emotional response that may not be an accurate representation of what's actually happening.

A wounded inner child is like a toddler throwing a temper tantrum. It can be difficult to reason with the toddler and show them their shortcomings. The only thing the toddler cares about is expressing how they feel and getting what they want.

By giving the inner child attention and responding to its outbursts with compassion, you can begin the process of healing his or her wounds. Your inner child wants to know that somebody cares about the pain he or she has suffered and that their complex thoughts and emotions are valid. As the wounds heal, and you learn healthier ways to cope with triggers, the child won't feel the need to project negative thoughts and feelings anymore.

One of the barriers that get in the way of inner child healing is the inability to bring up past suffering from a subconscious level to a conscious level, where you can reflect upon and evaluate your thoughts and feelings. This isn't due to a lack of tools, since techniques like meditation, visualization, and journaling can help you access your subconscious mind. The issue has more to do with the internal walls you may erect that make it difficult to accept or spend time thinking about past suffering.

While it is understandable why you would build internal walls and protect yourself from confronting painful past situations, this type of coping mechanism also prevents healing from taking place. You cannot let go of something that you are still clinging onto for dear life. Healing involves facing the fears and failures of the past and the willingness to move on from that dark and lonely place.

If you believe you may have internal walls that are preventing you from fully embracing inner child healing, here are four strategies that can lower resistance and increase self-acceptance:

- **Become acquainted with your pain.**

Pain is not a curse word. It isn't something you ought to fear or distance yourself from. Every human being experiences pain, whether it is physical or psychological, due to the unpredictable nature of life.

Being ashamed of your pain causes you to disconnect with a vulnerable aspect of you that is crying out for nurturing and support. Instead of turning your back on your pain, the loving response would be to lean in.

Becoming acquainted with your pain is about displaying a commitment to understand your past and how certain events and experiences have left you with emotional wounds. The purpose isn't to blame anybody or retraumatize yourself but instead to acknowledge the tragic and painful situations that you have been through and show yourself compassion.

- **Show self-compassion.**

Self-compassion is an act of kindness directed to yourself. Most of the time, we think that kindness is an external job, something that must be shown to others. But true kindness starts from within. After all, how can we respond lovingly to others when we don't give ourselves the time of day?

Since the memories of the past can be filled with a lot of regret and shame, self-compassion is required to be able to sit with your limiting beliefs and embrace those uncomfortable emotions. You can also think of self-compassion as your defense against negative self-talk or internalized guilt.

The message that is repeated is simple: You are only human. There is only so much control you have over your world or only so much strength or courage you can display in a given situation. Like anybody else, you have good and bad days—neither of them should define who you are. Self-compassion is the reminder to continue challenging thoughts that promote perfection, self-doubt, self-sabotage, or a victim mentality.

- **Learn how to genuinely love who you are.**

If you were raised in an environment where you were not affirmed or given regular positive reinforcement, it is likely that you grew up feeling confused about who you are.

The easiest person to control is the person who doesn't have a strong connection to themselves. This not only makes you vulnerable to manipulation, but you can also become easily controlled by your own thoughts and behaviors.

One of the reasons you may have internal walls is that you don't trust yourself. The walls are there to provide an extra protective measure against outsiders because you don't trust your own judgment. The lack of self-trust is a limiting belief that controls your interactions with others. If you had a strong connection to yourself, there wouldn't be a need for this type of belief.

Self-love seeks to fill the holes that your parents could not fill as a child. The goal of self-love is to become your own source of positive reinforcement, so that you don't depend on the inconsistent validation of others.

Another component of self-love is self-awareness, which is the ability to deeply know yourself. If you have ever had a deep romantic connection with someone, you will know that real love is built over time. The more you get to know a person, the stronger your feelings become.

Self-awareness facilitates self-love by strengthening the connection you have with yourself. How can you sincerely say that you love yourself if you are detached from your personal life experiences?

- **Give yourself permission to play.**

Finally, you can lower your internal walls and increase self-acceptance by giving yourself permission to play.

It might be strange that you would need permission to play, but many adults sometimes forget that their imagination and playful nature doesn't die during puberty. It lives on inside of them, appearing as flashes of inspiration, youthful energy, innovative thinking, and the search for adventure.

Tapping into your imagination allows you to access the subconscious mind and raise your level of consciousness. You are able to embrace ideas that are contrary to the norm, which might challenge your conventional thinking.

This is necessary during the work of inner child healing because the messages your inner child may convey won't always be conventional. For example, he or she might express the need for others to always say they are sorry when they hurt his or her feelings. The chances of this happening all of the time are slim, but your inner child may not be able to consider the practicalities.

Nevertheless, by using your imagination, you can find creative ways of fulfilling this need. Perhaps what the inner child is actually seeking is to feel respected. You can help them feel respected by setting firm personal boundaries and being unapologetic about what you need. This way, you are more likely to surround yourself with people who can take accountability for their wrong actions and apologize.

Giving yourself permission to play is also about making time for having fun. What you consider fun at your age may look different from what you consider fun at seven years old. But what matters is that you are embracing the free-spirited nature of a child that can calm your anxiety, reconnect you to your heart's desires, and allow you to live in the most authentic way.

Three Steps to Heal the Inner Child

Your inner child is activated whenever you think, feel, or sense things that remind you of your childhood. Surprisingly, this happens frequently because you are always encountering people, places, and situations that trigger memories and emotions.

You may be wondering how inner child therapy can help you heal your attachment style. By healing your inner child, you can positively change your response to anxiety triggers that arise in relationships.

Instead of reacting to your impulses—which is how the wounded inner child responds—you can seek to understand the underlying problem or unmet need that is being communicated. Plus, you are given an opportunity to validate and show compassion toward the wounded child, instead of turning your back on them.

Before we go into the three steps to heal your inner child, it is important to clarify that the inner child isn't always throwing a tantrum. Just think back to when you were a kid: Were you angry all of the time? You may have been upset when your needs were not met, which for an anxious person is occasionally.

Therefore, as you heal your inner child, remind that little girl or boy about the happy moments of childhood, when they felt most alive, creative, and connected with others. Let your goal for inner child healing be about getting back that child-like innocence and playfulness or reconnecting to lost aspects of yourself.

There are three steps to healing your inner child: connect, communicate, and nurture. Take a closer look at each step. What type of relationship dynamic does it remind you of? Can you see the similarities with a traditional parent-child relationship?

At the center of inner child healing is the process of reparenting, which can be described as providing yourself with the nurturing you didn't get as a child. Bear in mind that there is no passing blame in this process. For instance, your focus shouldn't be on reminding yourself about the shortcomings of your caregivers. Instead your attention should be on validating your needs and building inner trust by responding appropriately.

As someone with anxious attachment, reparenting yourself can also heal neediness, people-pleasing, and codependent behaviors. All of the love and attention you previously looked for in other people, you learn to source from within. You become the highest authority figure in your life that sets the standards, holds you accountable, and helps you correct mistakes.

Now that you understand the expectation of inner child healing (i.e. learning to become your own parent), it is time for us to go through each step and practice a few exercises.

Step 1: Connect

If you didn't have a close or healthy bond with your parents, you may not be familiar with the role and duties of conscious parents. Before you can connect to your inner child, you need to think about what type of parent you would like to be.

A basic definition of a parent is a man or woman who births and raises a child. However, this definition doesn't really tell us about the attitudes, beliefs, and acceptable behaviors of a parent. Thus, you will need to create your own definition of what a parent is, what their values and beliefs are, and how they relate to their child.

To make this exercise more explorative, you can study a few individuals (fictional or real) who display positive parenting qualities. Think about their lifestyles, daily interactions with their children, and communication styles. After doing some brainstorming, write down your definition:

Recognize that as you connect, communicate, and nurture your inner child, you will do so using the approach detailed earlier. This will ensure that your inner child gets to experience what unconditional love feels like. Not only will this help you during the healing journey, but it can also begin to positively change your attachment style.

So how do you connect to your inner child? The best way to connect to your inner child is to immerse yourself in childhood memories. Your childhood memories are rich with meaning, symbolism, emotions, and wisdom. Moreover, your memories get you as close as possible to the source of pain, where your triggers and destructive beliefs are rooted.

Reflection exercises can help you recall moments from your childhood. For instance, you can complete journal prompts and describe specific events, conflicts, transitions, or relationships from your past. The aim is to strictly follow the prompt and only write about one aspect. This allows you to fully focus on the details and connect to what your inner child felt at that specific moment.

Here are a few journal prompts to get you started:

1. Describe your earliest birthday party that you can remember. How old were you? Who was in attendance? How do you remember feeling throughout the day?

2. Think about a family home you frequently visit in dreams or have many memories of living in. Describe the experience growing up in that house. Who lived there? What type of family dynamic did you have? What parenting roles did your parents take? Where did you spend most of your time?

3. Recall a childhood memory where you approached your parents (you can choose anyone) for help. How old were you? What was your problem? How did you ask for help? What was the response you were given? How did you walk away feeling?

4. Recall a childhood memory where you let your parents down. How old were you? What mistake did you make? What was the impact of your mistake? How did your parents react? How did you walk away feeling about yourself?

5. Think back to your earliest memory of feeling love. Who showed you love? In your opinion, how would you describe that type of love? Is it similar or different to your current understanding of love and how so?

Reflection exercises aren't the only way of connecting to your inner child. Another way is to engage in activities you enjoyed as a child. For example, if you want to connect to your four-year-old self, you can play Legos, doodle, or get your hands dirty in the garden.

If you want to connect to your 16-year-old self, you can dress up as them, listen to your favorite music albums from that time, or meet up with high-school friends you are still in contact with. Naturally, as you immerse yourself in the experiences of the younger version of you, you will be able to connect with the thoughts and feelings that were going through your mind at the time.

Connecting with your inner child doesn't need to happen only when you want to communicate. Sometimes you may feel like distracting yourself from your current life situation and returning to happier times in your life. Or if you suffer from abandonment issues, you may simply want to check-in with your inner child and remind them that you still care.

Step 2: Communicate

The second step in the inner child healing process is to communicate. This step usually confuses people because the inner child isn't a real human being. But communicating with the inner child is simply about talking to yourself.

Sometimes your inner child will respond through gut feelings. Take a moment to reflect on what you are sensing, then write down the message. Other times your inner child may respond through synchronicities, such as seeing signs, numbers, and symbols that answer whatever question you had posed to them.

Bear in mind that your inner child may not communicate as eloquently as you do. Since they are a child, their thoughts and feelings may be scattered, spontaneous, or incomplete. Instead of showing frustration at the confusing messages you get, learn to seek clarity.

For instance, if you receive a one word answer, you can ask your inner child to explain what they mean. If they aren't good with words, perhaps they can explain with a picture or direct you to a specific place, person, or memory that might help you piece together what they are trying to communicate.

Remember to communicate with your inner child using the approach to parenting outlined in Step 1. Speak to them how you believe a parent should speak to a child and notice how they respond to you. Here are a few questions or prompts that you can ask your inner child to get the conversation started:

1. How was life growing up?

2. Who did you admire as a child? What did you love about these people?

3. What is the best memory you have of your mother?

4. What is the best memory you have of your father?

5. What do you still find difficult to accept about your living conditions as a child?

6. What do you still find difficult to accept about your relationship with your parents?

7. What were you afraid of as a child?

8. Can you remember your childhood dreams and aspirations?

9. Did you feel supported as a child?

10. Are there any secrets you are still holding onto from your childhood?

Even though communication with your inner child doesn't have to happen all of the time, it is important to first connect before communicating. Additionally, you can switch up the tone and subject of your conversations regularly. For instance, some conversations can be upbeat, and others can be serious and heartfelt.

Remember that your inner child is still a child, and they may not enjoy having emotional and long conversations all the time. If your inner child is opposed to having emotional conversations, try bribing them with playtime or some type of reward they might like!

Step 3: Nurture

The final step is to nurture your inner child. This is an ongoing process that doesn't stop after you have healed the inner child. At some point in your childhood, nurturing suddenly stopped or was withheld by your parents. This causes a lot of trauma that continues to be felt in your adult relationships.

When you commit to reparenting your inner child, you make an agreement to be consistent with your affection and nurturing. Consistency is what you yearned for as a child and therefore what your inner child needs most.

To provide consistent nurturing, you need to be aware of what your inner child needs, what their love languages are, and how they desire to be supported. There is no point in performing acts of service when your inner child craves quality time or physical touch. Thus, it is recommended to spend enough time exploring your needs and desires.

Two basic needs that children have, which inform every other need, are security and unconditional love. Your big task is to find out the specific ways in which you feel safe and loved. Remember that you are going to be the sole person responsible for responding to these needs, so avoid thinking about how other people can show up in the same ways.

Here is a list of ways to respond to your need for security:

- Set healthy boundaries.
- Be selective about who you allow into your space or home.
- Hold yourself accountable to personal goals.
- Get regular medical examinations and invest in your mental health.
- Be careful about how much you reveal about yourself online and be selective about the content you watch.
- Prioritize your career by developing a career development plan and hold yourself accountable to it.
- Save and invest money.

Here is a list of ways to respond to your need for unconditional love:

- Refrain from being judgmental about your past or current experiences.

- Spend quality time by yourself.
- Live an active and healthy lifestyle (e.g. eat a balanced diet, get sufficient sleep, adopt a spiritual practice, etc.).
- Improve your self-talk and be quick to challenge limiting beliefs.
- Listen to and validate your thoughts and feelings.
- Find hobbies and side interests that help you alleviate stress and anxiety.
- Commit to continuous learning by reading books, taking online courses, listening to educational podcasts, etc.
- Join a community of like-minded people, so you can deepen your sense of belonging.

Nurturing your inner child also involves increasing positive thoughts and feelings about yourself. You can heal your inner child by helping them become the confident and self-assured individual they have always wanted to be.

Increasing your inner child's confidence will also teach them to be more resilient when experiencing unpleasant situations. For example, if your attachment anxiety is triggered during the early stages of a romantic relationship, being confident can make your inner child less reactive in that situation.

True confidence takes time to develop, but these daily or weekly prompts can strengthen your sense of self-worth. Each time you respond to these journal prompts, identify something new that you haven't mentioned before.

1. I am proud of myself today because...

2. Something interesting that I learned about myself today was...

3. One person who supported me today was...

4. Today, I forgive myself for...

5. One strength that I displayed today was...

6. One weakness that I noticed and embraced today was...

Key Takeaways

- The inner child is the memory of your younger self that is ingrained in your subconscious mind. It has survived all of the pleasant and unpleasant experiences of the past, but it hasn't necessarily processed and healed from them.
- A wounded inner child makes its presence felt through emotional triggers, self-sabotage, unwanted thoughts, and unhealthy patterns of behavior. The tendency for most people is to ignore the unmet needs that are being communicated in those moments.
- Inner child healing involves showing yourself the love and attention

you were robbed of as a child. This is known as reparenting, and it consists of three steps: connecting, communicating, and nurturing deeper aspects of yourself.

- Reparenting is a lifelong journey that can help you source affection and validation from within and reduce the amount of anxiety you feel in relationships. Learning to respond to your own needs takes time, but with practice you can become better.

Develop a Strong Sense of Self

Step 3: Reconnecting With Yourself

"It's like everyone tells a story about themselves inside their own head. Always. All the time. That story makes you what you are. We build ourselves out of that story."

— PATRICK ROTHFUSS

This chapter talks about:

- The importance of developing a stable sense of self and complications that can get in the way
- How to wage war against your insecurities by winning the battle over your mind
- Steps to rewrite your life story and become your own person

The Root of Insecurities

A small child starts to develop a sense of self from the age of two. This is usually when they become conscious of being a living, breathing, human being, separate from others. As they grow older, they become aware of their thoughts and emotions, and how different stimuli affect how they feel.

This development is hampered when the child isn't able to fully grow into themselves. For example, a child who is not affirmed, nurtured, or given autonomy to think and feel how they like ends up being afraid of continuing to work on finding themselves.

We have discussed in great detail the impact of ambivalent-insecure attachment on child development. However, what we haven't fully looked at is the effects it has on building a strong sense of self.

If you grew up with inconsistent parents, you were unable to fully gain their undivided attention and affection. This unfortunately created deep rooted insecurity, which impacted how you perceive yourself.

As a child, your parents made up your entire world, but you were only a part of theirs. Subsequently, their absence or emotional neglect meant that you felt alone and unwanted most of the time.

These strong feelings might have caused you to believe that something was inherently wrong with you, that perhaps if you were another child or had a different personality or temperament, you would have a stronger connection with your parents.

Whether these limiting beliefs are true or not is not the focus. The focus is on how those beliefs justified self-destructive behaviors, which ultimately made you reject and abandon yourself too. In other words, you internalized the inconsistencies of your parents, felt ashamed of who you were, and unconsciously turned against yourself.

What many people don't understand about insecurities is that they breed self-hatred. Indeed they may start out as petty criticisms, comparisons, or self-doubt, but very soon they become perceptions that inform how you see yourself.

A child that grows up with insecurities, as a result of unmet needs, becomes an adult that feels like they are not good enough, despite being competent and responsible. They are constantly haunted by the idea of being outed as a fraud (imposter syndrome) or exposed for their vulnerabilities, which will result in being rejected once again.

Another interesting behavior of children who grow up with anxious attachment is the tendency to engage in self-destructive behaviors. This occurs due to unwanted thoughts, which trigger unwanted emotions and behaviors.

An example here could be an anxious woman who is afraid of commitment because she believes that nobody would love the 'real' her. To avoid inevitable heartache, she pulls back from partners when the relationship starts to develop, shortly after the honeymoon phase ends. The outcome? She returns to her single status and misses out on the opportunity to be genuinely loved for who she is.

Other ways that anxious people self-destruct is through binge eating, binge drinking, reckless sexual encounters, shopping addictions, pursuing troubled men or women, or staying in toxic relationships. In essence, they are drawn to any kind of behaviors that might reinforce their fears of rejection and abandonment.

Bonding With Yourself

The best way to address deep rooted insecurities is to develop a genuine relationship with yourself. Doing so will allow you to see yourself for who you are, outside of the trauma and pain you experienced as a child.

This goes beyond our traditional understanding of self-awareness, which is to be aware of your thoughts and feelings. Developing a bond with yourself is about confronting the inner critic once and for all and winning the battle over your mind.

Whether or not you are aware of it, there has always been a battle over your mind. This battle is known as social conditioning, which is the programming of people to think and behave in certain ways through the use of positive and negative reinforcement.

Your family and friends, public education system, community, media, and public figures have implicitly or explicitly participated in the programming of your mind to think and behave in certain ways. Depending on your life circumstances—like the relationship with your parents, the community you grew up in, and the messages you internalized from the media—you are wired to perceive reality in a particular way.

What this means is that your perception of yourself is rigged, and this isn't by any means your fault. It is the result of social conditioning, and the many beliefs and unconscious messages you have internalized from your environment.

Thus to win the battle over your mind and develop a genuine relationship with yourself, you will need to confront your social conditioning. This will involve reflecting on the most influential forces in your childhood, assessing the types of beliefs or messages they transferred to you, and rooting out negative programming that may affect how you see yourself and the world today.

Challenge Harmful Social Conditioning

It is a disheartening realization to know that your ideas and beliefs about life aren't entirely your own. For many decades, you have been surviving off of other people's rule books or society's definitions of "normal," and you have neglected your own truth.

A basic example of this is how you model some of the behaviors you witnessed growing up. For example, if you grew up eating dinner around a table, you might continue to eat dinner around a table even now. Or if arguments at home were resolved using the silent treatment, you may continue to resolve conflict in the same manner.

Before you completely rule against social conditioning, it is important to note that not every type of social conditioning is harmful. Just imagine how difficult it would be to get through school if there weren't specific rules, structures, and codes of conduct put in place, or how unhealthy workplaces would be if there weren't any expectations enforced. Rules dictated by external parties like parents, schoolteachers, or bosses at work aren't *all* bad, but there are some that do more harm than good.

The best way to know whether society's imposed rules or expectations are harmful is to tune into how they make you feel. Remember the inner child? That subconscious memory of your younger self? He or she intuitively knows what is good for you and what isn't. Connect with them and ask the tough questions, like which childhood messages were problematic and caused a lot of internal pain. Your inner child may bring up a few commonly accepted messages based on what you were exposed to as a child. Such messages may include things like:

- Children need to be seen, not heard.
- Girls don't play with boys.
- Crying is a sign of weakness.
- Money will buy you happiness.
- People who grow up in poverty won't amount to anything.

You can also ask your inner child specific questions based on different social aspects of your life, such as:

- **Language:** What did you learn about language and communication as a child? What were you allowed or forbidden to say? What were some of the expectations around sharing thoughts and emotions?

- **People:** What did you learn about people as a child? Who were you taught to trust and distrust? How was human nature described to you? How did you look at people who were more fortunate and less fortunate than you? What were some of the expectations around personal boundaries and interaction with other people?
- **Religion:** How was religion introduced to you as a child? What was your understanding of religion? What were some of the expectations you had to follow?
- **Career:** How was the subject of work brought up as a child? What were you taught about the purpose of work? What kinds of expectations around work were imposed on you?
- **Gender:** What did you learn about your gender as a child? What were you allowed or forbidden to do? What were the future outlooks for a boy or girl? What type of standards were you taught to uphold?

Apart from inner child work, another way to challenge harmful social conditioning is to consider the effects of maintaining the status quo. In other words, what has it cost you to live your life based on someone else's rule book? In order to connect to a deeper part of you and feel fulfilled in your relationships, your lifestyle must align with your needs, values, beliefs, and desires. You must be engaged in activities that both excite and challenge you, feel passionate about your work, and gain value from your close relationships.

In the space provided, write a personal letter to your younger self, validating the pain they must have felt not being able to express themselves and follow their heart's desires. This isn't a forgiveness letter, although if you feel you owe that young boy or girl an apology, you can give one. The purpose of this letter is to acknowledge the opportunities of self-expression that have been missed while following the status quo.

Become Your Own Person

If you intend on winning the battle over your mind, you will need to learn how to become your own person. Fortunately, you are an adult now and can choose how to live the rest of your life. You aren't obliged to live according to any individual, group, or society's manual, except your own.

As liberating as this sounds, it can also bring about a lot of anxiety. As someone who developed anxious attachment as a child, you tend to care a lot about what people think and say. For many years, other people's beliefs or judgments have helped you make sense of your own reality. This habit was born out of the need for survival and trying desperately to maintain connection with emotionally unavailable people. However, to become your own person you will need to fight this habit and work on seeking validation from within (more on changing habits later in the book).

These are some of the strategies you can practice to develop a sense of autonomy and claim the right to think and feel the way you like.

- **Expect to be misunderstood.**

Conforming to the status quo is the only way to gain mass approval. The moment you start to become your own person, it is inevitable that misunderstandings will arise. When others are confronted with ideas or thoughts that are foreign to them, their natural instinct is to reject them. Think of this as a survival response, a way to save themselves from unwanted information.

Your attachment anxiety can be triggered when you sense rejection from others, but in those moments remind yourself that people tend to judge or criticize what they don't understand. This doesn't make you a bad or undesirable person. It simply means that there is a clash between you and the other person's or group's worldview.

- **Surround yourself with "yes" people.**

To avoid constant debates or conflict around your choice of lifestyle, what you believe, or the goals you are pursuing, surround yourself with more supporters than detractors. As you are learning to become your own person, it is important to strengthen your boundaries. Distance yourself from people who tend to undermine your values, question your decisions, or make you feel guilty for standing up for yourself. Positive environments will nurture you and provide the emotional safe space you need to practice expressing needs and wants.

- **Trust your gut instinct.**

Your gut instinct is intuitive knowing that something is right or wrong. Unlike the brain, your gut instinct isn't based on facts but rather on emotional and experiential truth. How do you know what's good for you? You simply do, and undeniably so. Practicing inner child work can help you trust that inner source of wisdom and intelligence that helps you make the right choices.

- **Dare to fail.**

Most of the harmful beliefs we learned as children are based on fear. We were told to avoid certain things, stay away from certain people, or strictly live a certain way because our parents were afraid for us or projecting their own fears. To break free from the limitations of fear, be deliberate about failing at things. Take risks that you know have a 50/50 chance of working out, then embrace the outcomes. The aim of deliberating failing at things is to challenge those childhood beliefs or messages you learned about failure and to take the opportunity to positively redefine what failure means to you.

- **Stand on principles.**

Principles are the set of values and beliefs that form the foundation of who you are and what you do. They show what you deeply care about and the quality of life you desire. Standing on principles is about anchoring everything you do on specific values and beliefs. Everything you do becomes intentional, and nothing is done "for the sake of it." A great way to practice standing on principles is to ask yourself what value or belief you are honoring with each task you perform on a daily basis. For example, what values do you honor when you take your children to school, go to work, or practice meditation? If you can't anchor a task on a specific principle, reconsider its importance in your life.

Rebuild Your Self-Esteem

An important aspect of learning who you are and being comfortable in your skin is building healthy self-esteem. We can define self-esteem as the opinion you have about yourself or your overall worth. Depending on how high or low this opinion is, you can display high or low self-confidence.

When you go out into the world, you will come across different kinds of people who have different motives in getting to know you. Some people may be drawn to your personality and intend on starting genuine relationships. Others may be interested in what you have or what you do and seek to learn or take something from you (the intention isn't always manipulative).

Then there are those who have dark personalities (i.e. narcissists, psychopaths, etc.) who are drawn to you because they seek to exploit your weaknesses. When encountering these types of people, one thing they will all want to know is who you are. Some are curious because they desire to connect and build strong bonds, while others are curious because they want to know whether you have high or low self-esteem.

In general, the higher your self-esteem, the more stable your sense of self. It is much harder for people to mistreat you when your self-esteem is high because you can draw boundaries, reaffirm your values and standards, and cut ties with unsafe people, if necessary. In other words, you don't come off needy, insecure, or seeking approval from anybody.

Growing up with anxious attachment, a healthy self-esteem is perhaps something you have had to work on over the years. Due to the dynamic of the relationship with your parents, you may not have received positive reinforcement as a child, which reminded you of your sense of worth. As an adult, you can fill that void by affirming yourself and developing positive self-talk.

There are four components of self-esteem that you can work on to improve the opinion you have about yourself. These four components are discussed in detail.

Self-Confidence

Confidence is having faith in something or someone. When you display self-confidence, you show others that you believe and can depend on yourself. In order to truly feel this way, you must find reasons to believe that you carry value. For instance, you might reflect on the contributions you make in the lives of others, the progress you are making to heal from past trauma, or the aspirational goals that give your life meaning.

Here are some reflection questions you can answer to work on your self-confidence:

1. What do you do well?

2. What personal qualities help you get along with other people?

3. What positive coping skills have you picked up and significantly improved over the past few years?

4. If you had to sit down with your younger self, what is the one thing that would make them feel proud about who you are today?

5. In what ways have you positively touched other people's lives?

Identity

Identity refers to the knowledge you have about yourself. The best way to get to know who you are is to raise your level of self-awareness. In other words, it is the willingness to introspect and identify your beliefs, fears, needs, talents, and characteristics. You can also learn more about your identity by understanding the different roles you play in life and how they reveal aspects of who you are. For instance, you may be a mother, entrepreneur, and caregiver for your parent. Each role has its own foundation of beliefs, fears, needs, etc.

Here are some reflection questions you can answer to discover your identity:

1. Describe who you are in a few sentences.

2. Does your current lifestyle support who you are and what you desire?

3. What matters most to you?

4. What are your greatest fears?

5. What are you holding on to that you need to let go of?

Competence

The third component of self-esteem is feeling competent in what you do. As much as it is important to have a high opinion of yourself, it is also important to know that others are positively impacted by you. Competence is about gaining skills and knowledge so that you can make a meaningful contribution to the world. The higher your competence, the more secure you will feel in your relationships because you have tangible evidence of your value. Moreover, you will demonstrate greater resilience when confronted with challenges, since you have a toolkit of useful skills and abilities to support you.

Here are some reflection questions you can answer to work on your competence:

1. What are some personal challenges you have overcome recently?

2. What risk have you taken within the past year or two that has paid off?

3. Describe the ways you have grown within the past five years. Which areas of your life have you seen the most improvements?

4. What are your greatest physical or mental limitations right now?

5. Describe the way you resolve conflict. How might you improve your approach?

Sense of Belonging

Humans are social creatures who thrive on a sense of community. It is important for us to feel supported and validated at home, work, and within our social circles. We also have a tendency to define ourselves by the people we enjoy being around most. We see our loved ones as a mirror reflection or extension of who we are.

You don't need to have a large support network to feel a sense of belonging. The point is being able to identify a few people whom you trust and can depend on. In some cases, these people may not be friends or family; they can be medical doctors, gym instructors, church leaders, or colleagues.

Here are some reflection questions you can answer to deepen your sense of belonging:

1. In your own words, what does it mean to belong?

2. Identify values that you believe are important in a relationship.

3. What kind of support do you desire from friends and family?

4. Describe the ideal work environment that aligns with your values.

5. How do you maintain close relationships and show up for your loved ones?

Working on these four components of self-esteem can help you better understand who you are and what kind of environments and relationships positively impact your well-being. Treat the process of building your self-esteem like an ongoing exercise so you can keep track of your growth and personal transformations. For instance, on a regular basis, you can challenge yourself to perform one behavior that boosts your self-esteem. Examples include making time for a hobby you enjoy, saying one kind thing about yourself, or showing a random act of kindness to a stranger, friend, or coworker. These small behaviors will help to build self-confidence and reaffirm your identity, competence, and sense of belonging.

Rewrite Your Life Story

The reason why you need to challenge harmful social conditioning and work toward becoming your own person is so that you can reclaim your life story!

If I had to ask you right now to briefly summarize your life story, what would you say? Would you tell me about the worst years of your life? The complicated nature of your relationship with your parents? Or about the many failures you have faced? How much of your story would focus on the happy moments of your childhood? The people who actually showed up for you? Or the achievements you have won?

When you haven't yet processed the trauma, limiting beliefs, and harmful conditioning from the past, the story you tell about your life tends to be quite depressing. You may find it difficult to look beyond the pain and feel grateful for overcoming the hardships.

A negative life story affects how you see yourself in relation to other people. For instance, you might see yourself as broken, unlucky, hopeless, or not good enough. Just imagine what kind of energy you bring to relationships when your life story sounds like this. If given the chance, would you feel comfortable working alongside or being friends with someone who carried this heavy energy?

Part of connecting to yourself and being unapologetic about who you are involves rethinking how you perceive your life. When your life story changes, your attitude and mindset will follow. Bear in mind, you will still face challenges. However, the difference is that your perspective on challenges will be more encouraging, allowing you to demonstrate resilience through hard times.

You may be curious about how the process of rewriting your life story works. The aim is to identify the current narrative that replays in your mind, then adjust the storyline to position yourself as the hero—the man or woman who courageously escapes the strongholds of the past and paves the road to a positive future.

There are three main elements of rewriting your life story: introspection, cognitive restructuring, and visualization. Introspection helps you recognize what stories you are telling yourself and whether or not they are serving your greater good. Cognitive restructuring helps you challenge harmful stories that may have emerged as a result of experiencing hardship.

Visualization helps you envision the positive outcomes that could come from your life story, despite how negative it may have been. For example, while you may have suffered emotional neglect as a child, the positive outcome is that you are more sensitive and compassionate toward loved ones as an adult.

Here is an example of how rewriting a story would work, using the story of a young woman named Angela.

Introspection

Angela was determined to change a few life stories that were keeping her stuck in the past. The first was a story about the relationship with her mother as a child. One day, she sat on her bed and began reflecting about why she felt resentful about the way she was raised. She wrote down a few notes in a notebook and came up with the following story:

"I was raised by a single mother who worked two jobs. She left to go to work early in the morning while I was asleep and returned home past my bedtime. I never saw much of my mother; therefore I never felt her warmth. She didn't do what normal mothers did, like give me hugs, brush my hair, or take me shopping. All she cared about was whether I had done the chores, finished my homework, and stayed away from boys. I know what it means to have a mother who provides, but I don't know what a mother's love feels like."

Cognitive Restructuring

After doing a lot of introspection and identifying the story she would like to rewrite, Angela was ready to challenge the perception she had held for so long.

She decided to ask herself a series of questions:

1. What makes you believe your mother didn't show love?
2. How do you define love?
3. How do you believe your mother would define love?
4. What were your expectations of your mother at the time?
5. What were your mother's expectations of you at the time?
6. What might have pushed your mother to have the kind of attitude that she did?

Angela thought that these questions would be easy to answer. However, what she realized while writing about that period of her life is that she had only interpreted the events from her perspective. She hadn't stopped to consider her mother's reality and the stress that was driving her to step out of her nurturing role and provide for her family. The more she empathized with her mother, the easier it was for Angela to see the bigger picture.

Visualization

Angela's final task was to visualize the positive outcomes that came as a result of going through her situation. However, before she could do that, there were a few facts about the story that she wanted to keep, despite how sad they were. These included:

- never seeing much of her mother
- never feeling her mother's warmth as a child

- not knowing what a mother's love feels like

With these facts put aside, she could close her eyes and spend time envisioning how the situation might have positively impacted her life. In other words, what advantage would being raised in that situation—with that type of parent-child dynamic—give her?

During the first session of her visualization, nothing came up. Her confidence was slightly shattered, and doubt started to creep in. Perhaps there were no positives that could come out of her story.

She decided to take another visualization session, but this time she invited her inner child to join. Both of them sat quietly together and journeyed deep into the mind. Suddenly, Angela had a revelation.

She was currently working as a daycare teacher, looking after children in her house. Most of the children came from single parent households, and nearly all of their parents knocked off late from work.

Angela was the substitute parent that spent more than eight hours, five days a week, with these children. For the first time in her life, it made sense to her why she chose this specific career and why it felt so fulfilling to her.

In essence, by caring for children, she was healing her inner child and closing the void she felt as a child. Even though she couldn't change the fact that she never saw much of her mother or never felt her mother's warmth, she was able to nurture children who were possibly going through the same experience as she did when she was a child.

After going through these three steps, Angela adopted a new perspective about her relationship with her mother. She admits that they didn't have a traditional mother-daughter relationship, but she empathizes with the struggles her mother was facing at the time and understands how that may have distracted or detached her from the responsibility of caregiving.

Key Takeaways

- Due to anxious attachment and other developmental factors, you may have struggled to build a healthy sense of self.
- What you needed was a consistent display of affection and positive reinforcement, but unfortunately the relationship with your parents brought on deep rooted insecurities.
- Some of the ways in which insecurities from childhood manifest in adult relationships are not being comfortable with who you are and constantly feeling the need to prove your worth.
- Rewriting your life stories and learning to question how you were conditioned to think and feel are the beginning of connecting to a deeper part of you.

Ask for What You Need

Step 3: Reconnecting With Yourself

"From what I've seen, it isn't so much the act of asking that paralyzes us—it's what lies beneath: the fear of being vulnerable, the fear of rejection, the fear of looking needy or weak. The fear of being seen as a burdensome member of the community instead of a productive one."

— AMANDA PALMER

This chapter talks about:

- The role of attachment in being comfortable to ask for help
- How fear-based stories can discourage you from expressing your needs
- Five steps to communicating unmet needs with confidence

Why Is It Difficult to Ask for What We Need?

It is always the case, specifically for someone with anxious attachment, to be the one giving support rather than the one who asks for it. Have you ever wondered why that is so?

To understand where the resistance comes from, let us perform a meditation together. Settle yourself in a quiet room and follow the guidelines mentioned:

- Get into a comfortable position and relax your muscles. Allow everything to hang loosely but keep your back straight.
- Close your eyes and take a few deep breaths. Complete the box breathing exercise by inhaling through your nose for five counts, holding your breath for five counts, then exhale out of your mouth for five counts. Repeat this exercise by inhaling for five counts for three more rounds.
- Take a long breath and hold. As you exhale imagine that you were being transported back to your childhood. Go as far back as your mind is willing to go, so you can access your early memories.
- Take a few moments to orient yourself in this time period. Acknowledge how old you are, where you live, and your family situation at home.
- Visualize your younger self walking up to your dominant parent. Approach your parent slowly and tune into what that little boy or girl is thinking or feeling. Are they nervous or stressed? And how come? What thoughts are going through their mind as they approach their parent?
- Once they approach the parent, visualize your younger self making eye contact. As they look into their parent's eyes, what emotions do they sense? How comfortable are they feeling at that moment?
- Next, visualize your younger self asking their parent for something. Perhaps they are asking to go to the mall, bake cookies, or go on a play date with a friend. Tune into what the child is feeling at that moment, what thoughts are running through their mind.
- Take a few deep breaths and visualize your younger self walking back slowly, until they no longer see their parent, or the house, or the neighborhood.
- Open your eyes and record your experience.

The reason why the meditation ended without hearing your parent's response is because your thoughts and emotional experience is what mattered. As a child, asking for what you needed wasn't a problem. The difficulty was in anticipating your parent's reaction and deciding to place yourself in a vulnerable position where you could be rejected.

Depending on the thoughts and emotions you felt while completing the meditation, bringing yourself to ask for help as a child was stressful. Your parent may not have been the easiest person to approach, and maybe their responses were unpredictable.

Either way, you unconsciously learned that it is better to suppress your needs than give up control and risk being disappointed. This is why asking for what you need is so difficult as an adult.

Fear-Based Stories About Asking for Help

Riding on the back of the previous chapter, what stories are you telling yourself about asking for help? What makes you so resistant to express your needs and seek assistance from others?

Take a moment to think back to early beliefs or messages you internalized with regards to asking for what you need. These are some of the common fear-based stories children create about asking for help:

1. "I'm selfish for asking for what I need."

Did you ever feel uncomfortable for having needs and then guilty for expressing them to your parents? Perhaps you felt entitled, as though you were asking for a lot and putting a strain on your parent.

2. "They will think less of me if I ask for help."

If asking for help came with shame and humiliation, it is understandable why you avoided it. To prevent rejection or feeling vulnerable, you always pretended that everything was alright.

3. "I don't want to bother anyone."

Did your parents have a tendency to guilt-trip you whenever you asked for help? Even if what you were asking for was a basic need (i.e. asking for something to eat), they blew it out of proportion and made it seem like you were asking for too much. This fear-based story can lead to the first—believing that you are selfish for asking for help.

4. "Asking for help creates uncertainty."

You may have had intimidating parents who didn't put you at ease when asking for what you need. Or you may have been raised by unpredictable parents whose "yes" today is "no" tomorrow. The inability to anticipate the outcome of asking for help brought about too much anxiety, so you preferred not to ask at all.

5. "Asking for help takes too much energy."

Think back to when you were a child. Did you have to spend a lot of time brainstorming, planning, and rehearsing how you would ask for what you need? All of this preparation may have led you to believe that asking for help is draining, which felt even worse when your requests were denied.

Even though there may be some truth to these stories, they are nonetheless limiting because they prevent you from expressing your needs regardless of the outcome. Moreover, these stories serve to confirm the deep sense of rejection you may feel inside, which makes asking for help feel dangerous.

How Not to Ask for Help

With any request, there is a possibility of being turned down. That is simply the nature of asking for help. It would be unfair to expect people to say "yes" or avail themselves every time you need a helping hand.

Rejection sensitivity tends to make hearing "no" seem like the worst possible outcome. But it isn't. No is a boundary that informs you when another person has reached their personal limits. It protects them from overextending themselves and later feeling resentful about it.

Therefore, when you hear a no, avoid thinking that there must be something wrong with you. On the contrary, the boundary has nothing to do with you but everything to do with how the other person is choosing to take care of themselves.

The possibility of being turned down shouldn't stop you from communicating your needs, especially when you are committed to responding to the needs of others. You owe it to yourself to ask for the love, support, and encouragement you generously show others.

Albeit, asking for what you need is not as simple as you think. There are so many opportunities for misunderstanding when asking for help. In most cases, it isn't so much what you ask for that raises eyebrows, but how you ask for it.

People tend to remember how you made them feel, not what you said. The emotional feedback they get from you can determine how they feel about your request. A typical example is a parent yelling at their teenager for not completing house chores. Their intention is to motivate the kid to get up quickly and start on them, however the manner in which the request is communicated has the opposite effect.

Have you ever found yourself asking for what you need, then having to debate and defend why you need it? You may have been caught off guard by the aggressive response to your request because all you wanted was a simple yes or no. But what if I told you that the outcome could have been different if you communicated your needs better?

Here are some of the common mistakes that people make when asking for what they need:

1. Being overly understanding

Every relationship benefits from demonstrating empathy. It is only when you can fully step into another person's shoes that you can understand their worldview. However, when you overdo empathy, it can make it difficult to express your needs with clarity and conviction.

For example, you might need support from your partner because you are going through a hard time but hesitate to ask for it because you know how defensive they can be. You think about all of the ways in which they can misinterpret your need as a sign of not being good enough as a partner. Since you don't want to upset them, you decide that you don't really need support as much as you thought (which of course isn't true).

2. Being apologetic

Another mistake people make is to apologize profusely before, during, and after they have made a request. It might sound like this, "I'm sorry to bother you, but I really need you to send me the proposal before Friday. I'm sorry, I wish we didn't have such a short deadline."

There is a difference between apologizing for a mistake or inconvenience caused, like saying you are sorry for arriving late or asking for a favor at short notice. However, when you are respectful of other people's boundaries and are well within your rights to ask for help, there is no need to apologize.

To the person listening to your request, being overly apologetic makes you sound unsure of yourself. They are more likely to question why you need the help because you don't show any sense of conviction.

3. Using disclaimers

Many of us believe that if we make the request seem more attractive, the other person will likely agree to help us. This is why we tend to add disclaimers and other embellishments to our requests. A typical disclaimer might sound like, "I hate to have to ask you for this, but..." or "Don't get upset with me, but..."

The issue with using disclaimers is that they project a lack of confidence and, in some cases, can become self-fulfilling prophecies. For example, mentioning the idea that someone might be upset with what you are going to ask can negatively impact how they receive the news. The thought of being upset or inconvenienced has been planted in their mind, and now they have no other choice but to react with frustration.

4. Using reverse psychology

Have you ever exaggerated the size of a favor to make the other person believe that it isn't that big or difficult to perform? This is a classic example of reverse psychology, which is technically a form of manipulation.

For example, you might say, "I have such a huge favor to ask you. May you please pick up tomatoes from the grocery store on your way home?" or "This issue is going to require an expert, and I don't have the money for that right now. Do you know anyone who could quickly assist me?"

Since asking for help using reverse psychology is passive-aggressive, there is a chance that the other person may not catch on to what you are hinting at. When they do, they may get frustrated at the double message, which doesn't clearly communicate what you need.

5. Playing the victim

Another incorrect way to ask for help is to play the victim, such as sharing your personal struggles or how unfairly others have treated you. The reason why many people don't respond favorably to supposed victims is because they fail to take responsibility for their lives.

While mistakes happen and everyone faces their own fair share of suffering, it isn't right to use negative past experiences as bait to get others to respond to your needs. It is far more respectable to show a sense of independence and accountability, so others are confident that their support will make a positive difference in your life.

Five Golden Rules When Asking for Help

Now that you know what not to do, here are a few golden rules when asking for what you need. These are direct and assertive tips that you can practice whenever you make requests.

Rule 1: Commit to the request. Asking for anything requires confidence and conviction. It is important to show the other person that you are serious about having this need met, even if they end up turning you down. Showing commitment to the request conveys self-respect, and when you respect yourself, others are obliged to respect you too.

Rule 2: Understand the weight of the request. Be mindful of the gravity of what you are asking for. Consider who might be impacted, how much time and energy may be required, what skills may need to be deployed, etc. When you consider the impact, you can be more realistic and considerate of the next person.

Rule 3: Silence the inner critic. Before making a request, take a moment to silence the inner critic. Remind yourself that the outcome isn't about you. While you are in control of asking for your needs to be met, you have no control over how the other person might respond. Complete a short breathing exercise or meditation to calm your mind before approaching the individual.

Rule 4: Leave your expectations at the door. Don't attach yourself to any particular outcome. For instance, you might prefer being assisted with Option A, but the individual might only be able to assist you with Option B. What matters is that you are receiving help, meaning that your needs are being met—regardless of how it may look. A great way to manage your expectations is to regularly meditate on what you are grateful for. Allow the spirit of gratitude to be evident in the way you live and approach life.

Rule 5: Believe in yourself. Do you believe that you deserve to be helped? This question is of utmost importance because it shows whether or not you are open to receiving help. If you don't believe you are worthy of having your needs met, you may not be as confident and assertive in making requests, which unconsciously sabotages your opportunity to receive help. Spend time working on improving your sense of self-worth, so you are able to stand up for what you need.

BLOOM

There are times when asking for what you need is easy and other times when it feels uncomfortable. For instance, you may not have any trouble asking a friend to drive you to the airport, lend you money, or look after your pet for a few days. But whenever your needs involve communicating boundaries, the same cannot be said.

It is understandable why you get hesitant to set limits with loved ones or express unmet needs. The process of communicating your needs reveals your inner thoughts and feelings, which makes you feel vulnerable. You would like to assume that your close friends and family know how to respond to your needs without you having to remind them or that what you need is common sense, thus when others cross your boundaries, they are doing so deliberately. Unfortunately, these assumptions aren't true.

Communicating your need for space should be as easy as communicating your need for an apology or respect. This is because all of these needs are connected to your core values. When your loved ones honor your needs, they are essentially honoring you, and the opposite can be said when your needs aren't met. Therefore, as a sign of self-respect, you have every right to express unmet needs, including those that you would classify as embarrassing. Despite how awkward it may feel defending your needs, it proves how much you value them.

With that being said, there are five steps that you can follow when communicating unmet needs. These steps are summarized in the acronym BLOOM, which stands for

- Branch
- Label
- Open
- Own
- Make

What follows is an outline of the steps and how you can practice them.

B: Extend an Olive Branch

Whenever you are approaching someone for a serious conversation, such as expressing unmet needs, there is always a possibility of conflict arising.

To put the other person at ease, you can start the conversation by extending an olive branch. This can be a simple sentence or two that allows them to feel seen. For example, you might say, "Thank you for making time to listen to what I have to say."

On the lines, practice different ways of extending an olive branch. Write a few sentences that you can use in real life situations.

L: Label the Feeling

It isn't common to start a conversation by putting your emotions on the table. However, emotions tend to be what gets in the way of addressing the real issues. It is best to lay down your feelings from the get-go and allow the person time to process your emotional experience throughout the discussion.

Since the emotions are what you feel inside as a result of your unmet needs, use "I feel" or "I felt" statements to show ownership and avoid projection or passing blame. An example of an "I" statement would be "I have been feeling embarrassed whenever you put me on the spot in front of our friends."

Think of a few scenarios in the past where you were offended by friends or family. Based on those scenarios, create some "I feel" statements.

O: Open Up

Most people stop at expressing how they feel, but that doesn't provide enough context to allow the other person to empathize. It is important to really think about the impact of having an unmet need, beyond the temporary emotion that is triggered.

You can choose how much information you are comfortable sharing with the person about your personal needs. For example, if you are addressing a friend you don't know very well, you might say "I know you don't have bad intentions, but I have experienced bullying in social circles before, and it typically followed the same pattern."

If it is a friend you trust and feel comfortable opening up to, you might show more vulnerability by saying "I know you don't have bad intentions, but whenever you do that it triggers anxiety from being bullied by ex-friends." It is important to use your discernment when deciding how much to share so that you don't feel overly exposed.

Using the examples from the previous steps, choose a few experiences to open up about. Imagine that you are speaking to someone you don't know very well and someone whom you trust.

O: Own Your Ask

The fourth step is to make a request. Fortunately, you have already learned a lot about making requests, but a great tip to remember is to show conviction. You can show conviction by being clear and direct about your ask.

Mention step-by-step what you would like the person to do in order to fulfill your needs. Ideally, they should leave without feeling confused about what you want. Here is an example: "Moving forward, I would like for you to not make jokes at my expense, even if you think they are harmless."

Remember that conviction isn't the same as rudeness or arrogance. You can be firm and direct, while being considerate of the other person's feelings. Avoid making threats, snide remarks, or impolite statements that might cause the person to stop listening or caring about what you have to say.

On the lines, practice making requests with conviction. Look at each request and ask yourself if you would be comfortable being told the same thing.

M: Make It Specific

The final step gives you an opportunity to clarify what you need. In other words, making real life examples so that the person knows what you specifically want. When making examples, ensure that they are relevant to your relationship dynamic. Use situations that occur on a daily basis. Here is an example: "When I say, 'making jokes at my expense,' I mean using my personal stories or comments that I have made as something to mock in front of other people."

Using the responses from the previous step, take the opportunity to provide more clarity by offering examples:

If we had to put these five steps together, we would have the following:

"Thank you for making time to listen to what I have to say. I have been feeling embarrassed whenever you put me on the spot in front of our friends. I know you don't have bad intentions, but I have experienced bullying in social circles before, and it typically followed the same pattern.

Moving forward, I would like for you to not make jokes at my expense, even if you think they are harmless. When I say, 'making jokes at my expense,' I mean using my personal stories or comments that I have made as something to mock in front of other people."

Can you sense how clear, confident, and committed that request was? This is the goal that you will work toward as you learn to be more vocal about unmet needs.

Key Takeaways

- Every human being has needs, but some hide them better than others. Your openness or resistance toward asking for what you need has a lot to do with how responsive your parents were as a child.
- Take a moment to reflect on where the resistance is coming from. Think deeply about the fear-based stories you may be telling yourself about expressing your needs.
- Remember that there is a right and wrong way to ask for help. Some of the wrong ways include being overly empathetic, using disclaimers, or practicing reverse psychology. The right ways involve committing to your ask, leaving your expectations at the door, and believing in yourself.
- Communicating unmet needs can be difficult, but you owe it to yourself to stand up for the things that matter to you. The BLOOM five-step framework can teach you how to clearly and assertively express unmet needs and what you desire moving forward.

Which Direction Are Your Habits Taking You?

Step 3: Reconnecting With Yourself

"We change our behavior when the pain of staying the same becomes greater than the pain of changing. Consequences give us the pain that motivates us to change."

— DR. HENRY CLOUD & DR. JOHN TOWNSEND

This chapter talks about:

- How childhood attachment patterns continue into adulthood, and how to confront them
- The science behind habit formation, as well as discovering why unhealthy behaviors bring rewards to the brain
- How to use the NLP pain and pleasure principle to break unhealthy behavioral patterns

You Are What You Repeatedly Do

Tabitha was raised by strict, emotionally unavailable parents who had high expectations for her to live up to. She was often ridiculed for crying, expressing fears, or asking for help. This caused her to mature very quickly and develop a thick exterior.

As she grew older, Tabitha developed an unconscious preference for men who were emotionally unavailable. She interpreted this as being introverted and mysterious, but this was far from the truth.

Her boyfriends were incapable of holding emotional space for her. Whenever she would express how she felt, they would somehow change the topic or trivialize what she was going through. Tanya would get upset, close herself in the room, and come out when she was feeling better. Eventually, she married one of these men and experienced the same cycle of emotional invalidation in her marriage.

Pete, on the other hand, was raised by overprotective parents. He was an only child, and his parents treated him like a young prince. The only issue was that Pete was never allowed to make decisions for himself. His controlling parents did most of the thinking and feeling for him until it was time to go to college.

At college, Pete discovered he had an unconscious preference for women who were domineering. These were the type of ladies who wanted to be involved in every aspect of his life. Occasionally, Pete would get frustrated and attempt to stand up for himself. However, his message would often come out unclear because he hadn't practiced sharing his thoughts and feelings as a child.

Pete grew to have a negative view of women and relationships in general. He saw women as controllers who didn't have his best interests at heart. But this didn't stop him from being attracted to women that reinforced the same patterns he saw growing up.

Have you ever found yourself feeling frustrated because you kept repeating the same unhealthy behaviors and getting the same results?

Like Tabitha and Pete, you may have a "type" that is reminiscent of the attachment with your parents.

Repeating the same patterns over and over again is not a conscious process that you can control. The cues happen on a subconscious level, which means that you often wake up during or after the pattern or cycle has taken place. The best way to break unhealthy patterns is to understand how they were formed in the first place, then reprogram your mind to accept healthier patterns.

The Science Behind Your Habits

How many times have you looked in the mirror and said the words "This is the last time?" At the moment, you sincerely believed that you were bidding farewell to toxic behaviors and venturing on a new and healthier path. After a week or month, you somehow found yourself performing the same behaviors.

Was the mirror speech just an act? Or could you have overlooked a crucial component of behavioral change-habit formation? We can define a habit as a behavior carried out consistently over time. The part of your brain that is responsible for habit formation is known as the basal ganglia, which also assists with other brain functions like emotion processing and pattern recognition.

The reason for having a separate region of the brain that assists with forming habits is that without learned behaviors, the brain would be too overwhelmed with processing new information each day. Just imagine if you had to learn how to brush your teeth, hold a knife and fork, or drive your car every day, as though you hadn't done it before. How different would your life have been?

As much as you need habits to progress in life, there are some that don't serve you. These tend to be unhealthy habits that reinforce unwanted thoughts, emotions, and behaviors. Habits related to past trauma, emotional triggers, limiting beliefs, or low self-esteem can be classified as unhealthy and unproductive.

The type of habits you need to live a fulfilling life and build meaningful relationships should be helpful and encouraging. But breaking unhealthy habits isn't as simple as looking into a mirror and announcing that you quit. In order to break unhealthy habits, you need to make changes to the brain.

Fortunately, the brain is capable of learning and unlearning behaviors through a process called neuroplasticity. This process typically happens naturally as you are exposed to new experiences, however you can activate the process through what is called self-directed neuroplasticity (retraining your brain to create and enforce new patterns).

The Pursuit of Pleasure

The science behind how the brain forms habits is quite interesting. The main idea is that the brain is wired to seek pleasure and avoid pain. This very simple programming is what has kept our human species alive. Actions that bring pleasure are seen as safe and beneficial, while those that bring pain are seen as threatening and undesirable.

You can test this biological instinct in your own life by reflecting on the tasks you most enjoy and those you put off or conveniently forget about. You can also consider how long it takes for you to learn and memorize tasks that you enjoy compared to tasks that you dislike.

The brain has a sneaky way of persuading you to spend time doing pleasurable activities. Whenever you complete a task that you enjoy, you are rewarded with a good feeling. The good feeling is a release of the brain chemical dopamine, which has the same sedative effects as morphine. The release of dopamine motivates repeating the same pleasurable behaviors, over and over again, until eventually they become habits.

Nevertheless, there is a catch. As evolved and sophisticated as the brain is, it cannot differentiate between healthy and unhealthy behaviors; it can only tell the difference between behaviors that bring pleasure and those that bring pain. Essentially, this means that unhealthy behaviors which bring pleasure can become habits.

You might be wondering to yourself how something bad for you can make you feel good. For some reason, that idea sounds contradictory. Let us return to the examples of Tabitha and Pete to answer this question. If you recall, both Tabitha and Pete had attachment issues that trace back to childhood. Tabitha had emotionally unavailable parents, and Pete had overprotective parents.

Neither Tabitha nor Pete felt secure in the relationships with their parents. In fact, they spent the majority of their childhoods suppressing needs and finding different ways to cope with the inconsistent parenting. But shockingly, in their adult relationships, they played out the same attachment patterns!

Why on earth would Tabitha and Pete feel attraction toward partners who reinforced the same unhealthy relationship dynamics they experienced as children? Wouldn't they want something better for themselves? The truth is that despite how unhealthy their childhood attachments were, they felt familiar. For 18 years or so, their brains were trained to accept hot and cold behaviors. They learned to accept that unrequited love is normal, and a mutual give-and-take is abnormal.

Therefore what felt "safe" were partners who would love them the same way they were loved as children, and what felt "threatening" were partners who would challenge their understanding of love—even if challenging the pattern was for their own good.

As someone who grew up with anxious attachment, what you perceived as normal interactions and bonding may not be what is healthy for you. However, the patterns have already been formed in your brain, and until you change them, you are wired to continue practicing habits that feel "safe" even if they are destructive.

It would be easy to just look in a mirror and declare the patterns gone. But that isn't enough to break a habit and create new patterns. You will need to go through the process of self-directed neuroplasticity and retrain your brain to distinguish between behaviors that bring pain and those that bring pleasure.

Rethinking Pain and Pleasure With NLP

Neuro-linguistic programming (NLP) is a type of therapy that seeks to retrain your mind on how to think. It consists of three components:

- **Neurology:** Understanding and recognizing the mental processes and patterns of the subconscious mind.
- **Linguistic:** Using language to make positive suggestions to the subconscious mind.
- **Programming:** Approaching the mind like an internal operating system that can be updated whenever it receives new inputs.

As mentioned earlier, the best way to break unhealthy habits is to update the patterns that inform your behavior. This can be done through self-directed neuroplasticity using therapies like NLP.

Currently, your internal operating system (brain) is programmed using a specific "language." It can only understand messages that are processed in this specific language. Whenever you try to introduce messages using a foreign language, it simply rejects the suggestion. Therefore, before you can switch languages, you must spend time teaching your brain how to recognize the new language.

Perhaps your current language reinforces unhealthy behaviors that aren't bringing the results you desire in life. While reading this book, you have discovered a better language that you would like to teach your brain, which promotes healthier behaviors. NLP can help you make suggestions to your subconscious mind that can effect changes on a neurological level.

One of the most powerful ways to make suggestions to the subconscious mind is to use an NLP technique known as the pain and pleasure principle, or leverage. The aim of the principle is to motivate positive behavioral change by using both pain and pleasure.

In the previous section, we discussed the brain's natural response to pain and pleasure. It has been biologically programmed to avoid pain and seek pleasure as a way of survival. However, NLP teaches that both pain and pleasure can be beneficial to improving overall well-being.

For example, the pain of surviving a difficult childhood can create a desire for a peaceful and healthy lifestyle, or the pain of loneliness can motivate you to seek companionship. The motivating factor behind pleasure is obvious. You are drawn to aspirational goals because they promise an idealistic life.

Central to the pain and pleasure principle are emotions. Your emotions about certain situations are what drive you to seek change. Unpleasant emotions are just as effective as pleasant emotions because they create a strong desire. For example, being afraid that you can't trust anyone can generate enough motivation to work through your trust issues. In other words, even negative sensations or experiences can be used as leverage to change the way you think and approach life.

The trick, however, is to increase the intensity of your emotions to the extent that they create urgency, such as the need to take action NOW. Going back to the example of trust issues, unless you feel really grieved that you are unable to trust people, you might not be motivated to take the steps to heal. Connecting to the "why" behind your emotions can also help to increase the intensity and make the problem feel very real and serious.

Think back to the times in your life when you were driven to take action because of the fear of losing someone, being evicted from your home, suffering financially, or jeopardizing relationships that were most important to you. Even though that fear was extremely uncomfortable, you were able to make swift decisions and step outside of your comfort zone. This enables you to break out of habits and engage in new behaviors.

The benefit of using the pain and pleasure principle when breaking unhealthy habits is that it doesn't require you to have discipline. All it requires is for you to want something so badly that you are driven to disrupt existing behavioral patterns.

While discipline is an excellent skill to learn, it requires a lot of conscious effort. For instance, the way to increase discipline is to do those things that you dislike, over and over again, regardless of how you feel. When using this approach, your brain (which is constantly looking for a dopamine hit) will resist many times, making the process uninspiring.

The pain and pleasure principle works in a subconscious way and doesn't require you to think about doing those things that you dislike or that seem hard. Your only focus is to spend time intensifying your emotions (positive or negative) so that you feel a passion or strong pull to commit to change.

There are three steps you can practice to work on breaking unhealthy patterns using the pain and pleasure principle.

Step 1: Objectively Observe Your Current Behavioral Pattern

Before you begin making suggestions to the subconscious mind, take the time to assess the behavioral pattern you would like to change. This can be done through meditation or journaling. The aim is to reflect on the habit, when it is triggered, how it manifests, etc. Do your best to be as neutral and objective as possible, so that you can see the full picture without being clouded by emotions.

You are welcome to use the lines for journaling.

Step 2: Tune in to Your Feelings

Now that you are familiar with what is happening, it is time to charge your mind with emotions. You can choose whether to focus on the pain or pleasure associated with the habit.

For example, you might focus on the pain of losing something/someone or ending up in a worse state if you continue reinforcing the pattern. Or you can focus on the pleasure of being physically, mentally, and emotionally freed from the pattern.

It can also help to ask yourself deep questions associated with the pain or pleasure. Here are a few questions that can help you intensify the pain:

- What are the consequences of repeating this pattern for another 5–10 years?
- What will you lose if you don't change?
- What opportunities will you miss out on if you don't change?
- How much worse has the pattern gotten over the years?
- Here are a few more questions that can help you intensify the pleasure:
- How would you feel if you successfully overcame the habit?
- What opportunities would you qualify for after breaking the habit?
- How different would you feel about yourself and your relationships?
- What would your life look like in 5–10 years if you chose to break the habit right now?

Spend several days or weeks on this step. Repetition is key when it comes to making changes on a subconscious level. It won't take one round or one day to change deeply ingrained patterns, but rather several attempts.

Step 3: Interrupt Current Unhealthy Pattern

While you are diligently working on intensifying your emotions, try to catch yourself whenever you are triggered to reinforce the current unhealthy pattern. The earlier you identify the trigger or behavior, the easier it will be for you to interrupt the pattern.

Interrupting the pattern is about finding a positive distraction to shift your focus on something else. For example, when you are triggered to withdraw from your partner during an argument, you can interrupt the pattern by singing lyrics to a song, smiling while looking at your partner, or anything that might reduce the urge to carry out the existing pattern.

Continue to distract yourself until you notice the urge has gone. Thereafter, proceed by carrying out your desired behavior, which might be expressing how you feel in a calm and respectful way. Reward yourself after successfully completing the desired behavior as a way of hinting to your brain that the new behavior is pleasurable and worth learning.

Another positive distraction that can help you build a secure attachment style is practicing self-care. We can define self-care as behaviors that seek to enhance your well-being and overall quality of life. These might include things like scheduling daily check-ups with yourself, working out, staying connected with close friends and family, and practicing gratitude. You can interrupt an unhealthy pattern by turning to the simplest form of self-care you can perform at that moment. Reward yourself for completing a desired behavior.

The pain and pleasure principle is not a magical tool. You will need to put in the effort to engage your mind and make strong suggestions. Once again, repetition is the only way that your brain can learn new patterns and habits.

Key Takeaways

- Unhealthy habits can make you feel powerless and compromise the quality of your relationships. But when you begin to understand that your brain's job is to recognize and reinforce patterns, you can feel more empowered to change how you think.
- Habit formation is an essential function of the brain that is controlled by the basal ganglia. Behaviors that are associated with pleasure are rewarded with a release of dopamine, which motivates repetition.

- Unfortunately, the brain cannot tell the difference between healthy and unhealthy behaviors; it only knows what feels painful or pleasurable.
- NLP's pain and pleasure principle can help you unlearn harmful patterns and program your brain to recognize healthier patterns. This is done by increasing motivation and urgency and intensifying both painful and pleasurable emotions.

Strive Toward Secure Attachment

Step 3: Reconnecting With Yourself

> *"In essence, if we want to direct our lives, we must take control of our consistent actions. It's not what we do once in a while that shapes our lives, but what we do consistently."*
>
> — TONY ROBBINS

This chapter talks about:

- What a secure attachment feels like, and why love is the central component
- How to find people with the right companions who make you feel emotionally safe
- How to shift from codependency to interdependency and cultivate positive relationships

What Does Secure Attachment Feel Like?

The goal for overcoming anxious attachment is to adopt a secure attachment with loved ones. This goal is ambitious, but it is possible with the right interventions, like the ones shared in this book.

While working toward healing your attachment style, it is worth familiarizing yourself with what secure attachment feels like. After all, if you are unable to picture yourself being securely attached, you may experience trouble staying motivated to change toxic behavioral habits.

Before we go into an explanation of what to expect when you are securely attached, let us begin by completing a meditation to tune into the frequency of unconditional love. Follow these instructions (you can record the meditation yourself and listen to it if you like):

1. In a quiet area, find a comfortable place to sit and allow your body to hang loosely. Keep your spine lengthened and take deep and slow breaths.
2. When you are feeling calm, close your eyes and mentally picture your inner child (represented in a child's body) walking toward someone, real or fictional, who embodies love. This could be your grandmother, favorite pet, or a spiritual entity.
3. As your inner child gets closer, tune into what they are thinking and feeling. Don't rush the walk toward this loving figure. Take your time and connect with your inner child's excitement, nervousness, or whatever they might be going through.
4. Picture your inner child finally reaching the loving figure. What is the first thing that little boy or girl says? How do they behave around this figure? How do they express themselves?
5. Shift your attention onto the loving figure. Notice how they respond to your inner child. Do they smile, laugh, or play along? How do they make your inner child feel about him or herself? Play out the sweet interaction between the two in your mind.
6. Picture the two of them looking at each other, preparing to go separate ways. How do each of them feel at this moment? What do they desire or wish to express to one another?
7. Watch as your inner child walks back slowly from where they came from. As they walk away, what are they thinking or feeling?
8. Take a few deep breaths, and when you are ready, open your eyes

and journal about the experience.

There are some who mistakenly assume that people who fall under the three insecure attachment styles are incapable of feeling genuine love. This assumption is often justified by the fact that these individuals had a rough childhood.

What they overlook is that the emotion of love is not necessarily tied to parents. Of course, in many cases, parents are the ones who expose a child to love, but they are not the gatekeepers of love. In the absence of parental love, it is possible for a child to develop loving relationships with other real or fictional entities or as an adult to grow to love themselves.

The fear of not being capable of loving others should not hold you back from opening yourself up to the possibility of love. All you need to do is look around you, and you will find people or things to love. If you are unable to develop a loving bond with another person, look to animals or nature, find hobbies and passion projects, or connect to your Higher

Power.

The reason why we are speaking at length about love is because it is what enables a secure attachment. In order for two people to be securely attached, they must be open and willing to love each other. This love will look different in a platonic, romantic, or work relationship, but the intention remains the same.

The best way to describe securely attached friends, family members, or couples is: two imperfect people who are comfortable in their own skins and create a space where each of them can express who they are without judgment. An emphasis must be made on "imperfect" because there is bound to be conflict within those loving relationships. But the presence of conflict doesn't compromise the safety they have built and continue to maintain.

Now to answer the question of what a secure attachment feels like. Quite simply, it can feel like the following experiences:

- feeling a boost of energy whenever you are in the presence of other person
- being more open to trying new experiences and stepping outside of your comfort zone
- feeling comfortable sharing ideas and opinions without second-guessing yourself
- letting go of the need to control outcomes; trusting in the integrity of the relationship
- being generous with your resources, but knowing when you have reached your limits (also, not being afraid to set limits)
- maintaining your individuality and celebrating the other person's uniqueness
- feeling an inner motivation to become the best version of yourself to develop the skills necessary to maintain your relationship

- being realistic about the shortcomings of the other person; recognizing when your shortcomings are causing pain in the relationship
- accepting the fact that your relationship doesn't need to be perfect, neither do you hold each other to that standard
- living for the present moment and fully embracing the state of your relationship right now
- being committed to change, if and when your behaviors threaten the sense of safety you have both established

Find Your Tribe

As someone with anxious attachment, you may identify as having a tendency to people-please, or at least this was something you dealt with in the past. This habit stems from childhood, and it was often used as a strategy to get the attention of your parents.

Unfortunately, it has also gotten you into some sticky situations with friends and family, where you felt uncomfortable saying no or afraid to express your true personality. You may have also noticed that being a people-pleaser made you vulnerable to being used and abused.

As you work toward a secure attachment style, you will need to overcome the tendency to people-please once and for all. Since secure attachment is based on the willingness to love and be loved, you don't need to go out of your way to seek approval from others.

People who are willing to genuinely connect and develop a bond with you won't demand that you act in a certain way to get their attention. They encourage you to express who you are unapologetically and set boundaries when you have reached your limits.

Finding the right people and making the right associations can put your attachment anxiety at ease and allow you to open up without shame.

However, knowing who is right for you takes a lot of self-awareness because you need to look beyond who excites you in the moment and find people who make you feel safe.

For example, as someone with an anxious attachment, you would feel safe in a friendship or romantic relationship with someone who has a secure attachment style. In some cases, relationships with another anxious person can work, however both of you would need to be self-aware and willing to talk through the uncomfortable moments when you feel triggered.

Being friends with or dating someone with an avoidant or disorganized attachment style is a recipe for disaster. Since you need a lot of reassurance in a relationship, it is important to surround yourself with people who are emotionally available and are able to create a safe space for you to express your thoughts and feelings.

People with avoidant and disorganized attachment are uncomfortable with their own emotions, let alone those of others. They may unintentionally hurt you by dismissing your feelings or shutting down when they are upset.

Characteristics of Emotionally Safe People

The right kind of people for you don't have a particular face or body. They don't have to be the same race, age, gender, or socio-economic class as you either. But one thing is for certain: They must be emotionally safe.

Throughout the book we have discussed the importance of emotional safety in the parent-child relationship. The absence of emotional safety as a child meant that you found relationships difficult to manage as an adult. Now that you are ready to build secure relationships founded on love, it is important to train your brain to be attracted to emotionally safe friends, partners, coworkers, etc.

What makes someone emotionally safe is their ability to accept others for who they are. They don't wish for you to think or feel any particular way. Moreover, they don't expect perfection or for you to always be on your best behavior. Emotionally safe people allow you to be human, and that is what makes them suitable for you.

If you are interested to know what kinds of character traits to look out for that scream "emotionally safe," there are some to consider:

- **An emotionally safe person validates your feelings.**

A sign that you are in the company of an emotionally safe person is that you feel comfortable sharing details about your life and hard emotions that you are working through and becoming emotional in front of them. They respond by listening and allowing you to process your emotions.

- **An emotionally safe person admits to being wrong.**

To qualify as being "emotionally safe," you must be self-aware, which is being able to recognize your strengths and weaknesses. When you are in a relationship with someone who is self-aware and accepts their flaws, they are able to reflect on their actions, apologize for their mistakes, and make the necessary changes.

- **An emotionally safe person is willing to grow and learn.**

Still on the subject of self-awareness, an emotionally safe person knows that there are certain aspects of their character that need improvement. This is something they are able to admit and actively work on. They are also self-motivated to change because they understand the benefits of becoming a better version of themselves (not only to strengthen your relationship, but other relationships in their life too).

- **An emotionally safe person values trust.**

Trust is an important aspect of any healthy relationship. It is the agreement two people make with each other to always act in each other's best interest. An emotionally safe person honors the trust that you have for each other. They behave in ways that allow you to feel safe in their company and when you are apart.

- **An emotionally safe person takes full responsibility for their physical, mental, and emotional well-being.**

A sign that someone is emotionally safe is taking good care of themselves. They know themselves well enough to respond to their own basic needs. Additionally, they are proactive about addressing stress and other challenges life might throw.

For instance, to manage work stress more effectively, they might start going to the gym or improving their sleep routine. This doesn't mean that they don't need you, however they never make you feel like you are responsible for their well-being.

Work Toward Interdependence

One of the benefits of cultivating emotionally safe relationships is that you can lean on the other person without feeling dependent on them. This can be a breath of fresh air after many years spent feeling like you need people in order to be happy.

A word you might hear being used when referring to healthy relationships is interdependence. Interdependence is the ability to form an emotional bond with someone, while maintaining a strong sense of self. In other words, you are invested in building the relationship but don't allow the dynamic to consume your life.

People with secure attachment tend to display interdependence in their relationships. They are able to be vulnerable without becoming needy, and they respond to the other person's needs without overextending themselves.

The opposite is true for people with anxious attachment. Since close relationships brought about a lot of anxiety, they learned to cling on to people, outsource most of their needs, and become dependent on relationships for building identity or feeling a sense of purpose.

For some people it led to developing codependency, a type of relationship where an individual's thoughts and feelings become centered around the needs and behaviors of another person. Instead of wanting to connect and maintain a strong bond, a codependent person feels the need to keep the relationship intact, even when the dynamic starts to become toxic.

Part of working toward interdependence is learning the early signs of codependency in relationships, so you can take a step back and assess your boundaries. Some of the signs to look out for include:

- You get a boost of energy when others praise you and tend to feel down when your efforts aren't recognized.
- Your moods and behaviors change depending on how your close friend, partner, or family member feels at that moment.
- You neglect your own needs and plans to show up for loved ones and make sure that they are satisfied.
- You feel anxious making decisions without the other person's advice or consent.
- You adjust your thoughts and opinions based on the perspective your loved one or colleague takes.

It is possible to change a relationship dynamic from being codependent to interdependent. However, it will require commitment from both parties. If one party refuses to change harmful behavioral patterns, the dynamic cannot be interdependent. Remember, interdependence requires self-awareness and respecting boundaries, which must be reinforced by both people.

Nevertheless, this shouldn't stop you from working on yourself and overcoming codependent behaviors. While waiting for your loved one to get on the same page, you can start developing qualities of interdependence. What follows are a few practical ways to begin the shift toward interdependence.

1. Acknowledge your part.

The first step is to acknowledge some of the behavioral patterns you have reinforced in the past that have contributed to a codependent relationship.

Write down as many behaviors as you can recall and the impact they have on your relationship dynamic.

2. Get to know yourself.

For the next few weeks and months, prioritize getting to know yourself again. Each week, set up an activity that involves introspection or doing an activity that makes you happy. The aim is to rediscover who you are outside of the relationship, so you can begin to source strength from within.

Use the lines to plan out the activities and exercises that you will complete for the next week or month.

3. Practice making your own choices.

It is important to learn and be comfortable relying on yourself so that when others aren't available or willing to respond to your needs, you don't feel lost or abandoned. One of the ways to build self-reliance is to practice making decisions without seeking feedback from others. Trust in the fact that you intuitively know what is good for you; that you are capable of taking care of yourself.

Reflect on the people whom you lean on for support in decision-making. Write down a list of decisions you find difficult to make without them. For the next week, strive toward making these decisions alone. You are welcome to seek information from the internet or blogs but refrain from relying on people you know.

4. Invest in your social life.

The benefit of having a rich and vibrant social life is that you don't have to rely on a single relationship to meet all of your needs. For example, you might set up dates with friends whenever you feel like having emotional conversations, which can relieve a lot of pressure from your romantic relationship.

Take stock of your social life and write down what you believe is missing. Do you perhaps need more like-minded friends to do social activities with? Do you need to expand your definition of "social" and try out new activities? Or do you need to make your social life more of a priority?

5. Create positive communication rules.

Part of building interdependence is creating a relationship where two people can be themselves and express their own thoughts and feelings openly. In order for this to occur, there needs to be rules put in place to guide communication.

For example, in order to feel safe expressing your thoughts and feelings, you might need the other person to

- listen without interrupting
- validate your emotional experience
- reserve their opinion until you ask
- make time for check-ins and spending quality time together

They might also have rules of their own, which you would combine with your list. It is easier to hold yourself accountable for positive communication when there are clear expectations on how to engage with each other.

Accentuate the Positive

It is not a bad thing to seek happiness from a relationship. In fact, healthy relationships support your mental and emotional well-being and enhance positive emotions.

While conflict and challenges are unavoidable, they shouldn't be the center of your relationships. Remember that relationships that feel stressful trigger your body to shut down and find alternative ways to cope. When you shut down, emotional safety is compromised, and you cannot fully be open and present in the relationship.

As a child, you didn't have a choice of how your relationships turned out. You depended on your caregivers to provide the best care they knew how. But now that you are grown and can choose who to invite into your life and the type of relationships to invest in, it is worthwhile to choose people and relationships that accentuate the positive.

Since your well-being hinges on the connections you make, seeking out positive relationships should be a priority. One of the ways to know that you are in positive relationships is to assess how you feel in the presence of the other person, and whether you become more or less of yourself. Positive relationships are not meant to change who you are, but instead they create enough room for you to feel more deeply connected to yourself.

Here is a short assessment you can do by yourself, whenever you seek to reflect on the impact that your platonic, romantic, or professional relationships have on you. For each question, respond with curiosity about how you can accentuate the positives and develop a stronger relationship.

1. Do they bring out the best in you?

A positive person tends to have an optimistic attitude toward life and relationships. As a result, they can be encouraging and complimentary. This doesn't mean that they are unaware of your flaws, but they choose to focus and comment on your strengths and positive qualities.

Reflect on whether the other person brings out the best in you. Provide evidence to support this.

2. Can they fight well?

It is important to accept that people have a good and dark side. Yes, even the most compassionate people have character flaws. It is unfair to expect a friend, partner, or coworker to be positive all the time. However, the manner in which they respond to conflict matters.

Conflict is supposed to be an opportunity for learning who the other person is and what they want. It is a chance for both parties to express difficult feelings, seek clarity, and step into the other person's shoes.

The best way to tell if the other person fights well or not is to assess how you feel after an argument. For instance, do you avoid each other or are you able to change the topic and speak on something else?

Reflect on your arguments with the other person. Identify areas where you can both improve, such as how the fight ends or giving each other an opportunity to be validated.

3. Are you able to maintain your individuality?

A positive relationship is first and foremost a safe space to be yourself. One of the signs that you are in a positive relationship is being free to express your uniqueness. In other words, there are no expectations for you to be anyone other than you.

Reflect on how safe you feel being authentic in the relationship. In what ways does the other person respect your individuality?

4. Do you take turns supporting each other?

Healthy and positive relationships are about making sure both parties feel considered and supported. There is a constant switch in roles between the giver and the taker, which lessens the emotional burden on both people. For example, when one person has a bad day, the other person is able to support them without feeling taken for granted because when it is their turn to have a bad day, the other takes on the support role.

Reflect on the balance of give and take in your relationship. First examine how well you perform both roles, then consider how well the other person performs both roles.

5. Are you able to grow together?

Another predictor of healthy and positive relationships is the shared commitment to continuous growth. Both parties accept that there is room for improvement in their relationship, which motivates them to focus on personal development, so they can be the best version of themselves.

Reflect on how much growth is a priority in your relationship. How open are you to embracing change? Provide evidence to support.

Key Takeaways

- You may not have grown up with a secure attachment style, but with the right interventions you can work toward adopting this kind of dynamic in your relationships.
- Secure relationships are based on the willingness to show and receive love. That is what makes them feel safe and validating.
- It is important to remember that you cannot build secure relationships with people who don't feel emotionally safe, such as those who are avoidant or dismissive.
- Building secure and positive relationships takes time and intentionality. Find people who share the same level of commitment to become interdependent and seek to become the best version of themselves.

Conclusion

> *"To be fully seen by somebody, then, and be loved anyhow—this is a human offering that can border on miraculous."*
>
> — ELIZABETH GILBERT

Ambivalent-insecure attachment, or anxious attachment, is a type of emotional bond that a parent has with their child. It naturally develops due to inconsistent nurturing that leaves a child guessing whether or not they are lovable. This bond informs how the child interacts with other people and the quality of their relationships as an adult.

If you identify as someone with anxious attachment, it is important to remind yourself that you didn't get to choose to relate to others in that way. Your attachment style came as a result of early childhood neglect or trauma that ultimately changed how you view the world and other people. Nevertheless, the responsibility to heal and rebuild your sense of self rests on you.

There is no doubt that growing up with anxious attachment has made it difficult for you to express yourself and feel safe in relationships. Throughout your childhood, and even adulthood, you may have felt desperate to hold onto unhealthy relationships that felt safe but were unresponsive to your needs. Moreover, you may have been caught off guard by the constant attachment triggers that activate upon the slightest discomfort in your relationships.

Perhaps you have reached a stage in your life where you are unwilling to continue reinforcing the same anxious patterns anymore. You may be ready to invest in relationships that allow you to be unapologetically yourself. Alternatively, you may have a strong desire to experience true love, improve your relationships with colleagues, or strengthen family connections.

This book has provided you with plenty of strategies to overcome anxious attachment. The aim of these strategies were to help you address past childhood traumas and stories, challenge the limiting beliefs that distort your understanding of relationships, heal the wounded inner child and reclaim your sense of self, as well as to reprogram your mind, so you can reinforce positive relationship behaviors.

With the knowledge and practice that you have gained from reading this book, you are equipped to finally come face-to-face with yourself and make the necessary changes to build meaningful and positive relationships. Remember to treat the process of healing anxious attachment like a journey and be patient with yourself as you reawaken aspects of you that have been hidden or invalidated for so many years. You deserve to show yourself the same love you so generously give to others!

III

Codependency Recovery Workbook

9 Steps to Overcome Fear of Abandonment, Stop Pleasing People & Develop Healthy Relationships

Introduction

> *"Many of us live in denial of who we truly are because we fear losing someone or something—and there are times that if we don't rock the boat, too often the one we lose is ourselves."*
>
> — DENNIS MERRITT JONES

Codependency is commonly seen as one of the harmful behaviors that threaten healthy relationships and creates a dysfunctional dynamic. In codependent relationships, the couple, parent-child, or best friends take on two different roles: the sacrificial giver and the unapologetic taker.

The sacrificial giver downplays their needs at the expense of responding to the needs of the other. Due to a number of factors, such as their early childhood attachments, or preconceived ideas about love, they derive a sense of self-worth from proving themselves to others.

The unapologetic taker tends to also struggle with issues of self-worth, and relies significantly on the support, affection, and responsiveness of the other person to have a stable sense of self. The only difference is that instead of giving endless amounts of reassurance, they take as much as they can get.

Codependency isn't a new term, and many of us are aware of the damage of losing ourselves in service to others. However, as common as this relationship dynamic is, we often find it difficult to recognize the signs of codependent relationships, or realize what we can do to break the cycle.

Take my life, for example. Growing up, I thought that the codependent relationship with my mother was normal. From as early as I can remember, my mother suffered from bipolar disorder and would often require more caretaking, as opposed to providing nurturing and support. But this didn't seem out of the ordinary. After all, wasn't it every child's responsibility to take care of their parents?

It was only when I reached a state of burnout and suffered from depression in my teen years that I realized how unhealthy our mother-daughter relationship dynamic had been. The constant giving that felt like love was actually a sign of a lack of boundaries and deep-rooted insecurities. But since healthy displays of affection and nurturing were not modeled in front of me as a child, it wasn't an easy process confronting our dysfunctional relationship—and the codependent personality I had developed.

How to Use This Book

As a psychologist today, I see many clients who desire to learn how to break cycles of codependency. Fortunately for them, they have already recognized the dysfunctional pattern in their relationships, but they still lack the proper psychological tools to build a solid sense of self, separate their needs from others' needs, and strive for independence rather than codependence.

As part of their therapeutic intervention, I take them through the codependency recovery plan, which consists of nine steps to gradually heal from this relationship dynamic and prioritize their well-being. The nine steps include:

- Chapter 1: Define Codependency
- Chapter 2: Understand the Risk Factors
- Chapter 3: Recognize How Codependency Looks in Different Relationships
- Chapter 4: End the Terror of Obsessive Thinking
- Chapter 5: Put Yourself First and Set Boundaries
- Chapter 6: Learn the Art of Assertive Communication
- Chapter 7: Improve Your Relationship With Fear
- Chapter 8: Decide to Stay or Leave
- Chapter 9: Celebrate This New Chapter

The purpose of this book is to teach the above steps from my own experiences with codependency, and what I have learned over the years as a trained psychologist. By the end of the book, you will be able to explain what codependency is, how the dynamic is formed, and implement various strategies to break free from the cycle and prioritize self-growth and mutually supportive relationships.

The key to fulfilling relationships, as I have learned, is to cultivate psychological safety and create a space where both parties feel comfortable to show up as they are. Unconditional acceptance of the other is the secret ingredient that keeps two imperfect people connected and thriving within their relationships. Get ready to learn what it means to feel psychologically safe in your relationships and be empowered to express who you are, openly and freely!

Define Codependency

"Once they have been affected—once "it" sets in—codependency takes on a life of its own. It is similar to catching pneumonia or picking up a destructive habit. Once you've got it, you've got it."

— MELODY BEATTIE

What Is Codependency?

Historically, the term *codependency* was used to describe the relationship dynamic between substance abusers and members of their family. Codependent behaviors were synonymous with supportive behaviors, even though they were simply an act of enabling the behaviors of the addict.

There is nothing "supportive" about codependent relationships. At the core, you have two individuals who do not have a stable sense of self, and as a result, they rely significantly on each other to fulfill their physical, mental, and emotional needs.

Codependent relationships tend to be intimate and long-lasting, like any other healthy relationship. However, due to both individuals defining themselves based on their relationship, the attachment formed is not liberating, nor does it support trust, individuality, or accountability.

The pair will do whatever it takes to stay together, even if it means overlooking boundaries, forgetting about their individual interests and needs, and turning a blind eye to dysfunctional behaviors.

This leads to the next point. To sustain a codependent relationship, both parties need to play a different role. One person becomes the giver and the other the taker. How the roles are chosen depends on a number of factors, such as the personality of each person, how each defines love and attachment, as well as what each person's core needs are.

The giver, for example, is typically an empathetic person, who defines love by the measure of caretaking they can offer another person. They may also believe that they are responsible for "fixing" others or making them happy. The giver feels anxious when their loved one is upset or distant, and may blame themselves for their loved one's bad moods or unloving behaviors. Deep down, the giver fears being abandoned, and they will do whatever it takes to protect the relationship.

On the other hand, the taker is typically an insecure person, who defines love by the measure of validation they can receive from another person. They may display a sense of entitlement in relationships, believing that they deserve to be loved, protected, and nurtured. It is common to find that takers suffer from some sort of mental health condition, whether it be a form of addiction, mood disorder, or personality disorder.

Due to their condition, they lack the awareness required to recognize the excessive giving and self-sacrificing behaviors of the giver, or the desire to set healthy limits and practice reciprocity.

It is important to mention that codependent relationships begin with good intentions. Both the giver and taker are attracted to each other because of how each person is able to respond to the other's core needs. The giver fears being alone and, therefore, needs the presence of the taker to feel secure. The taker fears being unlovable and, therefore, needs ample amounts of validation from the giver to feel secure.

What makes codependent relationships unhealthy is the level of denial that both parties will go to in order to keep the relationship together. This tends to open the relationship up to all sorts of dysfunctional behaviors and abuse, which can lead to anxiety, low self-esteem, depression, and a sense of helplessness.

What Codependency Is and Isn't

Codependency is often misunderstood as relying on your loved one to respond to your needs. The truth is there is nothing wrong with having needs, communicating them, and taking turns to respond to each other's needs.

What makes a relationship healthy is the level of emotional interdependence that exists between a couple, parent and child, or best friends. Emotional interdependence is a term used to describe the capacity of both individuals to empathize and emotionally lean on one another. It is normal and healthy, for example, to need quality time, words of affirmation, acts of service, physical touch, and gift giving from your loved one, and for them to expect those same needs to be met.

Individuals in codependent relationships don't show a lot of emotional interdependence. The relationship is normally skewed toward prioritizing the needs of one person—the taker—causing inequality and dependency. Furthermore, the giver tends to regard their needs as being less important and urgent than the needs of the other person.

Unlike healthy relationships where both individuals find value in the union, codependent relationships are often kept going by the giver. The giver invests so much time and energy in maintaining the relationship, to the detriment of their health, career, and social relationships.

For example, the giver is less likely to have hobbies, a strong support network, or personal goals outside the relationship, whereas the taker may enjoy a full and enriching life outside the relationship.

Below are a few more patterns that the giver may display in a codependent relationship:

- **Being in denial of the state of their relationship.** The giver may struggle to recognize or accept what they are feeling. Even when they can sense that the relationship dynamic is unhealthy, they might distort reality, like believing it is selfish to not respond to every need of the taker.
- **Having a low self-esteem.** The giver has a deep fear of standing on their own. This fear makes it hard for them to make decisions, express their thoughts and feelings, or ask for what they need. Moreover, they may have a low sense of self-worth, and doubt that anybody may find them worthy of receiving love.
- **Compromising on their needs to a fault.** There are limits to how much you can give in any healthy relationships. In most cases, the limits are determined by your own physical and emotional boundaries. Since the giver doesn't have firm boundaries, they tend to compromise their values and engage in people-pleasing behaviors to avoid rejection or the taker's aggression.
- **Display controlling behaviors.** The giver derives a sense of satisfaction from taking care of others. However, if they are not careful, it could lead to controlling behaviors, like insisting on others taking their help, trying to persuade others to accept their ideas, using sex to gain acceptance, or finding other covert ways to influence others.
- **Avoiding behaviors that might bring shame or rejection from others.** Due to the deep-rooted fear of rejection, the giver may avoid

actions that could open them up to being ridiculed, shamed, or judged by others. For instance, they might avoid emotional intimacy in relationships, or attempt to hide their emotions altogether because emotions are perceived as a sign of weakness.

- **Struggling to enforce healthy boundaries.** Both the giver and taker may struggle to recognize, respect, and enforce boundaries in their relationships. From the giver's perspective, they may not insist on boundaries out of fear of backlash from the other person. They may have a hard time asserting themselves and calling out bad behavior when it happens.
- **Insisting on taking care of others.** It is normal to have the desire to take care of loved ones, but not to the extent of worrying about them, or obsessing about how they choose to live their lives. In some cases, the giver is groomed into the role of caretaker as a child by their parents. For example, affection may be withheld whenever the child doesn't respond to their parent's needs. They may grow up believing that something bad will happen if they don't devote themselves to taking care of loved ones
- **Struggling to communicate openly.** Codependent relationships naturally breed a lack, or poor communication. From the giver's perspective, they may fear expressing their needs, and end up using passive ways of communicating with others. Even when they are frustrated, the giver would much rather internalize their anger, and blame themselves, rather than confronting the issue at hand.

The Stages of Codependent Relationships

Codependency doesn't form overnight in a relationship. It often unfolds in a number of stages, which could take years to fully develop. There are generally three stages of codependency: the early stage, middle stage, and late stage. When the patterns of codependent behavior are not addressed, the dynamic of the relationship becomes progressively worse. Understanding each stage of codependency can help you identify some of your codependent traits and just how enmeshed you are in your relationship.

Below is a breakdown of the three stages of codependency:

The Early Stage

The first stage is very difficult to identify because it looks like any other loving relationship. Both parties display a lot of affection toward each other, and are able and willing to respond to each other's needs. The subtle difference between the parties is in how they define the relationship, and how they view each other.

The giver, for example, will likely fantasize about the taker. If they are in a romantic relationship, the giver will believe that they have found their soulmate, whereas if it is a parent-child relationship, the giver (could be the child or parent) will have an immense amount of admiration for the other person.

The taker may care about the giver too; however, they are more likely to have a balanced view about the relationship and the other person. They are aware of the giver's pleasant and unpleasant traits, and will therefore see them realistically.

Naturally, both parties in the codependent relationship will start to spend less time with their friends or family, or lose interest in many of their hobbies. The difference between the giver and the taker, though, is that after some time, the taker will regain a sense of individuality and reconnect with their friends or family. The giver, on the other hand, will not.

The Middle Stage

By nature, healthy relationships are built on reciprocity. What this means is that both partners take turns giving and taking. It isn't necessarily a titt-for-tatt scenario, but more so the awareness of how much each person contributes to the well-being of the other.

Codependent relationships do not have a strong foundation of reciprocity. This becomes more noticeable during the middle stage. The major factor to look out for here is the amount of time and effort both parties invest in the relationship.

It is common to find the giver making more compromises for their needs and lifestyle than the taker. They may not always enjoy being the one who is always bending their boundaries; however, it is seen as a small price to pay for maintaining the relationship.

The taker, who may be self-absorbed or oblivious to the needs of their loved one, may start to request certain treatment or norms in the relationship. They may not always stop to empathize with the giver and recognize just how much they are already investing into the relationship. Expecting unconditional love, nurturing, and cooperation becomes an unrealistic expectation for the taker.

To maintain the status quo of their relationship, the taker may develop unpleasant behaviors, like constantly nagging or guilt-tripping their loved one, in order to have their needs met. In extreme cases, some takers may even go as far as using manipulation tactics to keep their loved one constantly focused on their well-being.

Not all people in codependent relationships are ignorant of the power imbalance and lack of reciprocity. For instance, the giver may notice that their needs always take the back seat, but how they respond isn't the same as someone in a healthy relationship. Instead of sitting down with the other person, sharing their concerns, and setting boundaries, they might fight back with passive-aggressive tactics, like giving the silent treatment or performing subtle acts of sabotage.

When questioned by outsiders about the state of their relationship, they might lie to protect the taker from any backlash. Alternatively, they may withdraw from friends and family or find mind-numbing distractions or obsessions to avoid doing something about their unhealthy relationship dynamic.

The Late Stage

When codependency issues are left unaddressed, they may start to affect the giver's physical and mental well-being. Some of the mental health conditions related to codependency include anxiety, depression, and bipolar disorder. On a physical level, givers can also suffer with a host of issues like chronic migraines, loss of appetite, gut problems, insomnia, and eating disorders.

It may come as a surprise to learn that the taker's health suffers too—but not in the way you might expect. Due to the power imbalance in the relationship that favors the taker, they might develop a sense of superiority, entitlement, and hostility when they are being challenged. These are typical characteristics of narcissistic personality disorder, but may also make them vulnerable to other personality disorders.

Four Stages of Codependency Recovery

To avoid reaching the late stage of codependency, it is important to develop a strong sense of self. Throughout this book, you will learn how to do this by learning useful techniques and practicing various exercises.

Whether you are in the early, middle, or late stages of a codependent relationship, please be encouraged that you can retrain your mind on how to relate to others. The secret to this is undertaking the four stages of codependency recovery.

On the following pages is a look at what you can expect at each stage.

Stage 1: Abstinence

You can think of codependency as being similar to an addiction, except the "substance" you are addicted to is another human being. Therefore, the first step in recovery is spending some time away from the other person and refocusing your attention on your personal growth.

If spending some time away is not possible due to family commitments or financial obligations, you can practice detaching from the other person, which might include letting go of the need to control them and feeling personally responsible for their well-being.

The goal of abstinence is to create enough separation between you and the other person, so that you can discover your own beliefs, needs, and feelings. This process isn't easy, regardless of how long you have been with the other codependent person.

In some cases, it may even feel dangerous if the relationship has become abusive. Speaking to people who have recovered from their codependency issues may give you the courage it takes to initiate the separation and focus on yourself.

Stage 2: Awareness

The second step is to reflect on the nature of your relationship. Being separated from the other person will give you enough space to reflect on behaviors you may have never questioned before, like how they insist on having their needs met, but don't respond positively when you make requests.

Be on the lookout for denial or blaming the other person for the state of the relationship. Remember, it takes two to tango. As a giver, there was something that attracted you to the taker, as well as something in them that was attracted to you. The awareness stage is about identifying those internal wounds and beliefs that caused the codependent dynamic in the first place.

Stage 3: Acceptance

At the heart of codependency recovery is acceptance. This could be the acceptance of reality as it is, and the fullness of who you are. For example, one of your personality traits as a giver is being a people-pleaser. This might not be a trait that you have accepted about yourself. The lack of acceptance means that you cannot fully comprehend what being a people-pleaser means or looks like for you, and as a result, you are unable to address people-pleasing behaviors.

Acceptance also involves learning to be enough for yourself. This isn't an easy milestone to reach, since being in a codependent relationship taught you to define who you are based on what others think about you. It will take time to be comfortable being disliked by other people, who may not approve of your opinions, how you live, or the boundaries you create.

Stage 4: Action

The final step is to take action. It isn't enough to gain so much insight about your previous relationships and areas of self-improvement, without putting what you have learned to practice. The three B's—beliefs, behaviors, and boundaries—will be the test to see how much you have understood about yourself.

Taking action will encourage you to step outside your comfort zone, like exploring new types of self-care, getting to know different types of people, or finally living the lifestyle you have always dreamt of. These new experiences will help you get to know yourself better, and positively affect your self-esteem.

Closer to the end of the book, we will take another look at the four stages of codependency recovery, and focus on how you can practice them to manage obsessive tendencies.

Exercise: Are You a Giver?

Even though you have shown interest in the topic of codependency, you may still be wondering whether this relationship dynamic fits your experience. To gain more understanding about the symptoms of a giver, complete the short codependency quiz below.

Read the questions and put a tick inside the columns "Yes" or "No." Please note that the questions refer to a "partner," however, they apply to other types of close relationships too (i.e. friends, parent-child, siblings, etc.).

Questions	Yes	No
Have you ever skipped work to spend time with, or attend to, a false emergency of your partner?		
Has being in the relationship caused you to withdraw from friends and family?		
Have you ever lied to avoid your partner's negative reaction?		
Have you ever manipulated people to do what you want?		
Has being in the relationship caused you to lose sight of your interests and goals?		
After resolving an argument with your partner, do you try to get even?		
Has the thought of leaving the relationship crossed your mind?		
Do you turn a blind eye to your partner's bad habits, addictions, or obsessions?		
Have you ever borrowed your partner's money to get them out of a situation they could have prevented?		
Are you secretly harboring resentment for your partner?		
Has your relationship contributed to the decline of your physical and mental well-being?		
Have you ever felt unlovable?		
Do you often extend yourself to respond to other people's needs, but don't get the same support in return?		
Do you believe that your partner cannot survive without you?		
Would you rather deny your own needs to make others feel comfortable?		
Do you suppress strong emotions because you are afraid of receiving backlash?		

If you have answered "yes" to five or more of these questions, you may display symptoms of codependency in your relationship.

Understand the Risk Factors

"Codependency doesn't acknowledge that we actually feel what others are experiencing and want it to stop because it hurts us too."

— JENNIFER ELIZABETH MOORE

What Causes Codependency?

Life is full of ups and downs. If we all took a moment to think about our pasts long enough, we could write down a list of positive and negative events that we have witnessed or been a part of.

But not everybody responds to life's challenges the same way. Perhaps the most obvious reason for this is because we are all exposed to different types of stressors. Nevertheless, even in cases where two people experience similar adverse experiences, how they make meaning of them won't be the same.

Why is this important?

Codependency is a relationship dynamic that only some people form. It isn't necessarily true that growing up in an abusive household or suffering with a mental health condition will make you codependent on others. Therefore, the likelihood of developing codependency or not has more to do with each unique individual, and how they cope with stressful events, and make meaning of their life experiences.

The remainder of the chapter will explore various risk factors of codependency. There is sufficient research to prove that these factors can make you more vulnerable to developing codependent behaviors. However, once again, being vulnerable to codependent behaviors doesn't mean that you will end up adopting this kind of dynamic with others.

Consider each risk factor and think about how they may have played a role (or continue to play a role) in your life.

Trauma and Codependency

Trauma is defined by the American Psychological Association (APA) as an emotional response to a painful life event (APA, 2021). Your body's reaction to trauma is to activate the stress response, also known as fight-flight-freeze mode.

Immediately after the traumatic event, depending on the circumstances, it is common to either become emotionally reactive (e.g. having anger episodes), withdraw from others and enter isolation, or go into a state of shock and denial.

The long-term effects of not getting into a therapy room and addressing the trauma immediately afterward, is the devastating impact on your mental health. How trauma affects your mental health may vary, but some of the common side effects include developing an anxiety disorder, depression, post-traumatic stress disorder (PTSD), or low self-esteem.

Early detection of these mental health conditions, and following a treatment plan, can reverse whatever emotional damage that may have started forming. However, the frightening reality is that many people don't seek help, but instead continue with life as normal.

Take a moment to imagine what "life as normal" might look like for someone who has unaddressed trauma. Would they *really* be able to continue as though nothing happened? It is highly unlikely. Depending on what kinds of traumatic events they were exposed to, various aspects of their life could change. This might include the collapse of their stable belief systems, to be replaced by fear-based beliefs. Or the lack of secure attachments to people, which would lead to unhealthy relationships.

For example, someone who experiences childhood trauma, particularly growing up with absent or abusive parents, may struggle with closeness when they are older. Even how they look at relationships might change, and instead of seeking mutual respect, support, and affection, they might seek validation. Anyone who can give them the attention they were deprived of as a child could be considered "the one," regardless of other relationship qualities they may be lacking.

This is how codependent relationships form. Two people who have lost sense of, or have never experienced healthy and secure relationships, create a trauma-bond as a way to cope with unresolved pain from previous life experiences. They find comfort in each other because they are familiar with dysfunctional relationships, and the various coping mechanisms that highly stressed individuals adopt to protect themselves, like people-pleasing, using manipulation tactics, or having porous boundaries.

The lingering trauma within codependent relationships doesn't mean that there is a lack of love. Just like any couple or parent-child relationship, there is a positive attraction or connection felt by both individuals. However, being in love doesn't make the parties any less vulnerable to being abused. In fact, the idea of "being in love" may in some cases make it difficult to address harmful behaviors or violations of boundaries.

Getting Behind the Trauma Bond

The term *trauma bond* was coined by Patrick Carnes, in 1997. He described it as an adaptive, dysfunctional attachment that emerges in the presence of shame, a perceived threat, or exploitation in order to survive (Lancer, 2022).

The bond is characterized by a power imbalance between the abuser and the one being abused. What attracts them to each other is surviving a history of trauma, but there is not much depth to their connection apart from that. The abuser is the dominant partner, who finds ways to belittle, manipulate, or control the other person. One of their favorite tactics is to play on the other person's fears and insecurities, like making an empty threat to leave the relationship whenever they are not getting their needs met.

Of course, the trauma bond doesn't start out abusive, and neither does the abuser make their intentions to seek control known in the beginning. At most, the relationship might feel unstable and unpredictable, with a mix of good and bad days. Over time, bad behavior becomes normalized, but at this point, the one being abused has accepted the status quo of their relationship.

Moreover, the pattern of abuse is typically followed by a pattern of intermittent positive reinforcement, which "trains" the person being abused to accept rewards after enduring abusive behavior. An example of this would be the abuser being extra affectionate and generous following their abuse. This creates a neediness in the other person, to always chase an elusive fairy tale of what their relationship could be, even though it is evident that the abuse will not end.

Research has shown that intermittent positive reinforcement conditions the brain to seek rewards, even when the rewards stop coming. This can explain why severing the trauma bond is so difficult. Even though the relationship is full of mostly lows, the potential of the relationship becomes an addiction. The hope of feeling loved by the abuser feels just as strong as if that love was actually there.

Givers can be vulnerable to creating trauma bonds. Their loyalty and incessant need for closeness is what causes them to keep seeking to win back the love of the taker. The more they lean toward the taker, the faster the taker runs in the other direction. But before the giver loses complete hope, the taker returns to offer them a taste of what genuine devotion feels like. This temporary display of affection is enough motivation to keep the giver chasing after the taker, not realizing that the cycle of detachment and reconnection will continue again.

Mental Illness and Codependency

Codependency is not a recognized mental illness, although it is seen as a condition sharing similarities with other personality disorders, like dependent personality disorder (DPD), post-traumatic stress disorder (PTSD), and borderline personality disorder (BPD).

Some of the mental health challenges that are linked with codependency include:

- stress
- anxiety
- depression
- low self-esteem
- emotional reactivity

The absence of a medical diagnostic criteria means that people who suffer with this condition are normally diagnosed with DPD instead, even though codependency isn't the same as DPD. The first for this being this way is the nature of relationships formed under the two conditions. Codependency, for instance, is characterized by dependent behavior focused on a specific individual, unlike DPD that is characterized by dependent behavior displayed to anyone in general.

The second reason why the two conditions aren't the same has to do with how the parties inside these relationship dynamics interact with each other. With DPD, there isn't always an enabler (i.e. the taker). There could simply be one person, the giver, who feels compelled to take care of their parent, child, friend, or loved one. Furthermore, this dynamic isn't always abusive. There can exist interdependence in the relationship, but the dependent person may feel anxious about being separated from their partner, or have doubts about taking care of themselves.

In contrast, a giver in a codependent relationship may show extreme devotion to the taker, to the extent of neglecting other responsibilities or relationships. Their identity and sense of self-worth revolves around the taker, and because the taker won't refuse the engulfing affection, the cycle of codependency continues.

Being In a Relationship With a Mentally Ill Person

Another way that codependency can develop is when one person in the relationship suffers with a mental illness. For instance, a child who takes care of their mentally ill parent may eventually take over their responsibilities, or a spouse who struggles with alcohol problems may need a lot of support and motivation from their family.

What makes it difficult to identify codependent behaviors when caring for a mentally ill loved one is because there is a natural attachment formed between you. You desire to express affection or seek validation from the ones you care about the most, and this makes it harder to know when you are extending yourself too much.

Even in healthy relationships, caretaking is seen as a form of love, and in some cases, an unavoidable task. For example, if your partner had depression and struggled to get themselves out of bed, most of the household responsibilities would fall on you. It isn't so much that they don't want to help you perform tasks around the house, it is that they physically cannot.

The only difference between caretaking in healthy relationships and codependent relationships is that there are clear boundaries enforced in the former. Whenever one person has reached the point of exhaustion from fulfilling the other's caretaking needs, they express a boundary. This can be as simple as saying "no."

The giver in a codependent relationship doesn't feel like enforcing boundaries is an option. They feel responsible for making sure their partner is happy and cared for, at all times. When they are unable to respond to their partner's needs, perhaps due to exhaustion, they may feel a sense of personal inadequacy. "How can I be so selfish?" they might think. Essentially, there are no limits to the amount of caretaking a giver can perform, which is what causes the power imbalance in their relationships.

Attachment and Codependency

John Bowlby's attachment theory explains the parent-child bond (referred to as an attachment), which starts forming inside the womb, but becomes noticeable when a child is about six weeks old (Cherry, 2022). By then, the child is able to show a preference for primary and secondary caregivers, and as the months go by, they develop a strong attachment to a specific caregiver (in most cases their birth mother).

The reason behind a child forming an attachment is that without the nurturing of other human beings, their physical and emotional survival would be on the line. They are quite literally dependent on their caregivers to create environments of safety and nourishment to avoid feelings of stress and anxiety.

When a child shows physical signs of distress, like crying, they are signaling for their caregiver's attention. They could be tired, hungry, or frightened, and desire for their parents to help them stabilize their nervous system and fulfill their needs. The close proximity to their caregiver, and knowing that their physical and emotional needs matter, is what develops a sense of security in the child, and makes exploring their identity and the world around them feel safe.

A caregiver who is absent (whether physically or emotionally) and misses several opportunities to respond to their child's needs, is seen to the child as someone who is unreliable. Without the security of a present and responsive caregiver, the child feels compelled to suppress their needs or look for other ways to get their caregiver's attention. This is what makes them vulnerable to developing codependency issues later on in life, and believing that their sense of self-worth is tied to the amount of validation they can receive from others.

Before we go into the discussion about the different attachment styles, grab a pen and write down responses to the following questions:

1. Can you remember the earliest memory being held by your parents? What did that experience feel like?

2. How would you describe the bond between you and your primary caregiver (the person who spent the most time taking care of you)?

3. Looking back to your early childhood, do you believe that your safety and affection needs were met?

4. Try to visualize your five-year-old self. What did that little boy or girl need to feel protected and cared for?

5. Based on the relationship with your primary caregiver, what kind of child were you? For example, were you extroverted, withdrawn, untrusting, temperamental, or confident?

Anxious Attachment

It is possible that you learned codependency as a result of how you were raised. Your physical and emotional needs may have been neglected, or fulfilled on random occasions, which taught you that love is conditional. Love felt like it had to be earned, rather than provided willingly.

The idea of love being conditional may have even led to harmful beliefs about intimacy and closeness with others. For example, you may have grown up believing that you needed to act a certain way to be accepted by others. Or being yourself and unapologetically expressing your needs may have felt unsafe, due to your caregivers dismissing your emotions, or overriding your right to choose how to experience reality.

Your early childhood ideas and beliefs about intimacy and closeness can be traced back to the type of attachment you formed with your primary caregiver, and reflected in your intimate adult relationships. Out of the four attachment styles outlined by the attachment theory, anxious attachment best describes how your codependent issues may have come from.

Anxious attachment develops during childhood as a response to inconsistent parenting. This means that your primary caregiver may have been physically present, but couldn't always recognize or respond promptly to your needs. Overtime, the patterns of inconsistent parenting created a strong need for your caregiver's affection, as well as a fear of losing or being separated from them.

A common behavior of a child with anxious attachment is crying uncontrollably whenever their primary caregiver leaves, like when the parents go to work or drop the kid off at daycare. While feeling nervous about being left alone is normal for most kids, it feels like abandonment for a child with anxious attachment.

Other common behaviors that are typical to inconsistent parenting are attention-seeking behaviors, like being completely silent, throwing tantrums, deliberately behaving badly, or being excessively clingy. The inconsistency can also cause confusion about what to expect from the caregiver in the future. As a result, the parent-child relationship can feel unpredictable and the child may struggle to feel comfortable in the presence of their parents.

Anxious attachment can follow you into adulthood and affect how you relate with others, particularly intimate partners. Since receiving love came with conditions when you were growing up, you may be drawn, or even seek out, people who are emotionally unavailable. As much as you try to avoid these types of lovers, the relationship dynamic feels familiar to you. Moreover, there is a part of you that believes you *can* earn the other person's love and inspire them—through your generous giving—to reciprocate your affection.

In exchange for responding to your partner's needs, you might desire for them to give you constant reassurance that they are not going to leave. When you are not given this reassurance, you may feel anxious, jealous, or suspicious of their motives. Remember, anxious attachment causes a fear of abandonment, and perhaps the worst thing that an intimate partner could do isn't necessarily treat you badly, but instead decide to seek affection from someone else, or end the relationship altogether.

The question about whether your partner loves you might constantly run through your mind, making you more vigilant for any signs of rejection. When you notice them becoming distant, for reasons unrelated to you (e.g. increased workload, personal family issues, or working on personal goals), your response may be to lean in, and dedicate more of your time and energy serving them. It is also normal for childhood attention-seeking behaviors to come up, which can create conflict in your relationship.

Addressing anxious attachment requires different kinds of interventions, many of which we will discuss later on in this book. However, for now, you can practice recognizing and accepting uncomfortable emotions that may be triggered by perceived disregard, avoidance, or rejection.

Emotions are messengers that arise inside your body to communicate how you are feeling about a particular experience. They are neither good nor bad, but instead show up to help you interpret what you are sensing. Whenever you sense a strong emotion arising, practice taking a powerful pause. Stop what you are doing and be still. Interrupt any thought that might cause your emotion to grow even stronger. Simply whisper to yourself, "not right now."

End the powerful pause when you feel calm, then begin to interpret your emotional experience. With curiosity, reflect on what you felt and put a name on it. For instance, was the emotion anger? If so, how could you tell? Did you feel your chest tightening or heart racing? Did you have an urge to yell or hurt your partner in some way?

Go a step further and think about what message the emotion came to deliver. In other words, based on the context of the situation, how come you felt angry? What happened that might have triggered this specific emotion? When you have gathered enough insight, complete the following sentence:

I feel [emotion] because [the reason behind the emotional trigger]. For example:

- I feel angry because my partner spoke to me in a way that felt unloving.
- I feel disregarded because I spent the night cooking for my mother, and she didn't show any appreciation.
- I feel embarrassed because I expressed a need to my friend, and they shut me down.

Recognizing and accepting your emotions may not heal your anxious attachment; however, it can help you learn how to be compassionate and responsive to your own needs.

Dysfunctional Families and Codependency

There is no such thing as a picture-perfect family. By nature, families fight as much as they fiercely love and protect each other. Parents and children will clash, and sometimes go days without speaking to one another. But that is how intimate relationships tend to be.

With that being said, there are some families that are dysfunctional, meaning that one or a few members within the family behave in ways that negatively impact the well-being of others. Some of the problems that might cause the dysfunctional dynamic include joblessness, depression, addictions, or personality disorders.

To better understand what dysfunctional families look like, we can compare them to how functional families are arranged. The table below provides common differences.

Functional Family	Dysfunctional Family
Enjoy spending time together, despite being of different ages and having different responsibilities.	Feel uncomfortable in family members' company, and tend to live separate lives.
Both parents and children honor rules and boundaries, but at times are willing to negotiate.	There are no clear rules and boundaries between parents and children, or that hold each family member accountable for their actions.
Parent-child bonds are built on mutual respect and acceptance of individual preferences.	Parents tend to show favoritism amongst children (i.e. the smartest or most agreeable child gets preferential treatment), or present respect as something that children need to earn.
Children receive unlimited and unconditional affection, and are raised in a safe environment where they can just be kids.	Children may feel unloved or neglected due to their parents' invalidating or harmful behaviors. Some children may also take on adult responsibilities at a young age, or be exposed to traumatic situations.
Family members are given the space to disagree with each other and have their own opinions, without feeling judged or intimidated.	Family members fear expressing their thoughts and feelings out of fear of upsetting one or few family members, which may lead to conflict.

Being raised in a dysfunctional family can make you vulnerable to developing codependency issues. The reason for this is that you were deprived of the one thing that every child deserves—emotional validation. The inability to receive empathy or unconditional love from your parents may have created an insatiable need to be accepted or feel wanted by others.

The lack of emotional validation also could have taught you to hide your needs and emotions. Back then, this may have been the only way to cope with feeling dismissed, criticized, or neglected by your parents. In adult relationships, the same behavior can cause you to attract abusive people, who continue to make you feel dismissed, criticized, and neglected.

What makes codependency seem "normal" to someone who grew up in a dysfunctional family is the fact that they were conditioned to accept unhealthy patterns of bonding and affection as being the standard behavior. For example, someone who wasn't allowed to voice their concerns or share opposing views, will most likely grow up to become someone who finds it difficult to assert boundaries with others. It isn't because they don't see the need for boundaries, but rather they weren't taught that asserting boundaries is okay.

Another example is someone who was raised in a dysfunctional family where anybody who wasn't a family member was seen as an outsider, and met with suspicion. They may have been taught to conceal family secrets and never show any signs of disloyalty to the core family. In adult relationships, they may struggle to speak out against abusive or unfair treatment from others, as this may be considered being disloyal. Moreover, shutting out friends and family from the relationship can create an unhealthy dependency on their intimate partner.

Before we move on to discussing different roles in a dysfunctional family, grab a pen and answer the following questions about your family:

1. Do you remember family members abusing drugs or alcohol growing up?

2. Were you raised by a parent who suffered from a mental illness?

3. Was it normal for family members to go for long periods of time without speaking to each other?

4. Was it normal for family members to yell, insult, mock, or physically attack each other?

5. Were there secrets in your household that were kept hidden from non-family members?

6. Were there some topics that were kept off limits in your household, such as mentioning negative emotions or bringing up a family member's abusive behavior?

7. Were you robbed of your childhood by assuming adult responsibilities at an early age?

8. Did many family conflicts revolve around one family member's dysfunctional behaviors?

9. Were one or more family members emotionally, physically, or sexually abusive?

10. Did you often dread seeing or being in the presence of one or more family members?

If you answered yes to one or more of these questions, it is likely that your codependency issues are, to some extent, a result of your family upbringing. This realization can be comforting because you at least know where you may have learned some of your behavioral patterns.

Six Dysfunctional Survival Roles

In order to cope in the dysfunctional environment and maintain relationships with each other, family members tend to adopt survival roles. You can think of survival roles as the substitute identities that each family member creates to preserve their sanity and prevent as much psychological harm to themselves as possible.

These survival roles can be adopted by parents and children; however, they have more negative long-term effects on children. It is also common for family members to adopt more than one role, or switch between roles whenever there are changes in the family. Nonetheless, the longer a substitute identity is maintained, the easier it is to integrate it to the real self, thereby causing semi-permanent personality and behavioral issues—including codependency.

Below are six types of survival roles you are likely to find within a dysfunctional family:

1. Addict

The addict can be a parent or child that develops a substance or behavioral addiction. This may be the best way they know how to cope with stress or difficult life changes. For example, after losing a job, the parent might develop a drinking problem as a way to cope with financial burdens. Or as a way to cope with being emotionally abused by their parent, the child may develop a food addiction.

The addict is oftentimes the one whom family conflict is centered around. Due to their addict behaviors, they may play the role of a victim or rebel. The constant turmoil they create within the family is fueled by their ongoing addiction.

2. Co-addict

The co-addict is usually the closest person to the addict. They might feel like they know the addict better than anyone else, and therefore enable most of their harmful behaviors. It is common for the co-addict to have codependency issues, since they seek approval and desire to "stay in the good books" of the addict.

When they are a parent, the co-addict can take the side of the addicted parent over the children. Their undying devotion to the addict is something they never want to be questioned, even when it means turning a blind eye to abusive behaviors. When the co-addict is a child, they might tolerate any kind of treatment from their addicted parent, despite the harm it may cause to them. They may even view their parent from an idealistic point of view, creating an almost godlike image that cannot be challenged.

3. Peacemaker

The peacemaker tends to suffer from chronic anxiety. They are on constant alert for any signs of conflict, and quick to find ways of defusing it. What's interesting about the peacemaker is that they aren't loyal to any particular family member, which allows them to observe family dynamics, various personality traits of members, and lead with empathy when seeking to resolve conflict.

Due to their calm and understanding approach, they are able to get through to the addict and the co-addict, and make them aware of the impact of their behaviors on other family members. Of course, this may not lead to changed behaviors, but it can cause temporary reconciliation.

The peacemaker is vulnerable to codependency issues because, as part of their caretaking responsibilities, they often prioritize the needs of others and suppress their own needs. Children who are peacemakers tend to become adults who subconsciously seek partners they can take care of, such as people with mental health or chronic physical illnesses. The desire to attempt to save others from experiencing the consequences of their actions is something that the peacemaker will find very difficult to switch off.

4. Golden child

The golden child is the one who is given preferential treatment by the addict. In the addict's eyes, this particular child can do no wrong. The reason why this child is chosen over the others is due to their desirable qualities. For instance, they may be born with a unique talent, look extremely beautiful, or show above average competence at school.

These are all qualities that the addict sees as reflections of their own desirability. In other words, the golden child is not praised because of how phenomenal they are, but because of how good they make their parent look.

The golden child grows up believing that they are only good when they are achieving something. As such, they may grow up to be perfectionists, people-pleasers, or adopt different personas depending on who they are around.

5. Mascot

The mascot is typically one of the younger kids in a family, who is born into an already dysfunctional environment. Similar to the peacemaker, they can also suffer from chronic anxiety; however, they deal with it by finding ways of making the atmosphere at home lighter.

For instance, they will always use humor to defuse a tense situation or distract themselves from confronting strong emotions. Every time they are able to make other family members laugh, they feel an even greater responsibility to provide humor during stressful situations. Consequently, they are never able to express their thoughts and feelings with others because of the clownish personality they have created.

Children who are mascots are likely to grow up as people-pleasers who calm the fears of others through humor or other light-hearted behaviors. This can easily put them in a caretaker role, where they can use their "clown skills" to make their loved ones feel comforted.

6. Lost child

The lost child copes with the dysfunction at home by isolating themselves from other family members, and taking care of their own needs as much as possible. They are most likely to be labeled as the "rebel" or "black sheep" of the family because of their deliberate refusal to play along with the unhealthy patterns of behaviors that exist.

A lost child may grow up to have self-esteem issues, see themselves as a victim, or look for people who can take care of them. Instead of attracting needy people, they are often the one who displays needy or clingy behaviors in adult relationships.

As mentioned above, the consequences of being part of a dysfunctional family are mostly felt by children. From the time they are born, children raised in these types of homes lose touch of what is normal and healthy. What is important for them is surviving the treacherous environment they are born into, and this leads to developing survival instincts that make them feel safe.

We have explored four risk factors that can make you vulnerable to developing codependency. These are trauma, mental illness, attachment issues, and being raised in a dysfunctional family. Once again, it is possible to have experienced any of these risk factors and not develop codependency issues. Nonetheless, it is still good to reflect and assess the role and impact of past experiences, including your childhood upbringing, on how you relate and form bonds with others.

Recognize How Codependency Looks In Different Relationships

"The child lacking a sense of welcome, joyous belonging, gratuitous security, will learn to hoard the limited supply of affection [...] When the gift of belonging with is denied, the child learns that love means belonging to."

— SAM KEEN

Recognizing Codependency in Different Relationships

Codependent relationships won't all look the same. In some relationships, the roles of giver and taker may not be so obvious, perhaps due to the nature of the relationship.

A good example would be the relationship between an employee and a manager. An employee signs a work contract to carry out certain tasks and responsibilities. It is perfectly acceptable for the manager to offer direction on how to complete these tasks and responsibilities, but when they are constantly looking over the employee's shoulder, redoing completed work, or being overly "helpful," they may start to micromanage.

If neither the employee nor manager know what the signs of codependency look like, they both might accept this controlling relationship as being normal. Think of a time when you felt like a powerless employee under the leadership of a dominant boss. Were you aware that you were part of a codependent relationship?

The following section will look at various real-life examples of codependent relationships, beyond the common romantic relationship. However, before we go into each example, it is important for you to learn the basic signs of codependency, as these are the red flags that show up early into any kind of relationship. These signs include:

- One person has the need to prove themselves to another.
- One person's self-worth is tied to how useful they can be to another.
- One person unconsciously apologizes constantly to another.
- One person decides to withhold their opinions to maintain peace in the relationship.
- One person has the tendency to avoid confrontation.
- One person has the tendency to ignore or downplay their own needs and desires.
- One person feels an excessive need to help, save, or fix another.
- One person feels guilty doing something for themselves.
- One person agrees to doing activities they don't enjoy to please another.
- One person experiences an overwhelming fear of rejection or abandonment.

While the context of your codependent relationship may be different, you will be able to notice a few of the signs mentioned above. When this happens, you have the opportunity to turn things around and restore a balanced power dynamic between you and the other person.

Codependency in Romantic Relationships

Two people enter a romantic relationship out of the desire to be together. The unspoken expectation is that both people will strive to respond to each other's needs. For as long as the couple continues to balance the amount of giving and taking, the relationship can remain mutually beneficial. But as soon as one person develops an over-reliance on their significant other, codependency issues can emerge.

The common myth about codependency in romantic relationships is that someone who is independent cannot develop codependency issues. The underlying belief behind this myth is that being self-sufficient prevents neediness.

The truth, however, is that independent people can find themselves entangled in codependent relationships. They may be completely self-sufficient, but have an unhealthy desire to be needed by others. This unhealthy desire is what attracts an independent person to a needy and clingy individual, who doesn't mind giving them the validation and sense of control they seek.

Another common myth about codependency in romantic relationships is that developing this type of dynamic is a choice. In the past, you may have listened to people say to you, "Stop trying to rescue people!" or "Why do you care about someone who obviously doesn't care about you?" These kinds of sentiments imply that you have a choice in the matter, as though you can flick a switch and eliminate your caretaking tendencies.

However, the relationship between a giver and taker is far more complicated than that. The act of taking care of others to the point of sacrificing their own needs is not something the giver is conscious of most of the time. But even when they do notice the power imbalance in their relationship, it is something that brings much anxiety and shame, rather than changed behavior.

For many givers, the need to take care of others began at a young age, before they were even aware that they were behaving in that manner. It was a coping mechanism to deal with stress and maintain relationships with loved ones. In other words, caretaking was a survival instinct that made the giver feel safe, and provided a false illusion of being loved and accepted by their caregivers. The more they self-sacrificed, the better they felt about themselves.

This is why caretaking in codependent romantic relationships isn't much of a choice. Even in adult relationships, it is still a viable coping mechanism to deal with stress and feel some kind of connection to one's significant other. The giver's sense of self-worth is linked to how much love they can earn. Therefore, there are no limits to how much they can do for the man or woman they love.

Lastly, there is a difference in codependent romantic relationships between helping and enabling your significant other. Helping your partner generally refers to offering assistance or support. When they are upset, for example, you may offer to listen and empathize with what they are going through. The aim is to empower them to get out of the rut, so they can find a solution to their problem.

Enabling strives to keep your partner depended on your care and support. Instead of empowering them to solve their own problem, you create dependency by solving the problem for them, helping them avoid consequences, or telling them what they want to hear. As a result, your partner may learn to seek help from you whenever they find themselves in trouble, rather than relying on their own skills, insight, and experience to overcome challenges.

Based on the explanation offered above, here are a few real-life scenarios of what codependency looks like in romantic relationships:

Over-compromising

Tanya's partner expresses that they want to see more of her. This request comes after a conversation about her busy work schedule. During the conversation, she mentions how work is going to demand a lot more of her time because she is working on exciting career goals.

Unfortunately, her partner is less than excited to hear about the news, since it means that he won't get to spend as much time with her.

Out of fear of jeopardizing her relationship, Tanya makes an agreement to spend two nights out of the week at her partner's place. This compromise doesn't seem to satisfy him, citing that he feels like he is competing with her work.

To avoid further conflict about this issue, Tanya agrees to spend four nights out of the week at his place. This arrangement seems to be enough to get him off her back, but it also means that Tanya isn't able to devote as much time to her career goals as she had planned.

Dependency on their advice

Pete struggles to make up his mind when making decisions and often goes to his partner for advice on what to do. Every choice, whether small or large, gets approved by his partner before he can take action.

At the beginning of their relationship, this was quite a turn on. He loved the idea of his partner having so much of a say about important matters in his life. However, after some time, this feeling has been replaced with the fear of not getting his partner's approval on important decisions.

For example, their "no" feels ten times worse than any kind of rejection. It doesn't matter how excited Pete was about the plan, hearing "no" from his partner is enough to cancel whatever idea he had in mind.

Moreover, when his partner expresses disapproval about someone, like Pete's friend or family member, he regards their opinion as the truth, and assumes the same negative attitude toward their loved one. In Pete's eyes, his partner knows better than him, and is more capable of making good decisions on Pete's behalf.

Desire to be needed

Brandon enjoys playing the provider role in his romantic relationship. As such, he tends to attract women who desire to be financially taken care of. This doesn't bother Brandon like it would other people because he finds pleasure in being depended upon. Sometimes, he goes as far as setting restrictions on how much money to give his girlfriend, asking for receipts as proof of their purchases, or creating rules on how they are supposed to spend their money.

For as long as his girlfriend remains reliant on his financial allowances, Brandon maintains the upper hand in the relationship. He feels a sense of self-worth for being able to take care of his significant other, and less fearful about the possibility of his girlfriend leaving him.

Codependency in Parent-Child Relationships

Besides romantic relationships, codependency can also appear in parent-child relationships. Typically, the primary caregiver (in most cases, the mother) will form an unhealthy attachment with their child, to the extent of controlling the child's life. To outsiders, this parent-child attachment may seem normal and loving, but behind closed doors, the parent may be either overly-reliant or exert dominance over their child.

Since codependency in parent-child relationships can be so subtle, below are a few tell-tale signs to look out for:

- **Parent holds too much control.** The parent's self-worth thrives on their child's neediness. They seek to take away as much autonomy as possible from their child to keep them in a state of constantly seeking their physical, emotional, or financial support.
- **Parent does not respect boundaries.** The parent views their child as an extension of themselves, therefore they don't see a need to respect their child's boundaries. They may be overly invested in their child's private life, stalk them on social media, share their child's personal secrets with others, or refuse to take their child's "no" seriously.
- **Parent sacrifices other relationships to care for their child.** The parent may devote 24 hours, 7 days a week, to spending time and nurturing their child. Consequently, other relationships with friends and family may fall away. It is also common for the codependent parent to be a single mother or father, or have a strained relationship with their romantic partner.
- **Parent manipulates their child's emotions.** Due to the desire for control, the parent learns various tactics to get their child to behave exactly how they want. Instead of using aggressive strategies, like yelling or name-calling, which may not always get the child to act accordingly, the parent may learn passive-aggressive strategies, like using the silent treatment, projecting their feelings, stirring up guilt.
- **Parent believes that they are always right.** The parent finds it difficult to recognize when they are in the wrong and apologize for their mistakes. In their world, they are always right, and may feel personally attacked when confronted about their harmful behaviors.
- **Parent fears disciplining their child.** Due to the fear of rejection, the codependent parent fears setting boundaries with their child and correcting bad behavior. They would much rather prefer overlooking disrespect and preserving a good relationship with their child than enforcing discipline and risk being disliked by their child.

Codependency in parent-child relationships can lead to emotional abuse. The child may feel unsafe to express their genuine thoughts and feelings, which causes them to comply to the needs of their parent. When they reach adolescence, they may find it difficult to develop their own identity separate from their parent, or may feel uncertain about gaining independence, speaking up for themselves, or imagining a life where they don't need their parent's assistance.

Please note that codependent parents are not necessarily abusive; however, the excessive need for control can, in some cases, trigger personality disorders like NPD or BPD. For example, a codependent parent becomes manipulative when they play the victim in order to make their child feel guilty or lure them into taking care of them. Alternatively, a codependent parent displays narcissistic traits when they value their own feelings and comfort above their child's, and only seek control to keep the child in a submissive position.

Based on the explanation offered above, here are a few real-life scenarios of what codependency looks like in parent-child relationships:

Extreme focus on the child

Suzanne's world revolves around the safety of her child. Due to her own tumultuous upbringing, she is committed to providing her child with the utmost affection. She monitors several cameras around the house to track her child's movements. To rule out illnesses, her child's body temperature is kept at a specific level, and all inflammation-causing foods are banned from their home—including sugary treats like soda, candy, and chocolates.

As part of keeping her child safe, Suzanne has also implemented certain rules regarding who has access to her child, and how much time they spend with them. When her child is unhappy, she feels personally responsible for their moods. Her sole task in those moments is to give her child whatever they need to make them happy again. At times, Suzanne is unable to cheer her child up, and this makes her feel like an incompetent parent.

Guilt-tripping

Divina often shares her painful childhood memories with her child. She feels as though people from her past were never held accountable for the wrong committed against her. Having a child has been Divina's way of finally getting somebody to pay for the wrongdoings of those in her past. She expects her child to provide the care that wasn't given to her as a little girl.

Divina's child is too young to understand her mother's complex needs, and how to respond to them in the exact manner she likes. At times, her child rebels and attempts to draw a boundary. However, Divina quickly pulls out the victim card to garner sympathy. The end goal is to get her child to perform the various caretaking duties that are required. When her child complies, they are rewarded with positive reinforcement, like being given a hug or told how much they are loved.

Being overly emotional

Jaden doesn't respond well when her child refuses to do what she says—which in her mind is seen as a sign of disrespect. Instead of expressing how she feels and giving her child an opportunity to respond, Jaden becomes emotional.

Sometimes, she might yell and make verbal threats. Other times, she uses the silent treatment and withholding affection to show her disapproval. Whenever it seems like she is losing an argument, she tends to divert attention away from herself and recall a painful past experience that makes her cry hysterically.

All of these displays of emotion make it difficult for Jaden to listen during arguments and empathize with her child. Without properly listening, she can make the wrong assumptions about her child's intentions, like accusing them of being insensitive or spiteful. What's important to her at those moments is how uncomfortable, disrespected, or unloved she feels.

Codependency in Friendships

It takes more than shared interests to make a friendship work. Like any relationship, there must be a good balance of give and take. A friendship where one person is doing most of the communicating, organizing, or supporting can create codependency.

One of the ways of keeping a friendship healthy is to establish solid boundaries. These boundaries are what protect both parties' needs, values, and interests from being taken for granted. When there aren't clear boundaries between friends, the two can become enmeshed in one another, and lose their sense of individuality.

Enmeshment won't always feel like you are being suffocated by your friend. At times, it can be as subtle as thinking and feeling the same way as them. This should raise alarm bells, especially if you remember having unique opinions, beliefs, and goals before you started getting close with your friend. The mark of true friendship isn't about finding your "twin" or "better half" who can finish your sentences and physically feel your distress. True friendship is about creating a safe space where two unique individuals can express who they are and feel supported.

Besides a lack of boundaries, codependent friendships create a power imbalance, where one friend does most of the giving, and the other does most of the taking. Below are a few signs of codependency in friendships:

- **One friend seeks constant reassurance.** This friend might need excessive amounts of support through long phone calls, chronic texting, or asking for your advice on a number of different life circumstances. When there are brief moments of silence, they may suspect that something is wrong in your friendship.
- **One friend spends too much time fixing the other's problems.** Giving solicited and unsolicited advice can become a habit, especially for a friend who enjoys feeling needed by others. They will invest a lot of time and energy in analyzing their friend's problem, and offering solutions—even though they may have unresolved issues of their own.
- **When one person is upset, the other feels upset, too.** Codependent friends often share emotions because of how few boundaries they have around their emotional lives. After some time, their moods can be dictated by how the other person is feeling.
- **One friend feels energized, while the other feels drained after spending time together.** The taker tends to lean on their giver friend for emotional support. In true giver style, they will expend all of their time and energy to make sure their friend leaves feeling lighter and happier. The same supportive environment is not created for the giver, which often means they walk away feeling emotionally exhausted.
- **One or both friends relies significantly on the survival of the friendship.** Codependent friends don't typically have many other friends outside their relationship. They heavily rely on each other to fulfill a heap of needs. Both the giver and taker in the dynamic get something out of the friendship, which perpetuates the cycle of codependency.

Codependency in friendships tends to be glamorized and seen as a measure of how much the friends love each other. The truth, however, is that codependency creates an obsession with the other person, not a genuine affection toward them. It is seeing your friend as an object that you can use to satisfy your emotional needs, and not a human being who has unique desires and outlook on life.

There isn't any real respect and connection between codependent friends, even though it may feel like it. What keeps the friendship going is the transactional power dynamic, where both the giver and taker get something out of being friends with each other. When the codependent friendship ends, it is common to have doubts about whether the friendship was real in the first place—or if it was simply the result of one person being needy and the other person desiring to be needed.

Based on the explanation offered above, here are a few real-life scenarios of what codependency looks like in friendships:

Feeling emotionally drained

Hannah's friendship with Buella consumes most of her time and energy. During the week, the two of them text constantly throughout the day, and every weekend is spent together.

Over time, Hannah has noticed that her friend relies significantly on her for emotional support. Whenever she struggles to get out of bed, resolve conflict with her boyfriend, or deal with everyday stress, Buella's first instinct is to call Hannah.

Hannah feels guilty for needing time away from Buella, even though she knows that it will be good for her mental health. Since the friendship began, her needs have taken a back seat because of the amount of problems constantly arising in Buella's life that require Hannah's undivided attention. Nevertheless, she knows that if she continues to give unconditional support, she will soon reach the point of emotional burnout.

Support from one direction

TJ has always been an attentive friend, who intuitively knows how to respond to his friends' needs. He has built a reputation for saving his friends from the most outrageous situations, and making sure that they are taken care of. However, over the past few years, he has noticed that whenever he needs help, his friends are unavailable.

The first few times weren't a big deal. He was low on cash and needed a favor from close friends, who all politely declined. On another occasion, TJ asked one of his best buddies to fetch him from the airport the following week, but once again they were unable to assist him.

The most recent time, TJ was struggling with a difficult coworker and needed someone to vent to. He tried calling a few of his close friends, but only one picked up his call. When he began speaking, his friend found ways of turning the conversation to him, explaining a recent fight with a coworker. TJ never got the opportunity to open up and share his feelings. Instead, he ended up giving his friend advice on how to resolve the conflict with his coworker.

Jealousy over other relationships

Indigo and Sam are best friends. They work similar jobs, live in the same neighborhood, and enjoy the same social activities. Recently, Sam got into a romantic relationship. At first, Indigo seemed supportive, but after some time, she expressed feeling left out.

For the first time, Indigo doesn't get to see or talk to Sam every day. This adjustment hasn't been easy, since she depended on her friend for validation. Now that they hardly get to see each other, Indigo feels inadequate as a friend. She is upset with Sam for seemingly abandoning her, but also secretly yearns for the same bond Sam shares with her boyfriend.

As the giver, Sam tries to spend equal amounts of time with her best friend and boyfriend, but doesn't get it right all the time. She feels guilty, knowing that Indigo is having a hard time adjusting, and attempts to show her in different ways that their friendship will remain unchanged. What she doesn't realize is that the only thing that would satisfy Indigo is if Sam were single again, so she could have her undivided attention.

Codependency in Work Relationships

Codependency issues exist at work, as much as they do at home. Codependent workers step into a workplace and quickly make it their own. They feel personally responsible for achieving the mission of the company, or turning their department into a success.

On the surface, this seems great. After all, employees who are passionate and self-driven are every employer's dream. Unlike other employees, codependent workers don't need to be pushed or supervised to perform their job. They are typically high-performers and will deliver exceptional results from day one.

To get ahead in the company, codependent workers will go as far as studying their coworkers, from colleagues within their team to senior managers on an executive level. They want to know who does what, and how to appeal to each individual's needs.

Codependent workers will sacrifice their own personal time and energy to impress coworkers and develop good relationships with others. If they aren't careful, they can become overworked and burned out. However, to them, this is a small price to pay to stay on others' good books and advance in their career.

The ugly side of a codependent worker's personality is that they can be controlling. This controlling nature is often seen when things don't go their way. Remember that codependent people seek control from external sources to feel good about themselves. When they are not in a powerful position, they can feel insecure. Even if they are not the person in charge, it is common for the codependent worker to display leadership traits. They feel responsible for supervising their team members and making sure work tasks are carried out in a certain manner.

When their suggestions are not taken, the codependent worker can feel resentful, and find passive-aggressive ways of showing their annoyance. For instance, they might not share information that can assist team members in doing their job (a form of subtle sabotage), or they might privately complain to management about their fellow coworker.

Another explosive trait of a codependent worker is their emotional meltdowns at work. Due to the amount of responsibility they carry upon their shoulders, and the fear of sharing and releasing strong emotions, the codependent worker can experience frequent meltdowns. When they are overwhelmed, they can cry, yell, or criticize others. Since they do such a good job of covering up their frustrations, these meltdowns can seem like they came out of nowhere.

Most times, meltdowns are signs that the codependent worker needs a break. They may have been working tireless hours on a stressful project, managing difficult employees, and neglecting their own physical and mental well-being to produce quality results for the company.

Based on the explanation offered above, here are a few real-life scenarios of what codependency looks like at work:

Obsessive need for control

Joe manages a team of 20 employees. His sense of self is enhanced by the people he works with on a daily basis. Although the team is highly skilled and experienced at what they do, Joe feels the need to constantly watch over them, provide instructions, and assess progress on a weekly basis.

No detail or task performed by team members gets approved without Joe's input. Most times, he will scrutinize the work produced and offer suggestions to improve it. Employees sometimes feel discouraged when their quality work is sent back for further improvements. They believe that Joe's performance standards may be impossible to reach.

Joe believes that he is helping the team by teaching them how to pursue excellence. He was raised by parents who demanded a lot out of him as a child, which led him to become a high achiever. He envisions leading a team of high achievers, who are capable of delivering work that meets his level of satisfaction.

Friend and foe

Selena is a people's person and enjoys networking at work. She can strike up a conversation with anyone, and walk away having made a new friend. Her social skills have enabled her to gain the trust of several coworkers, including her manager and the top boss.

However, Selena has a secret. She isn't the fun, bubbly, and agreeable person that everyone has come to love. In fact, this persona is strictly put on for work purposes.

Behind the mask, Selena is highly critical of others and seeks to have the upper hand in every relationship. Over the years, she has studied human behavior and learned how to interact with different types of people, in a personal and professional environment.

Instead of openly disagreeing with others, she will find discrete ways of venting her frustrations. For instance, she might complain about one coworker to another, play the role of victim to gain sympathy, or use her close proximity to management to influence certain rules and policies at work.

Whenever Selena is accused of doing any of these things, she experiences an emotional breakdown. She fears being disliked or rejected by others, and therefore must have coworkers on her side at all times. Being emotional is her way of deflecting from her questionable behaviors and releasing the anxiety of being found out.

Self-sacrificing

Dorothy is a self-driven "boss babe," who is passionate about her job. However, she sets incredibly high expectations for herself to accomplish exceptional results, all the time!

In the office, she is the first in and last out, but continues to work even at home. Her work day doesn't really have a set start and end time because of the excessive amount of work she willingly takes on.

Dorothy makes it a point to tell others how busy she is. Part of the satisfaction of working hard is getting praise and recognition for her contribution. She feels compelled to share with others how great of a sacrifice she is making by working extra hours and missing out on personal commitments. When she isn't given the attention she wants, she may pout, complain, or play the victim.

It is easy for Dorothy to feel taken for granted by her coworkers when they don't acknowledge her sacrifices. What her coworkers don't realize is that all of her giving is done in exchange for constant validation. For as long as she feels seen and appreciated, she will go above and beyond for them—to the detriment of her own well-being.

Exercises to Become a Better Version of You

Healing codependent relationships is a lengthy process that requires several kinds of interventions, many of which will be outlined in the book. However, to support these interventions, you must start by empowering yourself!

At the end of the day, strategies are just strategies. What makes them effective isn't the step-by-step process, but the person who chooses to implement them. You are the x-factor that makes healing from codependency possible. When you are determined to heal your relationships, you give the various strategies new life.

Below are two exercises to become a better version of yourself within current relationships. Continuously practicing these exercises will open your mind to new ways of relating to yourself and others.

Exercise 1: Recognize and Express Your Needs

Perhaps when you were a child, you didn't feel safe sharing your thoughts and feelings with others, so instead you taught yourself how to deny or minimize your needs. Alternatively, you may have been raised by parents who made you feel inferior to them and constantly criticized or downplayed your needs.

In adult relationships, you can find yourself repeating the same parent-child dynamic; where you play the role of the invisible child and your partner plays the role of the overpowering parent.

To avoid this dynamic from repeating itself, it is important to remind yourself that having needs is not the same as being needy. The aim of adult relationships is to create a safe space where both parties take turns expressing and responding to each other's needs.

However, before you can feel empowered to express your needs, it is important to learn how to recognize what you need in the first place. The best way to recognize your needs is to acknowledge and embrace emotions. If this is an uncomfortable step for you, focus more on exploring what you feel than sitting with your emotions.

Bring your awareness to the physical sensations flowing throughout your body. Notice the parts of your body that feel light and tense. Focusing on your physical sensations can be a beginner-friendly way of teaching yourself to recognize comfortable and uncomfortable sensations. You can learn that comfortable body sensations, like calm breathing or relaxed muscles, make you feel light. In contrast, uncomfortable body sensation, like shortness of breath or stiff muscles, make you feel tense.

The next level is to associate physical comfort and discomfort with emotional messages. For example, when you experience a shortness of breath, what type of uncomfortable emotions might that sensation be signaling? Could it be signaling fear, anxiety, or nervousness? Or when you experience stomach pain, could it be signaling distress, sadness, or loneliness?

Continue to explore the various emotional messages that different physical sensations might be signaling. Write down your observations below. Note that there are no right or wrong answers.

Once you are able to recognize what you are feeling, the next step is to reflect on why you feel that way. Determine what might have happened to signal that particular emotion. Instead of focusing on the recent situation that played out between you and the other person, think back to experiences that have shaped what you deem pleasurable and threatening.

Ask yourself what early childhood conditioning might be at play. Could this situation have triggered childhood fears and insecurities? Did the other person say a word or speak in a way that took you back to experiences? Or did their actions bring back fears of being rejected or abandoned?

Exploring your experiences will help you make sense of why you are feeling emotional, and where your emotions possibly stem from. The more comfortable you are interpreting past experiences, the easier it will be to track your emotions. As you explore, write down memories that come up and how they impacted you below.

Now that you have explored your emotions, you are ready to acknowledge and express your needs. All emotions stem from met and unmet needs.

The feeling of calmness, for example, is proof that your need for emotional safety has been met. But feeling anxious, on the other hand, is proof that your need for emotional safety has not been met.

You can use pleasurable and unpleasurable emotions to identify met and unmet needs. Look at the list of emotions below and identify what met and unmet needs they reveal:

- sadness
- self-doubt
- happiness
- rejection
- feeling loved

When you are feeling strong emotions, recognize that you are suffering because of unmet needs. If your needs were being met, you would feel calm, open, and comfortable. You can think as far back as your childhood to identify unmet needs that could be triggered by present experiences. Once you are able to recognize the unmet need, the final step is to communicate it.

The best way to communicate unmet needs is to be clear and phrase your sentences in a way that makes your request easy to understand. Don't assume the other person can intuitively sense what you need, or how their behaviors may have affected you. You can follow the steps below to improve the way you articulate unmet needs.

To practice this short exercise, think about a common unmet need in any type of relationship (i.e. romantic, parent-child, social, or work relationship), then follow the steps.

- **Describe your observations**

Explain the pattern of behavior that you have picked up. Speak from your point of view, and try not to assume how the situation looks from the other person's side. Use "I" statements to state what you are noticing. E.g. I noticed that you don't acknowledge me when you come back from work.

- **Describe how you feel**

Let the other person know how you feel as a result of their actions. Once again, describe the emotional impact without making judgments or accusations. Use "I" statements to describe your experience. E.g. When you walk past me without greeting or giving me a kiss, I feel unimportant.

- **Be upfront about your needs**

This is your opportunity to express what you need from the other person. Remember that having needs is not the same as being needy. Someone who loves and respects you won't feel burdened by the idea of responding to your needs, especially when you do the same for them. Your needs matter to them because your happiness is what makes the relationship sweeter!

When stating your needs, be upfront. Describe in specific terms what you want them to start doing. E.g. I need you to acknowledge me when you get home by showing affection, like giving me a kiss or hug.

Exercise 2: Start Your Individuation Journey

If you were raised by a codependent parent, then it is possible that you skipped the individuation stage, which often begins in the teenage years. Individuation is the process of finding yourself, separate from your parent's identity. Think of it as a period of exploration where you grapple with different ideas about who you are, what you believe, and which direction you desire to go in life.

The process occurs naturally amongst adolescent children, but since codependent parents tend to be controlling, their children never get to discover who they are, or even form opinions that are unique from theirs.

Individuation has no age limits. It is a lifelong process that accommodates several personal transformations. Whenever you pick up a new life role or responsibility, you have the opportunity to continue the individuation process, and redefine who you are.

If you never undertook the individuation journey when you were younger, the good news is that you can start the process now! Psychiatrist Carl Jung presents five stages for undertaking the individuation journey. However, to prepare for this journey, he explains three aspects of your psyche which play a role in the process: the ego, persona, and shadow (Moulik, 2022).

The ego is the perception you have about who you are. It produces an identity (sense of "I") that makes you aware of being human. Your ego evolves over time, which means that the perceptions you hold about yourself are also likely to change.

The persona is the self-image created to showcase your identity. Unlike the ego, the persona is a mask that is worn to gain approval from others and feel a sense of belonging in a group or community. If you are lucky, your persona will reveal glimpses of who you are, but never the entirety of your being.

The shadow consists of the buried parts of who you are, which are seen as undesirable or unacceptable, according to society's standards. Many of your "dark" traits, like having a short-temper, being envious of others, or people-pleasing, are hidden in the shadow. Nonetheless, under significant stress, these repressed traits are triggered and reveal themselves through actions, attitudes, or dreams.

According to Carl Jung, these elements of the psyche exist in every human being. The challenge is to learn how to strike a good balance between them, so you can build a stable sense of self.

During the individuation journey, your ego, persona, and shadow will reveal themselves. You will get a chance to be acquainted with parts of you that are familiar, parts of you that come as a surprise, and also parts of you that are difficult to accept. Remember that both the acceptable and unacceptable parts of you make up the whole; you are neither completely good nor are you completely bad. You are a culmination of beliefs, mindsets, habits, and traits, which make you unique!

Consider the five stages of the individuation process, and answer the subsequent questions.

Stage 1: Suffering

One of the truths that Buddha taught was, "Life is suffering." By this he meant that in life, we will never be placed in perfect conditions. There will always be good and bad times, which provide both pleasure and pain, thereby causing us to never feel fully satisfied.

The journey of finding who you are begins in a place of suffering because only pain, rather than pleasure, can lead to growth. When you go through difficult times, where your picture-perfect reality is threatened, you get to discover who you are, and what you are truly made of. However, you must choose to learn from your suffering instead of defining yourself by it, in order to self-actualize.

Below are a few questions to help you learn from past suffering:

- What difficult memory are you avoiding?

- What story, belief, or attitude is tied to this memory?

- How is this story, belief, or attitude impacting your life?

- What would happen if you continued to hold on to the story, belief, or attitude?

- What would happen if you chose to let go of the story, belief, or attitude?

- What pain do you need to let go of to make peace with this memory?

Stage 2: Integrating Your Shadow

Once you have acknowledged the parts of you that are in pain, the next step is to accept the traits and behaviors that have been repressed for many years. Any thought, emotion, or behavior that is seen as undesirable or unacceptable is thrown into the shadow, so that your self-image is only made up of what you believe others might approve of.

If you grew up with a codependent parent, it is possible that some aspects of your personality or common childish behaviors were seen as unacceptable. Perhaps your parent didn't approve of you showing anger, being curious, embracing your sexuality, or having strong opinions. To avoid separation between you and your parent, you learned to hide these so-called undesirable parts of you in the shadow.

To fully heal from suffering, emotional wounds and unattended parts of you must be acknowledged and embraced as being a fundamental piece of your life story. You may not identify with some of those dark traits right now, but that doesn't mean that they cannot be brought to light and integrated into your psyche.

Integrating your shadow, also known as shadow work, is an act of self-acceptance (which we will explore in depth later on in the book). Instead of rejecting parts of you that were neglected as a child, you choose to act compassionately and embrace your imperfections.

Below are some questions to lovingly embrace your shadow:

- If you had to describe yourself to someone, which traits would you emphasize and which would you leave out?

- What are some of the family patterns you fear repeating in your adult life? How have these patterns shaped your life?

- In what situations do you feel less than others, equal to others, and better than others?

- What are some beliefs you have inherited from your parents? When were these beliefs introduced to you?

- Describe the earliest memory of feeling rejected by a loved one. What story or belief did you create after that moment?

- When was the last time you felt jealous of someone? What did they have that you wanted for yourself?

- How comfortable are you expressing anger? What are the overt or covert ways you show anger?

- Did you feel accepted for who you are as a child? How much of your true self did you feel comfortable showcasing to others?

- What emotions do you often avoid? How do you avoid them?

- Which aspect of yourself do you find most difficult to accept? What makes it so hard to accept?

Stage 3: Anima/Animus

So far, you have acknowledged past suffering and accepted repressed aspects of yourself. The third stage of individuation is to identify polarities, so you can embrace your "whole" self.

As a child, you may have been taught to be a "good girl" or "good boy," and given specific standards to uphold. However, authenticity is about being your genuine self, which consists of two polarities: anima and animus.

Jung describes the anima and animus as feminine and masculine energy that exists in each human being. Women tend to have more feminine energy than masculine energy, and men tend to have more masculine energy than feminine energy. Finding balance would therefore involve embracing the polar energy that is less active within.

Note that the energy you most resonate with doesn't have to be associated with your gender. For example, there are men who may have more feminine energy than masculine energy. They may feel comfortable around feminine qualities and expressions, and estranged from traditional masculine qualities and expressions. Finding balance for them would entail connecting more to the animus, masculine energy, since that is less active within.

Being fixed on one mode of being, such as embracing only feminine or masculine qualities, means that you constantly tap into the same part of you whenever you are confronted with new life circumstances. For instance, if you are a man, your default response to life might be to think logically, neglecting the emotional impact of the situation. As a woman, your default response to life might be to lead with passion, doing what feels right, rather than what makes logical sense.

Not accepting your polarities therefore means that one side of you is left dormant and cannot be activated to bring about a sense of balance. Below are ways that you can embrace the other half of you, and feel a deeper sense of wholeness.

If you have more masculine energy, connect to your anima by doing the following:

- Listen with the intention of understanding where the other person is coming from.
- Find a hobby, sport, or interest that you are passionate about.
- Tap into your sensual side by practicing romantic gestures.
- Nurture something, like a pet, plant, or child.
- Find creative ways to express yourself, such as drawing, learning a musical instrument, practicing a dance routine, or preparing a new recipe.
- Journal about your thoughts and feelings, or find a trusted therapist who you can talk to.
- Practice self-care by spending time alone, getting sufficient sleep, living an active lifestyle, and setting healthy boundaries.

If you have more feminine energy, connect to your animus by doing the following:

- Practice communicating assertively.
- Find someone to mentor (or find a leadership role in your community).
- Set meaningful goals and hold yourself accountable to achieve them.
- Practice being more self-sufficient (e.g. paying bills on time, improving time management skills, taking care of your household responsibilities).
- Learn a new practical life skill.
- Practice critical thinking, like weighing the pros and cons of a situation or making decisions based on factual evidence.

Stage 4: Wise Man

When you are free to express every aspect of who you are, there is a special kind of empowerment you feel. The inner void or disconnect is gone, and suddenly you are able to express all types of thoughts and emotions without any resistance. There are no hang-ups in displaying anger, joy, or sadness—or even recalling memories that trigger these emotions. You begin to appreciate the uniqueness of your life story and find meaning in your personal suffering.

According to Jung, the archetype activated during this stage is the wise man. When you think of a wise man, think of someone who has gained life experience and has a grounded approach to life. They embrace different views and opinions because they are not afraid of being wrong, or learning something new about themselves.

To assess how much you have discovered about yourself thus far, below are wise self-reflection questions to explore:

- What have you done, and continue to do in your life, that works for you? What are the signs that it is working?

- What negative habits are you aware of that you need to let go? What obstacles are preventing you from letting them go?

- Think of a childhood struggle that you have survived. What lesson or lessons have you learned from that struggle?

- Which relationships in your life feel safe and loving? What has it taken to create safety in these relationships?

- Which relationships in your life need more forgiveness? What would it take for you to practice forgiveness in each of these relationships?

Stage 5: Self-Consciousness

Self-consciousness is the pinnacle of wholeness. When you are self-conscious, you are aware of who you are and why you react to life the way you do. This doesn't mean that you are flawless, but instead that you are aware of your strengths and flaws. At this stage, you are able to practice self-compassion and accept both good and bad accepts of who you are. This in turn makes it possible to empathize with others and be less judgmental of their flaws and bad traits.

It takes going through these five stages to complete the process of individuation. As you can tell, this journey isn't one that can be completed overnight. It will take time to address past social conditioning, make sense of and acknowledge childhood traumas, heal emotional wounds, and eventually see yourself as an integrated being. Nonetheless, each step of this journey offers healing and helps you become a better version of yourself.

End the Terror of Obsessive Thinking

"Yes, I am a prisoner of sorts, but my prison isn't the house. It's my own thoughts that lock me up!"

— V.C. ANDREWS

What Does Obsession Have to Do With Codependency?

In the previous chapter, we looked at real-life examples of codependency in different kinds of relationships. While each type of relationship had its own unique dynamic (E.g. parent-child versus employee-employer), there was a common thread running through all of them—the obsession with the other person.

Codependency issues make it tough for the giver to be themselves. After all, who are they apart from their loved one? Instead of openly expressing who they are, they try to predict what the taker might want to hear or feel, and adopt those thoughts and feelings. Since their self-image is largely based on their role of serving the taker, the giver spends a lot of time thinking about what the taker needs.

It is natural to think about someone you care about a few times a day. When you eat lunch, you might wonder if they have eaten. Or when the weather changes, you hope they packed a jacket in their work bag.

Codependent people spend a disproportionate amount of time thinking about their loved ones, to the extent of getting distracted from their own work or life commitments.

The giver in the relationship might structure their lives around the taker. The decisions made about their personal life depend on what is good for the other person in the relationship. For example, a giver may turn down a promotion at work, if it means there will be traveling involved, and they will be forced to spend days away from their loved one. Or they may throw away a certain type of clothing (e.g. short dresses) that make their loved one feel uncomfortable, regardless of how they feel wearing the clothing.

The obsession to make the taker happy and comfortable stems from early childhood conditioning, where the giver received the following subconscious messages from their primary caregiver:

- "Your needs don't matter."
- "I am the number one priority in your life."
- "You are selfish for thinking about yourself."
- "You are responsible for taking care of the family."
- "Taking care of me is normal."
- "Expressing your feelings is not safe."

The subconscious messages written above explain the obsession that givers develop with takers. Since childhood, the giver was conditioned to believe that self-sacrifice was the only way to nurture important relationships in their life. Spending time thinking about their own needs brought about anxiety about the well-being of the other person. Would the parent be able to cope without their obsessive caretaking? Or would they react with anger and withhold love?

Characteristics of Obsessive Personalities

It is important to emphasize that codependent people don't choose to constantly worry about their loved ones. They are terrorized by involuntary and obsessive thoughts about their loved one's safety and happiness.

If they had a choice in the matter, they would invest most of that time and energy into building themselves up and responding to their own needs. But since prioritizing others was ingrained in them from a young age, they cannot help but possess obsessive traits.

An obsessive personality, medically referred to as "purely obsessional OCD" is a mental health condition recognized in the DSM-5. It is a variant of obsessive-compulsive disorder (OCD), and is characterized by "repeated, intrusive, and uncontrollable thoughts that usually have no outwardly related behavioral compulsions" (Christiansen, 2020).

Instead of displaying outward rituals, they develop mental rituals that involve reviewing information, over and over again. For instance, they might review past childhood memories, or recent interactions with others, and create stories about how that life event or interaction could have turned out differently. The stories could be centered around standing up to their abusive parents, expressing their love for a romantic partner, or planning their revenge on people who have hurt them.

Since codependency isn't yet recognized as a mental health condition by the DSM-5, doctors diagnose the patient with co-occurring conditions, like purely obsessional OCD. However, not every individual who suffers from codependency issues will develop this condition. Some may simply adopt obsessive habits or characteristics that cause them to worry about their loved ones constantly.

A few common obsessive traits found in codependent people include:

1. Exaggerated sense of responsibility

A giver believes that without their help and support, the taker won't survive. They have an urge to be the first one to respond to emergencies by sharing advice, taking on others' burdens, and trying their best to fix things. In a controlling way, they may even believe they are the most reliable or knowledgeable person to solve the taker's problems. Taking on so much responsibility can be draining. Even when they feel compelled to help, the giver is left feeling taken for granted.

2. Seeking others' approval

People-pleasing is an obsessive trait because it directs focus outwardly, by seeking to live up to the standards of others. Codependent adults grew up in households where one parent's needs took priority. As kids, they worked tirelessly to please their parent, especially when doing so would earn them affection. They become accustomed to putting other people's needs first and feeling a sense of pride or heightened self-esteem whenever they secure approval.

3. Poor boundaries

Obsessively worrying about another person is a sign of poor boundaries. Codependent people tend to become overly involved in their loved ones' lives, to the extent of being controlling. They struggle with issues of personal space, privacy, or being told "no." Whenever boundary lines are drawn, such as making a request to limit the number of calls per day, they may perceive the limit as a sign of rejection from their loved one.

4. Obsessing over societal roles

Codependent people need to show up correctly to the world, to avoid being criticized or abandoned by others. Consequently, they obsess over their societal roles, such as being a mother, husband, best friend, or boss. Getting these roles right is important for them because it provides a prebuilt identity they can hide behind, and use to feel responsible and good about themselves. When they fail at these roles, like breaking up with a friend, they can experience a lot of anxiety. Questions like, "Who am I without this identity?" or "Am I good enough?" expose their core fear of rejection.

5. Transactional approach to relationships

Relationships are a tool that codependent people use to find a sense of purpose and meaning. Saying that relationships mean everything to them, is an understatement. Not only do they throw themselves at every relationship (even new ones), they have high expectations for them to provide a sense of validation or meaning. In exchange for providing a sense of validation or meaning, the codependent person will provide extreme caretaking. They will hold onto those relationships, regardless of how unhealthy they are, for as long as they derive some sort of validation or value from being with the other person.

These obsessive traits are not a life sentence. You are able to recover from them, recognizing and seeking support. Later on in the chapter, we will revisit the four stages of codependency recovery, and look at how you can follow them to heal from obsessive tendencies.

Obsessive Love Disorder

Obsessive love disorder (OLD) is a condition that causes sufferers to become obsessed with a person whom they are in love with. Their primary focus is directed to their loved one, and will often go to great lengths to protect them.

Codependency doesn't cause OLD, however, it can make you vulnerable to it. Some of the early signs of the condition to look out for include:

- Being overly attracted to one person.

- Going from "complete stranger" to "romantic partner" extremely quickly.
- Constantly thinking about the other person throughout the day.
- Feeling the need to protect your loved one, even from their own friends and family.
- Seeing your loved one as your possession, someone who belongs to you.
- Feeling intense jealousy when your loved one interacts with other males and females.
- Constantly having doubts about your loved one's faithfulness or trustworthiness.

Similar to codependency, someone who suffers from OLD may struggle to take rejection. To avoid their loved one leaving, they create relationship rituals. For instance, the OLD person may call or text repeatedly during the day and get upset when their partner cannot be reached. Or they might expect their partner to share their location and whereabouts whenever they are not with them. These rituals are disguised as ways to develop closeness and intimacy. However, in reality, they are tactics used to monitor and control the other person.

The Difference Between Love and Obsession

In popular culture, the idea of someone being obsessed with a loved one sounds, well, romantic. The famous "ride or die" archetypal couple defines what many romantic relationships are like in this modern age. Two individuals enter a relationship (in most cases a codependent relationship) willing to sacrifice everything to prove their love.

The test of love, many believe, is seen in how much difficulty you are able to withstand in a relationship. There is an expectation to accept someone's flaws, and help them heal from their past trauma or present day challenges. While nobody enters a relationship being perfect, the modern understanding of love promotes codependency, and opens the door to obsession and abuse.

Due to movies, reality TV shows, and social media influencers, who glamorize codependent relationships, many of us have forgotten the difference between being in love, versus being obsessed with someone. So, what is love?

Love is a strong emotion that causes you to attach to someone else. You feel a powerful attraction or affection toward someone, and desire to take care of them. A loving relationship creates a physically and emotionally safe environment for two unique individuals to bond and feel accepted by each other. Neither of them try to dominate each other, or assume authority in the relationship.

Obsession, on the other hand, is the need to possess or control something or someone. Many times, obsession doesn't start out as a dark emotion. During the early stages of a relationship, the obsessed partner may display extreme passion. They feel enamored by the other person, and may even put them on a pedestal. Being with the person fulfills a core need, such as feeling worthy, validated, or powerful.

However, as the relationship progresses, the passion turns into possessiveness. The obsessed partner doesn't believe they can survive without the other person in their life, and will do whatever they can to make sure their partner remains dependent on them. Obsessive relationships also tend to have a power imbalance, which by the way is intentional.

In order to make it harder for the other person to leave, the obsessed person will seek dominance by controlling resources, limiting access to friends and family, or making all the decisions. Whenever their sense of control is threatened, they may experience extreme jealousy, paranoia, or become abusive.

Loving relationships shouldn't breed insecurities. They should feel like a refuge, where you can let your guard down and freely express who you are. The couple should seek ways of providing positive reassurance to one another, but never feel responsible for playing the role of fixer or rescuer. Both the act of giving and receiving love should be a choice. For instance, you should be able to choose to enter a committed relationship, respond to your partner's needs, and share aspects of your life with them.

Obsessive relationships don't provide couples with a choice to give and receive love. The obsessed person places expectations on their partner to fulfill certain needs. This creates a toxic situation, where the relationship revolves around one person—the one with greater control. It quickly stops becoming about two individuals feeling safe and accepted, and instead becomes about one individual seeking control and the other one feeling trapped and suffocated.

How to Treat Obsessive Love Disorder

OLD can be treated through taking a variety of interventions. The first step is to seek a medical diagnosis from a doctor. Since there isn't specific medication to treat OLD, you may be prescribed antianxiety medication (e.g. Xanax or Valium), antidepressants (e.g. Prozac, Zoloft, or Paxil), mood stabilizers, or antipsychotics.

You may benefit from taking psychotherapy, to identify and address obsessive thoughts, feelings, and behaviors, as well as understand the impact of your early childhood attachment on your current adult relationships. A qualified therapist will teach you positive coping skills to reduce obsessive thoughts, practice mind-body relaxation, and find healthy distractions.

You can also manage obsessive thinking by going through the four stages of codependency, which are outlined below.

Confronting Obsessive Thinking With the Four Stages of Codependency Recovery

In Chapter 1, we looked at the four stages of codependency recovery: abstinence, awareness, acceptance, and action. While these four stages are generally used to treat codependency as a whole, they can also address specific codependent behaviors that you seek to resolve, such as obsessive thinking.

Below is an example of how you can practice the four stages to reduce obsessive thinking:

Stage 1: Abstinence

Abstinence is about restraining from doing something that is habitual or enjoyable. In the case of obsessive thinking, you would make an effort to restrain from thinking about the other person altogether.

This may be difficult, especially because you have developed a habit of excessive thinking or worrying about them. However, just as you learned the habit by repeating specific behaviors, you can unlearn it by practicing different behaviors.

A great dialectical behavioral therapy (DBT) technique that you can practice to abstain from obsessive thinking is called "opposite action." The aim is to do the exact opposite behaviors of what your thoughts and feelings encourage you to do. For instance, if you feel the urge to text, switch off your phone for 30 minutes. Or when an urge to worry about the person comes up, distract yourself by doing a household chore.

Opposite action isn't a way of pushing down your thoughts and feelings. After all, you need to be aware of the obsessive thought in order to choose an opposite action. Instead of pushing down your thoughts and feelings, this technique creates enough distance between you and the stimulus, so that it is easier to deny your urges. It can also relieve stress and anxiety by encouraging you to get out of your head and do something completely different, as a positive distraction.

To practice taking the opposite action, write down a list of your common obsessive thoughts. For each thought, think about the most appropriate opposite action. This could be a positive behavior that you can practice whenever the obsessive thought comes up. Below are a few examples to assist you:

- Whenever you think "I need to take care of them," practice a self-care activity, like going for a haircut, meditating, or cleaning your living space.
- Whenever you think "I'm afraid they are going to leave me," reach out to a close friend or family member for a catch-up call or coffee date.
- Whenever you think "What will our future be like?" find a small goal-related task that you can perform to redirect focus on your future endeavors.

Now it's your turn. Use the examples above to come up with your own suggestions of opposite actions to take whenever you have obsessive thoughts.

Stage 2: Awareness

Awareness is about reflecting on the dynamic of your codependent relationship, and being willing to assess the pros and cons. By nature, codependent relationships are not healthy, but that doesn't mean there aren't any positive elements to it.

Human beings are wired to run toward pleasure and away from pain. This means that even the most toxic relationships offer some type of pleasure, otherwise there would be no incentive for maintaining them. It is important to be honest with yourself about why you obsessively think about your partner, and the fears or incentives that might be fueling your behavior.

Write down what kinds of fears and pleasures you get from worrying about them, putting their needs first, or doing everything possible to prevent them from leaving you. Do your best to examine your behaviors objectively, as though you were an outsider observing someone else's actions. As you seek to understand the intentions and possible benefits of your obsessive thinking, avoid judging or attempting to correct yourself.

Stage 3: Acceptance

Acceptance is perhaps the most difficult stage of codependency recovery because it involves being okay with who you are. For many givers, who were raised or learned from past experiences to put others' first, self-acceptance can trigger feelings of guilt and shame.

For instance, you might not believe you are deserving of love, hence, your need to obsessively think and worry about others. Or, alternatively, you might think that the only way to receive love is to seek validation from those you sacrificially serve. The beliefs and feelings you may have around self-acceptance can be tough to process and make peace with it.

To help you begin the long process of accepting who you are, here are a few journal prompts that you can work on:

- Where are you saying "yes," when you actually mean to say "no?" What makes saying "no" difficult?

- What is something that you are not allowing yourself to feel?

- What do you need that you are afraid to ask for?

- What can you forgive yourself for?

- What challenging conversation do you need to have with yourself?

- How can you stand up for yourself?

- Which aspects of your personality do you need to make peace with?

- Place your hand on your heart. What does your heart need?

- What can you let go of to significantly improve how you view yourself?

- Where do you need more support?

Stage 4: Action

Taking action is about displaying the proof of what you have learned, and the new beliefs, behaviors, and boundaries you are willing to establish in your life. Remember, taking action is never about proving something to anyone, particularly your codependent partner. It is not a way to gain more attention or change their behaviors.

You are positively changing your obsessive tendencies to improve your quality of life.

Fortunately, reducing obsessive thinking can be done by simply abstaining and finding other positive distractions. However, you may feel that taking some time away from the other person can help you think of them less. You have the right to ask for distance if you believe that will help you address obsessive tendencies. Asking for what you need is part of holding yourself accountable to your commitment.

Be strong and resolute when explaining why you need time away, and trust that you know what's best for you!

There are also a few tips you can practice to keep yourself accountable:

- **Get an accountability partner.** This is a person whose job is to follow up with you and make sure you are staying on track with the commitment you have made. An accountability partner can be a trusted friend or relative, or an unbiased third party, like a licensed therapist.
- **Make self-care a priority.** Activities that promote taking care of your needs can keep you from falling back into old habits of self-harm. Make taking care of yourself a daily practice through meaningful tasks like getting proper sleep, exercising, or surrounding yourself with positive influences.
- **Call yourself out when you are making excuses.** Be honest with yourself when you are covering up for bad decisions. In a loving way, seek to understand what's stopping you from sticking to your goal. Is it possible that you are afraid of the other person? Or don't have strong belief in yourself? Confront your denial with compassion and seek to resolve whatever is creating a barrier.
- **Create both short and long-term goals.** It is important to be goal-oriented when seeking to replace obsessive thoughts and behaviors. Divide your goals into short and long-term. Your short-term goals can focus on managing your obsessive thinking (i.e. stages one and two of codependency recovery). Then your long-term goals can focus

on turning new behaviors into habits, and addressing underlying psychological issues (i.e. stages three and four of codependency recovery). If you believe your life is in danger, your primary focus should be on getting out of the toxic relationship and finding a safe place.

- **Reward yourself.** Be the first person to recognize and celebrate your positive behavioral improvements. You don't need to throw a party; however, take the time to reflect on how far you have come, and how challenging (and meaningful) the journey has been for you. Reward yourself by continuing to prioritize your needs and living your life according to your terms!

Please note that obsessive thinking isn't something you can cure overnight. Like any kind of obsession or addiction, it takes a great deal of time and consistent positive reinforcement to learn healthier behaviors. Continue to practice the four stages of codependency recovery to slowly start changing the way you think and behave.

Put Yourself First and Set Boundaries

"Daring to set boundaries is about having the courage to love ourselves even when we risk disappointing others."

— BRENE BROWN

Early Childhood and Boundaries

Boundaries are the invisible lines that separate who you are and what you need, from who others are and what they need. They ensure your values, beliefs, and standards are protected from being violated or disrespected by others.

When you establish proper boundaries to govern different areas of your life, you are able to express who you are with others, without feeling threatened or violated. But in order to establish boundaries, you must first distinguish the difference between healthy and unhealthy behaviors.

This skill may not have been something you were taught as a child, especially if you were raised in a dysfunctional home. As a result, in your adult life, you may be confused about what you should and shouldn't tolerate, or how to speak against harmful behaviors done to you.

No child is born knowing anything about boundaries. The responsibility to teach children how to assert their needs is usually given to parents. Of course, young children will attempt to create their own boundaries by shaking their heads, pushing adults away, or crying. But eventually, as they get older, they will test their parents to see where the boundary lines are, and how much they can get away with.

For children to establish healthy boundaries and feel confident expressing their needs, they must be taught acceptable and unacceptable behavior. Parents create a precedent of what is the "norm" in the household by reenacting certain behaviors in front of their children, showing them what is allowed and forbidden.

In dysfunctional families, good behaviors are not recognized and rewarded enough, while bad behaviors are tolerated and never corrected. This can be confusing to children, who unconsciously learn that there aren't incentives for being good, or ways to hold others accountable for being bad.

Parents in dysfunctional families may also contribute to this confusion by being inconsistent in the types of behaviors they allow and forbid. In most cases, there could even double standards for what is acceptable for parents, but unacceptable for children.

For example, in alcoholic families, where the alcoholic mom or dad is the center of attention, it might be acceptable for them to throw tantrums, but considered unacceptable for their children to display the same emotional outbursts.

Or in families where parents are living with a mental illness, it might be acceptable for them to demand caretaking, but seen as unacceptable for their children to demand the same kind of support and nurturing.

The inability for children to learn and be clear on what is helpful and harmful behavior is what leads to codependency in adulthood—and makes it difficult to establish healthy boundaries. The same way codependent adults tiptoed around their parents and feared confrontation, in the same way they tiptoe around their peers and avoid asserting their needs.

The Need to Address Boundary Violations

Boundary violations are common occurrences for people with codependency issues. You might constantly feel like other people are taking advantage of your kindness, or being inconsiderate of your needs. However, since you are accustomed to placing other people's needs above your own, it is hard to share your true feelings with others, more so when your feelings are negative.

The inability or fear of establishing boundaries may cause you to tolerate any kind of treatment from others. When your feelings have been hurt, you might internalize the anger and frustration, and try not to make a big deal out of it. Most of the time, the people around you may not be aware of how their actions negatively impact you because on the surface, you don't show any signs of being upset or offended.

What is important to remember is that having needs and expressing them to others is natural and normal. Moreover, when people fail to meet your needs, you have the right to acknowledge that you are not receiving something that is important to you, such as respect, support, privacy, or affection. Knowing that you can count on people to respond to your needs is what makes relationships feel safe. Without that knowledge, you may struggle to fully warm up to people.

This also leads us to boundary violations. When a boundary has been violated, you might feel angry, exposed, betrayed, or disrespected. These powerful emotions signal that the relationship doesn't feel safe. In order to restore a sense of emotional safety, it is good to acknowledge what happened and how it made you feel. Express to the other person what boundary they crossed, and what they can do to prevent the same violation in the future.

This conversation is not easy, and in the next chapter, we will look at ways of navigating difficult conversation. However, for now, practice standing up for boundaries and explaining what you need from others. Look into the mirror and show a disapproving expression, or boldly say the words, "I don't like that!" The confidence will come naturally over time, but what matters most is seeing yourself draw the line.

Examples of Boundary Violations and How to Repair Them

Both strangers and loved ones will cross your boundaries. And most times, it may not be intentional. Your job is to learn how to recognize when your boundaries have been crossed, and find ways of regaining a sense of physical and emotional safety.

In this section, we will explore three types of boundaries: physical, emotional, and intellectual. For each, we will discuss what boundary violations look like and how you can address them.

Physical Boundary Violations

Your physical boundaries determine how physically close you desire to be with others. There may be forms of touch that you reserve for specific people only, and feel uncomfortable when others touch you in that manner. For example, kisses may be reserved for your spouse, hugs may be reserved for close friends and family, and with anyone else you prefer handshakes or social distancing.

Examples of physical boundary violations are being physically attacked, deprived of physical touch (i.e. when you are not given the affection you need), as well as when you are touched inappropriately by someone you haven't given consent to. Your body will send signals when physical boundaries have been crossed. For instance, you might freeze, hold your breath, get knots in your stomach, or feel the sensation of your skin crawling.

How to repair boundaries: Ignoring these signals can lead to distrusting your own senses, or perception of danger. After a while of not responding to these violations, you may not show any reaction whenever you are attacked, inappropriately touched, or not given the intimacy you deserve.

Paying attention to your body cues will help you identify when your personal space or body has been invaded, and take action to rebuild your sense of safety. Whenever you are around different people, practice noticing how you feel. How does your body react to being held? How do you feel standing close to them? If you are intimately bonding, what forms of touch make you feel good, and which ones make you feel uncomfortable?

Note that physical boundaries are set depending on how safe you feel around someone, and not the role they play in your life. For example, it is possible to feel unsafe around your siblings, even though you grew up in the same household. Don't be afraid to express discomfort when you are touched inappropriately by a close friend, family member, or coworker. Setting physical boundaries with them doesn't diminish the role they play in your life.

Emotional Boundary Violations

Emotional boundaries separate your needs from other people's needs. Think of them as the protective shield that prevents you from taking on other people's problems or emotions, and adopting them as your own.

The ability to establish strong emotional boundaries is rooted in childhood, particularly in the parent-child relationship. If you were given the space to share your thoughts and feelings, or have different opinions to your parents, then you may be able to take ownership of your emotions, while holding others accountable to theirs.

However, if you were not given the space to share personal thoughts and feelings, but instead were conditioned to think and feel like your parents, it may be difficult for you to determine how you feel about a situation. Whenever someone upsets you, you might feel confused about how to feel or react to the situation. Yes, you may feel angry, but struggle to express yourself, or take ownership of your emotions.

Another example of a poor emotional boundary is allowing others to project their emotions on you. For example, if your friend is upset for personal reasons, you allow them to take out their frustrations on you, through unnecessary arguments, unfair criticism, or other aggressive behaviors. Once again, the inability to draw an emotional boundary is rooted in childhood.

Perhaps you had a parent who was an alcoholic, suffered from bipolar, or had poor emotional regulation skills, and would take out their frustrations on you. Whenever they were upset, the mood in the house would change, and you would feel their wrath. If they were abusive, they may have even said hurtful remarks, like blaming you for their distress or misfortune.

In adult relationships, you might feel personally responsible to keep the other person happy. When they aren't happy, you may feel like you are not doing a good job being there for them. As a way to console the other person, you allow them to dump their emotions on you. The release feels good to them, but unfortunately leaves you feeling drained and responsible for issues that aren't yours to solve.

How to repair boundaries: When your emotional boundaries are violated, relating to others starts to feel unsafe. To protect yourself, you build high walls and defenses, rather than healthy boundaries. Connecting and creating meaningful relationships with people becomes a risk—even with good-intentioned people who desire to show you unconditional love and acceptance.

Emotional boundaries can be repaired by acknowledging your own feelings. If you were raised by parents who often belittled, criticized, or shamed you, being vulnerable and sharing your emotions may not have felt safe. This repeated experience could have taught you to hide, deny, or neglect your emotions, so that you wouldn't feel hurt again.

Acknowledging your feelings is about reopening that aspect of you that once existed as a child. It is about being re-acquainted with the full range of your emotions, and accepting them as valid forms of expressions. Journaling can be a great tool to help you put feelings on paper, and become reacquainted with your emotions. It can even expose recurring emotions and situations that trigger them.

Another aspect of acknowledging your feelings is learning how to affirm your emotional needs. Every human being has emotional needs, which must be maintained in order for relationships to feel safe. Examples of emotional needs include:

- acceptance
- affection
- safety
- trust
- belonging
- empathy
- validation
- kindness

- autonomy
- respect

If the needs above scare you, think about why that is. Could you be deprived of specific needs, and therefore feel apprehensive about asking for them? The relationship with your emotional needs is another theme that you can journal about. You may find that some needs were neglected during childhood, and consequently make you feel uncomfortable.

Nonetheless, not being familiar with your emotional needs, doesn't make them any less important. If you want a challenge, practice looking into a mirror and saying "I need…" followed by one of the needs above. Afterward, mention a sentence about why you need it. For example, "I need respect because I am a unique individual and desire to feel accepted for who I am."

Intellectual Boundary Violations

Intellectual boundaries protect your unique worldviews. They help you understand what you need, value, or believe regarding your life. Healthy intellectual boundaries are flexible enough to allow for learning new information, but assertive enough to interpret the new information based on your ideas and beliefs.

Being raised in a home where your thoughts and opinions are seen as valid, helps you build strong intellectual boundaries as an adult. However, when your outlook on life is too tightly controlled by those around you, you can become dependent on other people's opinions and worldviews.

A typical example is a child who is raised by a codependent parent and lives most of their childhood not making decisions about their life. Every aspect of their day, from when they are going to wake up to what they are going to eat, is decided by their parent. In adulthood, the child may struggle to make life decisions for themselves, and may rely on their parent's or romantic partner's help for most choices that adults would make alone.

Another aspect of an intellectual boundary violation is being told that what you think is wrong or unacceptable. In other words, having someone question your understanding of reality. Not only is this an invasion of your mental space, it can also become a form of manipulation. Gaslighting, for example, is a type of psychological manipulation where the abuser attempts to make you doubt or feel confused about your thoughts and feelings. This is done so that they can distort how you view reality and gain control over your mind.

You have the right to decide on what to think, and how you interpret the world. Be careful of people who make you feel as though your outlook on life is inferior, unrealistic, or something to be ashamed about. Your ideas and beliefs deserve to be treated with respect, and not judged or ridiculed.

How to repair boundaries: Damaged intellectual boundaries cause you to follow whoever is in charge, and adopt their thoughts and beliefs. This puts you in a vulnerable position where you mistrust your own beliefs and struggle to say no to others. Journaling can be a great tool to help you regain confidence in your own ideas. You can reflect on past events and write down your take on what happened and how you felt about it. The privacy and intimacy of journaling can also be a safe way to rebuild trust in your own thoughts.

Another way to repair damaged intellectual boundaries is to remind yourself when listening to others that you can choose to accept or discard what they say. Just because someone speaks with authority, uses a strong tone of voice, or inserts a lot of big words, doesn't mean you have to agree with their view of reality.

Remember, boundaries separate who you are from who others are. It is perfectly okay for others to express their opinions, but unacceptable for them to impose their opinions on you. Practice listening carefully to others and thinking about how much of what they are saying you agree with. If possible, offer your own opinions about the same matter, while creating enough room in the conversation for the others to assert their opinions.

We have looked at three types of boundary violations and how to repair them. The important message to take away from this section is that you are allowed to have needs and wants, no matter how different they may look from the next person's needs and wants. Being comfortable having needs and wants will improve the relationship you have with yourself, which in turn will positively influence the relationships with others.

Why You Should Put Yourself First

Boundaries are a form of self-care that you practice to ensure that your needs are considered in various relationships. They teach you how to show up as your most authentic self and prioritize your well-being.

You may have been taught that putting yourself first is a sign of self-centeredness. However, this is not the case. Selfish people tend to be completely self-absorbed, meaning they fail to regard the needs of others. They see themselves as being the only one, rather than being one of many.

Putting yourself first is a form of caretaking to protect your physical, mental, and emotional health. You show concern about your needs, just as much as you care about the needs of others. In other words, you choose not to neglect yourself at the expense of being present and supportive for other people.

It is understandable why you would feel awkward about the idea of putting yourself first. Perhaps throughout your life, you have been told to put other people's needs first. The result is a disconnect from your deepest needs and desires, which causes you to undermine yourself.

There are a few habits that you can practice to learn how to put yourself first, without feeling overwhelmed by the new attention you are giving yourself. These habits include:

1. Recognize you are worthy

In this superficial world, where everyone is constantly competing and comparing themselves to each other, it can be easy to forget your own self-worth. Make it a habit to remind yourself that you don't need to compromise your needs, desires, or beliefs to be accepted or respected by people. Use positive affirmations to sow uplifting thoughts in your mind. For instance, before going to sleep, close your eyes and repeat the following affirmations:

- I am proud of myself.
- I feel safe in this body.
- My life is getting better.
- I am full of love.
- I accept myself for who I am.

The important thing is to actually believe these affirmations to be true. If there is a part of you that doubts them to be true, journal about where that self-doubt is coming from, and why you find it difficult to see yourself in a positive light.

2. Have regular check-ins

Throughout the day, take two minutes to pause and check-in with yourself. You can do this in between tasks or when you feel a shift in your mood. Simply ask the question: *How are you doing?* And wait for your body to give an answer.

For instance, you might notice dryness in your throat, which signals thirst. Or stomach cramps, which could either be a sign of hunger or digestive issues. On an emotional level, you might notice feeling stressed (an equivalent physical sensation would be a migraine or heart palpitations), or sensing the urge to do something, like take a few deep breaths.

Each time you check in with yourself, there could be different physical and emotional sensations you notice. Some sensations may feel new and unrecognizable. Do a quick Google search of what you are noticing and see what comes up. The information offered could shed some light on what you are experiencing. If you don't have time to respond to your needs immediately, make a note of them and do your best to respond before the day is over.

3. Create a healthy routine

Responding to your physical, mental, and emotional needs is a time-consuming task. To keep up with your daily needs, establish a routine that is tailored according to your priority tasks. Examples of priority tasks would include:

- eight hours of sleep
- three healthy meals a day
- fifteen minutes of cardio exercise
- going to work
- spending time with your pets

Make a commitment, each day, to complete these tasks. Put them first on your list of to-do's, before responding to other people's needs. Avoid making plans during times when you are supposed to be performing your priority tasks. Politely decline the request or invitation, and suggest a more convenient time for you.

Exercise: Self-Care Checklist

Do you know you have a responsibility to take care of yourself? It isn't a luxury, or something that you do whenever you feel like it. The three principles of self-care state that:

1. Failing to respond to your own needs lowers your ability to trust yourself.
2. You are the only person responsible for taking care of yourself, and no situation can justify neglecting your needs.
3. The duty to help others cannot be performed without the duty of self-care.

The best way to improve your level of self-care is to make a checklist of all the needs that are currently being unmet, and for each of them, write down one or two activities you can perform to fulfill those needs.

When deciding on which activities to practice, consider what would be realistic for you, in terms of money, time, and effort. For example, if physical exercise is one of your needs, ask yourself if you are financially able to take out a gym membership, or how much time you can realistically devote to exercise each day. This will help you manage expectations and feel more committed to your practices.

To make your checklist, create a list of unmet needs similar to the one below.

Unmet needs	Activities
Sleep	
Nutrition	
Healthcare	
Physical exercise	
Physical intimacy	
Stress management	
Healthy boundaries	
Personal growth	
Companionship	
Personal time	
Spirituality	

For every unmet need, write down an activity that you can perform each day or week to fulfill that need. Remember to make the activities practical and realistic. Below is an example of a completed checklist.

Unmet needs	**Activities**
Sleep	Go to bed at 09:00 p.m.
Nutrition	Consume a whole foods diet
Healthcare	Schedule a quarterly check-up with your doctor
Physical exercise	Complete a 15-minute cardio workout video
Physical intimacy	Get a professional massage
Stress management	Journal for 15 minutes
Healthy boundaries	Say no whenever you feel like you are overextending yourself
Personal growth	Read a self-help book
Companionship	Join a support group online
Personal time	Take an hour for yourself
Spirituality	Take a 10-minute mindfulness meditation

Learn the Art of Assertive Communication

"To be passive is to let others decide for you. To be aggressive is to decide for others. To be assertive is to decide for yourself. And to trust that there is enough, that you are enough."

— EDITH EVA EGER

What It Means to Be a People-Pleaser

A people-pleaser is someone who feels compelled to seek approval from others. They are often not comfortable asserting their own thoughts and feelings, and look to others for reassurance.

Most times, people-pleasing is disguised as showing compassion for others or being considerate of others' needs. However, there is a difference between empathizing with others and being afraid of saying no. People-pleasers don't feel like they have a choice to turn the "nice" switch off. They feel obliged to do favors for others and extend themselves, until the point of exhaustion.

The desire behind people-pleasing is to feel accepted and loved by others. This desire is pure, and often rooted in the lack of acceptance and affection in childhood. To gain friendships and make social interactions a lot smoother, people-pleasers learn to adapt their behaviors to appeal to the people around them. For instance, they can be extraverted around extraverted people, and introverted around introverts. This is how they win people over and form close relationships.

One of the problems brought about by people-pleasing is the inability to share strong thoughts and feelings openly. Communication is filtered to portray a favorable self-image, and conflicting needs or emotions that could lead to disapproval (e.g. anger, stress, resentment, etc.) are hidden. It is therefore difficult to understand how a people-pleaser genuinely feels, what they need, or where their boundary lines are. Even when they are upset, they try very hard not to show it, to avoid any drama or conflict.

Some of the communication issues experienced by people-pleasers include:

- difficulty saying no to others
- taking on extra tasks, even when they are overworked
- overcommitting to social plans and creating excuses for non-attendance
- insist they are fine when they are emotionally distressed
- avoid confrontation or expressing opinions that might not be shared by the group
- agree to go along with plans they are unhappy about to avoid conflict

These communication issues can create a lot of stress for people-pleasers, and consequently lead to the following adverse behaviors:

- pressure to be happy and pleasant all the time
- anxiety about speaking up for themselves
- stress due to overextending themselves to others
- constantly feeling taken for granted

- low self-esteem due to feeling inferior to others

Codependency issues can put you at risk of developing people-pleasing behaviors. However, it is important to note that you can be a people-pleaser without having codependency issues. What makes the two traits similar is the obsessive need to help others, difficulty setting healthy boundaries, and the fear of communicating genuine thoughts and feelings.

If you identify as a people-pleaser, one of the most empowering decisions you can make for yourself is to learn how to communicate effectively with others, and say no when necessary. Like all the other strategies we have discussed so far, being an effective communicator takes skill and practice.

How Codependency Affects Communication

Due to the desire to feel needed, you might struggle to express genuine thoughts and feelings, especially when you believe they might upset the other person. Unlike other people, you have a low tolerance for conflict and cannot stand any kind of disagreement.

The desire to feel needed, coupled with the low tolerance for conflict, often means that you struggle to express anger and frustration, hold others accountable for bad behaviors, or communicate unmet needs. Nonetheless, when you are backed against a corner, you will eventually communicate—but not in a healthy way. Below are four common styles of communication seen in codependent people:

Passive Aggressive Communication

Passive-aggressive communication is a discrete way of expressing aggression without being caught. The aggression is seen through subtle, indirect sabotage or sarcasm. The aim is to appear cooperative, but secretly plot to frustrate someone who has hurt you. Since you feel powerless to confront them head on, you use less obvious ways of showing disapproval.

Resentful Communication

Harboring so much pain from unmet needs, betrayal, and disappointment from others leads to a build-up of resentment. In your mind, you sense there is an inequality in how others treat you, versus how you treat them. For instance, when resolving interpersonal problems, you might use exaggerations like "I always!" and "you never!"

Another tactic is keeping score of what you do for others. You might say things like, "I'm doing more work than you" or "I'm the only one who makes an effort." It is also common to blame others when you feel resentful. Instead of expressing how their actions make you feel, you might say "If you acted differently, this wouldn't have happened" or "You make me feel angry."

Immature Communication

Immature communication is when something is said in a childish way. Think about how a child would react when they are angry. They would make demands like "Do this for me right now!" or make hurtful, impulsive comments like "I hate you!"

A child is also still grappling with their emotions and is unable to separate how they feel from what is happening in the situation. For example, they will assume that just because they feel angry about the situation, like being told to do their house chores, their parents must have done something wrong. In some cases, this is true, but other times their emotions paint a different picture of what is actually happening.

Miscommunication Due to Unclear Needs

Communication is tough when you are confused about your needs, or when you know what you need but fail to articulate it. In relationships, this might look like indecisiveness, going back and forth on a decision, and not being able to reach some kind of resolution.

Another reason which might contribute to the miscommunication is feeling compelled to go along with other people's choices, then feeling lost when you decide to backtrack and do what feels right for you.

For example, you might agree to go on a date with someone, only because it was their idea, and they seemed really excited about it. However, as you spend more time thinking about the date, you realize that it isn't something you are up for. Backtracking on your decision and pulling out on the plan might cause the other person to feel confused and even offended. This makes it harder to follow your heart and do what's right for you.

Strategies to Communicate Assertively

Assertive communication is a way of expressing your thoughts and feelings, while being considerate of another person's thoughts and feelings. In other words, you confidently stand up for yourself, without becoming controlling or disrespectful. Many people confuse assertive communication with aggressive communication, where someone comes off as being pushy or argumentative. However, that is not what assertive communication is about at all.

The assertive communicator's goal is to create win-win situations. They walk into a conversation being mindful of their position, yet open to learn about the other person's position, and how both of them might find middle ground. They don't seek to make demands or manipulate others into following their lead. What they truly want is to be understood and seek to understand where the other person is coming from too.

There are a number of benefits to becoming an assertive communicator. Some of these benefits include:

- Gaining the confidence to express a range of thoughts and feelings openly.
- Feeling less anxious and unprepared to have difficult conversations with others.
- Improving the respect you have for yourself, which causes others to show deeper respect for you.
- Being able to make decisions on your own without requiring assistance from others.
- Feeling a sense of relief knowing that people around you are aware of your needs and boundaries.

Overall, becoming an assertive communicator improves the quality of your relationships. You have the ability to express your needs, set and reinforce boundaries, as well as resolve conflict in a firm, yet empathetic way. Below are five assertive communication strategies that you can practice, over and over again, to express your needs and wants in a positive and respectful way:

1. Use "I" statements

You cannot control how others treat you, but you can control how you respond to them. Using "I" statements, like "I feel" or "I think" shows ownership of your thoughts and emotions. Yes, the situation could have brought about the feeling of anger, but that feeling came from you. The beauty of assertive communication is being able to hold others accountable for their actions without blaming them for how you feel.

Here are a few ways of using "I" statements:

- I feel ignored when you come into the house and don't greet me.
- I felt uncomfortable with the way you spoke to me earlier.
- I get frustrated when you don't give me an opportunity to speak.
- I need you to make more of an effort to help around the house.

Please note that "I" statements can also be used to show appreciation and recognize positive behaviors. For instance, you might say "I feel happy whenever I spend time with you," or "I appreciate the concern you show for me."

2. Learn to say no

Saying no feels uncomfortable, but it is one of the easiest boundaries to set. If simply saying "no" feels too direct for you, there are other assertive ways of expressing disapproval, while being considerate of the next person's feelings. Below are a few suggestions:

- I'm busy right now. Can I call you later?
- I'm sorry, this doesn't work for me.
- I can't take on any new projects right now.
- I don't feel comfortable with this arrangement.
- My schedule is looking full this week. Can we postpone it for next week?

Finding indirect ways of saying no is fine, however, remember to be as clear as possible. Your statement shouldn't leave any room for the other person to assume you meant "yes" or "maybe."

3. Be open to feedback

Assertive communication is a two-way conversation. You start by stating your needs and wants, then allow the other person to share their opinions or expectations. The conversation continues to go back and forth, until you are able to reach a healthy compromise. It is therefore required to allow an opportunity for feedback, but most importantly, be open to hearing what the other person has to say.

Here are a few ways to express your openness to feedback:

- You have heard my perspective. I would like to hear yours too.
- From what I have shared, is there anything you would like to share?
- Based on what I have said, what are your thoughts?
- Is there anything you would like to add?

Be prepared to receive feedback that is contrary to what you want to hear. Remember to respect the other person's intellectual boundaries (their right to have unique thoughts and beliefs), even if you don't agree with them. You can gain more understanding about where they are coming from by asking open-ended questions like "When you say... What do you mean?"

4. Show empathy

Empathy is the ability to step inside someone else's shoes and imagine what they might be thinking or feeling. During a conversation where you are discussing needs or setting boundaries, being empathetic demonstrates a willingness to learn and understand the other person's perspective, so you can find a middle ground.

Some of the ways to show empathy in a conversation include:

- I understand what you are saying.
- I can only imagine how that feels.
- You are making a lot of sense.
- It sounds like you are having a difficult time.
- I can see that you are frustrated.

Acknowledging someone's experience doesn't diminish your request. It simply shows that you care about how a situation impacts them, rather than only getting your needs met.

5. Be mindful of your emotions

What makes assertive conversations effective is their ability to balance logic and emotion. On the one hand, you are clear about the offense committed or need that hasn't been met, and seek to find a solution or establish a boundary. But on the other hand, you are aware of the emotional impact of having your boundaries violated or not being on good terms with the other person.

To maintain the balance of logic and emotion, keep a watchful eye on your emotions. Do your best to monitor how you are feeling during the conversation, by checking-in with yourself and picking up on body cues. Becoming overly emotional will cloud your judgment and cause the other person to become defensive. The conversation will turn into a blame game, and neither of you will walk away feeling understood.

Whenever you sense that you are getting too emotional, excuse yourself from the conversation and take five minutes to cool down. Take three deep mindful breaths and return when you have regained a sense of control. If you notice the other person becoming increasingly emotional, suggest a break or postpone the conversation to another time. It isn't good for both of you to feel pressured to give a response or continue a conversation that is starting to feel aggressive.

Improve Your Relationship With Fear

"I think sometimes making yourself vulnerable before you are ready is exactly what can hold you accountable. Do what you fear."

— BRITTANY BURGUNDER

Is Fear the Real Enemy?

A few years back, I purchased an alarm system for my house. I remember being adamant to buy one that had the latest technology—I'm talking motion sensors and the works!

After installing the device, I didn't get any sleep for a week. Every night, upon activating the alarm, I would be woken up by loud sirens going off. Apparently the device was so sensitive that it could pick up on dust and leaves blowing past. I called the company and had my security settings adjusted so that I could finally get my peaceful night's rest!

Imagine if I decided to throw away my security system altogether because of how frustrated it made me feel. Would that have been the best decision?

Your relationship with fear is much like having an annoying security system installed in your body. Since you have a history of surviving adverse life experiences, your built-in security system is highly sensitive to potential threats. It may keep you up at night, cause you to lose focus at work, or make it hard for you to develop healthy relationships—all because of false alarms constantly going off!

Of course, you have options. Do you throw away the security system altogether and expose yourself to real and imagined threats, or do you attempt to adjust the settings so that you aren't constantly on high alert?

Feeling on edge and stressed all the time can be exhausting! Sometimes, it seems better to just disown your fears altogether. However, there is a biological benefit to feeling afraid. When you feel afraid, you are able to think on your feet, seek professional help, escape dangerous relationships, and identify emotional wounds that haven't been healed.

Disowning your childhood fears won't solve your relationship problems, neither will it make you feel safer bonding with others. The real issue isn't the fact that you are afraid, but that you haven't found ways of addressing your fears and getting the closure you deserve.

Fear isn't the enemy that you have made it out to be.

In fact, once you change your perspective, you will find that your fears once brought you a lot of comfort and security in a time when you didn't have anyone to turn to. However, now that you are ready to heal, you no longer need to hide behind the fear, or fear-based coping mechanisms. You can embrace your fears and accept them as being real experiences, without identifying with them anymore.

Are you ready to experience this kind of freedom?

Healing From Codependency Fears

Codependency and anxiety go together. You have a tendency of worrying about other people's emotional states or problems, without even realizing it. Whenever you sense another person's discomfort, you can feel upset or responsible for restoring their sense of balance. Taking on that excessive amount of distress upon your shoulders can trigger your body's stress response, bringing up personal childhood fears that may not have anything to do with their situation.

A common example that occurs in romantic relationships is feeling a sense of rejection when your partner is in a bad mood that is unrelated to you, or your relationship. Seeing them suffer in that way sends alarm bells ringing in your body. Your immediate thought is, "something is not right, and I am responsible for fixing it."

If you are unable to fix their mood by making them feel better, another thought might arise in your head, "They are feeling upset because of me." This second thought is a sign that a deeper fear—the fear of rejection—has been triggered by your anxious feelings.

You might wonder what is important to address first: your anxious feelings or the underlying fears that are triggered every time you feel anxious? If you are looking for a long-term solution, addressing your underlying fears can make it easier to cope with stress and manage your strong emotional reactions.

Addressing your core fears won't be easy, nor will it feel comfortable all the time. This is because you have spent many years running away from, or seeking to numb, your fears. Now that you are ready to confront them, you can be taken back to past childhood experiences that were painful to go through. However, as you courageously take this step to face your fears, remember that you are an adult now. You are no longer living the life of that younger version of you, and therefore you can reflect on their life experiences without reliving the past.

The following section will present a common childhood fear that is typical of people who are experiencing codependency issues: the fear of rejection. You will learn about the fear in more depth, so you can understand what exactly you are afraid of, then receive strategies on how you can start conquering the fear of rejection.

Conquering the Fear of Rejection

Rejection is a risk that doesn't pay off. What makes this experience painful, is the difficulty accepting things not working out. It takes so much courage to open up, step outside your comfort zone, and show vulnerability. For someone with codependency issues, putting yourself out there like this doesn't happen every day.

When your risk doesn't pay off, you are reminded of all the childhood risks that didn't pay off, like trusting your parents to provide a sense of security, opening your heart to a boy or girl who ended up breaking your heart, or seeking out work opportunities that ended in failure. There are few factors that make you more sensitive than others to things not working out. These factors include:

1. Childhood trauma

Unresolved feelings of experiencing rejection as a child can make you sensitive to rejection as an adult. Examples of adverse events that may have led to feelings of rejection include losing a loved one, living with a single parent (or witnessing a separation), being treated less than other siblings, or being raised by a parent who was unable to show unconditional love.

2. Low self-esteem

If you already feel worthless or inferior to others, then even the slightest amount of disregard, or someone saying no, can make you feel rejected. Moreover, having a low self-esteem can cause you to attract people who are dominant or seek dominance in a relationship. You may repeat much of the same attachment patterns exhibited in the relationship with your parents, and make it your mission to seek approval or affection from them.

3. Negative core beliefs

As a child, you make up stories about what the world is like, based on the kind of "world" created in your household. These stories become ingrained in your mind and become core beliefs. Negative core beliefs are disempowering stories that you have told yourself about the world and others. They might include things like:

- The world is a dangerous place.
- People can't be trusted.
- Love must be earned.
- People always leave.

In adult relationships, these negative core beliefs are triggered whenever you are stressed, feel anxious, or experience failure. Rooting out these negative core beliefs requires you to change the narrative.

It is possible to conquer the fear of rejection. But beware, it will not make you immune from experiencing rejection in the future. Unfortunately, rejection is a part of life. At some point or another, someone will disappoint you, or you may disappoint someone. It is unrealistic to think that every relationship will be healthy, or will satisfy every need.

Nevertheless, you don't have to allow the fear of being rejected to hinder you from building healthy relationships and learning to trust others. One way to conquer the fear of rejection is to address your limiting beliefs.

Overcome Your Limiting Beliefs

Limiting beliefs are negative assumptions about yourself or others that provoke certain fears, such as the fear of rejection. Depending on how strong your limiting belief is, it has the power to prevent you from pursuing career opportunities, building new relationships (or leaving unfulfilling relationships), or living the life you desire.

Limiting beliefs may be centered around how you view yourself and how you view the world. Beliefs about yourself can negatively impact your self-esteem and cause you to feel a sense of shame and rejection, as though there is something inherently wrong with you.

For example, you might think that you are:

- less intelligent than others
- socio-economically disadvantaged
- too old or too young to pursue certain goals
- too ugly to attract companionship
- too psychologically damaged to maintain a healthy relationship

Note that these beliefs don't need to be true for you to feel like they are. For example, you may be doing really well for yourself in life and have a strong support system, yet still have a nagging feeling like people don't like you.

But limiting beliefs about the world can be equally destructive, and cause you to lose hope or trust in humanity. They mostly focus on what you think people will or won't allow you to access, what other people think of you, or questioning what exists and what doesn't exist.

For example, you might think:

- People respond negatively to you because of your different personality.
- You can't access certain opportunities, like going to university or applying for your dream job because of previous life disadvantages.
- Life favors people who demonstrate specific traits that you may not possess.
- True love between two people doesn't exist.
- Human beings are selfish and will always find a way of disappointing you.

Overcoming your limiting beliefs takes introspection. You are the best person to ask the tough questions and challenge beliefs that you once created in your mind to make sense of the world.

Here are three questions that can help you confront and overcome your limiting beliefs:

What If You Are Wrong?

Has it ever crossed your mind that you could be wrong about your limiting beliefs? That they may be based on false assumptions, rather than facts? Limiting beliefs tend to create black-and-white outcomes. For instance, you are either ugly or beautiful, poor or rich, weird or normal. These black-and-white outcomes are not true representations of reality, nor are they fair conclusions to draw about yourself.

Bring up a limiting belief related to your fear of rejection. Ask yourself the question: *What if I'm wrong?* On the lines on the next page, provide evidence for and against your belief. Shift away from black-and-white thinking and try to present the full picture.

How Is This Belief Serving You?

What is the benefit of holding onto a belief that makes you feel afraid to trust yourself or others? You might think that there isn't any, but if that was the case, why would you continue to reinforce it? Beliefs are created to protect your perception of reality. They make life feel safer, or more bearable. Even limiting beliefs serve some kind of purpose.

Think about another limiting belief (not the same as the one above) related to your fear of rejection. Figure out what purpose it is serving in your life. Could there be some benefit of holding onto this belief?

What's the Alternative?

Your beliefs are not set in stone. As you grow and gain new insight about yourself, your beliefs can adapt to reflect your fresh outlook. There is always "another side" to a limiting belief. The other side is often a more fair and balanced perspective. It seeks to evaluate life without leaning too heavily on negative or positive outcomes.

An alternative doesn't need to be complicated. It can be as basic as substituting "can't" with "can" or "never" with "not yet." For example:

- "I can't maintain healthy relationships" turns to "I can maintain healthy relationships."
- "I will never know what true love feels like" turns to "I haven't experienced true love yet."

Tell yourself that you don't need to settle for your limiting beliefs. You have plenty of options on how you decide to experience life. If your belief isn't motivating enough, ask yourself: What's the alternative?

Think about a third limiting belief that you hold (different from the first two) related to your fear of rejection. Write down at least three alternative beliefs to replace it with.

Finally, choose at least one alternative belief to test. Spend a week reflecting on the belief, rehearsing it to yourself, and behaving in ways that support it.

Notice how natural and realistic it feels. If you find that it isn't a good fit or feels superficial, test another alternative belief. Do this until you find an alternative belief that resonates with you and feels as comfortable as a new pair of jeans!

The Power in Accepting Your Fears

In this chapter, we focused on one fear related to codependency. However, there are many others that you may be living with, such as the fear of criticism, failure, vulnerability, not being good enough, or feeling out of control. Overcoming your limiting beliefs can help you address these other fears too; however, another incredibly powerful strategy is to accept your fears for what they are, rather than disowning them.

Have you wondered what would happen if you accepted your fears? Is that even something you can imagine right now?

Coming to a place of acceptance is a journey. There are many pit stops that you make along the way, such as acknowledging and healing childhood traumas, rediscovering who you are separate from your wounded self, and finally embracing your life for the beauty and chaos that it brings.

Eventually, you will reach the point of coming to terms with your fears. This moment can be both exhilarating and terrifying. For the first time you can imagine a healthy life that isn't governed by trauma-informed coping mechanisms, but since you have never lived without fear, the thought of not having things to be watchful for is discomforting.

Nevertheless, what becomes clear to you is the need for healing and breaking old cycles, so you proceed anyway.

Accepting your fears feels like making peace with parts of yourself that you have been fighting against for many years. The war against yourself is finally over, and you can reconcile different aspects of you, and accept them as one united whole.

Unfortunately, there is not much more I can say about the experience of accepting your fears because there is no formula to reach that point, nor does the experience look the same for each individual. However, what I can say is that going through the codependency recovery journey and learning to view your life with greater compassion and non-judgment, can help you come closer to making peace with your fears. Do the inner work. It's worth it!

Exercise: Processing Fears With Inner Child Work

An ongoing exercise that you can practice as you continue the codependency recovery journey and process your fears is inner child work. The inner child is the unhealed aspect of your subconscious mind that is carried from childhood to adulthood. It remembers childhood experiences, both good and bad, and often seeks closure for unresolved emotional wounds.

Since the inner child isn't a real person, it seeks closure by bringing up painful memories or triggering strong emotions that lurk in your subconscious mind. You can imagine this as a real child who throws a tantrum to get the attention of their parents.

Likewise, your inner child is yearning for your attention. It knows that you are the only person who can go back in time and heal past wounds through acknowledging and releasing them. It also knows that you are old enough to re-parent that neglected part of you, and offer yourself the love and nurturing that you were deprived of.

On the following pages you can find a few exercises to begin the inner child work:

Describe Your Inner Child

Have you met your inner child before? If not, why not start off by getting acquainted with them?

The best way to connect to your inner child is to recall the earliest traumatic event. Your inner child was born after this event. Ever since then, they have been seeking support to heal from various traumatic experiences.

As you reflect the earliest traumatic event, try and answer the following questions about your inner child:

- How old is he/she?
- What is your inner child wearing?
- What expressions does your inner child have on his/her face?
- How is he/she feeling?
- What secrets is he/she keeping?

Describing your inner child will help you create a mental image that you can frequently bring up whenever you are seeking to connect with this part of you.

Affirm Your Inner Child

Your inner child felt most of the strong emotions you felt as a child: neglected, lonely, unworthy, or unloved. Since nobody reaffirmed you back then that you were safe, intelligent, creative, and worthy of affection, you can offer your inner child that kind of validation to silence some of their doubts.

To affirm your inner child, close your eyes and imagine yourself hearing the following statements, spoken in a soft, warm, and loving voice:

- I am happy you are alive.
- I need you.
- I love you.
- You are so special to me.
- I love every quality in you.
- You make me proud.
- Thank you for being you.
- You are safe with me.
- I enjoy being around you.
- You are important to me.

Identify which statements caused the strongest emotional reactions within you. Make a note below of those statements and reflect on why those specific statements mean so much to hear.

Explore Your Inner Child's Beliefs

Think of a hurtful childhood experience that involves your parents, and answer the following questions:

- Write down keywords to describe how the experience made you feel. E.g. scared, rejected, betrayed, judged, etc.

- Write down keywords to describe how your parents responded or treated you. E.g. cold, self-centered, moody, aggressive, controlling, etc.

- What words or comments did your parents make? E.g. "You are a burden!"

- What disapproving facial expressions or body language did your parents give? E.g. tight lip, frown, crossed arms, etc.

- What story did you come up with about yourself after the experience? E.g. I am difficult to love.

Decide to Stay or Leave

"Courage isn't having the strength to go on – it is going on when you don't have strength."

— NAPOLEON BONAPARTE

Can Codependent Relationships Work?

A common misconception people have about codependent relationships is that there is no love present at all. This idea is wrong. Like any other type of relationship (i.e. romantic, parent-child, work, or social relationship), there is some degree of intimacy that exists. Of course, unlike healthy relationships, this intimacy is often clouded by harmful behaviors that make one or both parties feel unsafe.

Therefore, when discussing the subject of ending codependent relationships, we must be sensitive to the fact that there may be genuine bonds between two individuals that aren't easy to break.

If you are at a crossroads, deciding whether to stay or leave a codependent relationship, understand that it is normal to go back and forth on your decision. Finally pulling the plug and deciding to go no contact with the person is never taken lightly.

Instead of applying pressure on yourself to make a quick decision, spend some time thinking about your options, and reimagining life without your partner, friend, family member, or colleague. It may also help to consider the possibility of your relationship actually working out, and how both you might be able to turn things around.

Here's a question you may have not asked yourself before: *What would it take to heal your codependent relationship?*

Seriously think about this question, and write a list of all the changes that you and the other individual would need to make.

Your list will have several points of behavioral changes that need to take place. Some of the changes will need to come from you and others from them. However, without both of you being able to recognize the need for change, the dynamic of your relationship will stay the same.

What's crucial to understand about unhealthy behaviors is that they don't disappear overnight. They are usually a symptom of harmful thoughts, beliefs, and attitudes that have existed for many years. Unfortunately, being aware of your loved one's problematic behaviors doesn't erase them either. They must go through the four stages of codependency recovery (i.e. abstinence, awareness, acceptance, and action) to begin confronting years' worth of maladaptive coping mechanisms.

Why is this important to note? Because as someone with codependency issues, you might fall into the trap of thinking you can fix or rebuild the other person. This assumption is not true. As heartwarming as your presence may be in their lives, staying in the relationship for the sake of "fixing" them will not correct their behaviors.

Not only do they need to recognize the need for change, they must also be open and motivated to change—and take the necessary steps to enforce the change (i.e. going to counseling). The action (as outlined in stage four of recovery) has to come from them, otherwise we cannot truly say they are motivated to change.

Something else that you may want to think about is whether the other person is mentally and emotionally fit for a healthy relationship. As mentioned throughout the book, it is common to find one or both people in a codependent relationship who are suffering from mental illness or substance abuse problems. What this means is that even if they might recognize the need for change and feel motivated to change, the simple fact that they are not well can make it difficult for them to go through the stages of codependency recovery.

Perhaps before thinking about saving the relationship, both of you can discuss getting on a treatment plan to address mental health issues. The other person's state of mind and quality of life should be one of the first interventions taken, if both of you desire to stay in the relationship.

With all this said, I do believe that codependent relationships can work. But there is a lot of time and healing that must take place in order for the dynamic to change. Both parties must recognize the need for behavioral changes, and be willing to take the necessary actions. Moreover, any current and underlying mental and emotional health issues should be dealt with first to ensure that the new dynamic built feels safe and healthy.

Signs That Your Relationship Is Harmful

While I agree that codependent relationships can sometimes work, there are cases when it is better to walk away. Of course, this decision isn't taken lightly, especially when there is a long history between the individuals. But when the relationship begins to negatively affect your physical, mental, and emotional well-being, there is more to lose by staying than leaving.

Below are a few signs that your relationship has become unhealthy, and possibly life-threatening:

- **Your partner/friend/relative/colleague constantly finds something to criticize you about.** Someone who is always finding fault in you can slowly damage your sense of self-worth. After a while of repeatedly listening to their negative or sarcastic words, you may start to take what they say as being the truth.
- **There is a noticeable imbalance of power.** There is a clear distinction between who has most of the control in the relationship. This creates an unhealthy union where one person feels superior and dominant over the other. The imbalance of power can also justify harmful, oppressive behaviors practiced on the submissive person.
- **Your partner/friend/relative/colleague is excessively jealous.** When their jealousy reaches a point where they seek to monitor your movements, request device passwords, control what you wear, or who you have access to, it is a clear sign of an abuse of power, and that the relationship has become toxic.
- **Your partner/friend/relative/colleague fails to take responsibility for their actions.** The lack of accountability is not a positive sign that any behavioral changes can take place in the near future. When they struggle to apologize and admit their mistakes, it shows a disregard for your needs and hurt feelings. In such an environment, it may be hard for you to feel safe and supported.
- **Your partner/friend/relative/colleague uses manipulation tactics to control you.** Did you know that any type of manipulation is a form of abuse? Even something that many people overlook like giving the silent treatment. Manipulation tactics are used to gain control over another person's actions or emotions. What makes them so dangerous is that over time they can cause mental and emotional damage (e.g. anxiety, depression, eating disorders, substance abuse problems, etc.).

Some of these signs may not be noticeable in your relationship. Or maybe the positive moments you share somehow make the bad times appear less damaging. To truly rule out any possible signs of toxicity in your relationship, spend a month documenting how you feel around the other person.

After spending time with them, record how you felt before, during, and after your encounter. Be honest with your assessments, and just write what you felt in your body. Try not to analyze your notes until the month is up. Thereafter, sit down with a trusted friend or licensed therapist and go over your records.

Five-Step Plan to Leave a Codependent Relationship

So you have decided to exit your codependent relationship? I applaud you for such an enormous display of courage. Even though your mind is made up, the process of leaving your loved one can feel terrifying and confusing. Below are five steps to prepare you to safely get out of a codependent relationship.

Step 1: Look in the Mirror

Before you get up and walk away, look at yourself in the mirror. Recognize the role you played in creating this unhealthy relationship dynamic, and acknowledge the various problems that have motivated your decision to leave. If there have been any wrongdoings that you have committed against the other person, write a forgiveness letter to them (you are not forced to share it with them). And if there were any wrongdoings you committed against yourself, write yourself a personal letter asking for forgiveness.

You are welcome to write your forgiveness letter below.

Step 2: Have the Difficult Conversation

If you feel safe enough to have the conversation face-to-face, then schedule an appropriate time where both of you can meet. If possible, meet at a communal space, like a restaurant, which is neutral and public.

Anticipate the conversation going in a multitude of ways, and have a plan for when tensions start running high. For example, if the other person starts to raise their voice, your plan might be to set a boundary. But if their behavior exceeds that and becomes more aggressive, you can plan on walking away and resuming the conversation via text or email.

Another option that might work for both of you is having a mediator, such as a counselor, present in the room while you are having the conversation. They may be able to assist in diffusing the tension and making sure both of you get equal opportunity to voice your thoughts and feelings.

Do you have a plan B for when the conversation doesn't go as expected? Write it down below.

Step 3: Focus on Self-Care

The weeks and months following the break-up are important days of self-care. Not only is putting yourself first a positive distraction, it is also a good way to start training your mind to accept the new norm. The four stages of codependency recovery will come in handy during this time—so will staying connected to your friends and family and seeking medical support for any physical, mental, or emotional issues.

Create a list of your favorite self-care activities that target your physical, mental, and emotional well-being.

Step 4: Continue to Read About Codependency

Even though the storm is over, and you are probably feeling a lot safer now, it is important to continue studying your codependency issues. If you are attending therapy sessions, this is something that your therapist can assist you with. Alternatively, you can purchase books, courses, or listen to videos that shed light on codependency, and the various ways to recover from it.

Step 5: Develop Your Sense of Self-Worth

The final step is an ongoing step that you will continue to practice (and be mindful of) throughout your life, and in the new relationships you form. Find ways to reinforce a positive sense of self-worth, like practicing self-care, cultivating self-acceptance, reinforcing healthy boundaries, setting aspirational goals, or making a meaningful contribution in the lives of others. There is no such thing as having "too many reasons" to love and value the person that you are!

So, will you feel healed after practicing these five steps? Maybe or maybe not. What is certain though is the fact that you will be in a better off position than you were when you left the codependent relationship. Remember, healing, like codependency recovery, is a journey that takes time and constant positive reinforcement to complete successfully.

Managing Post-Breakup Grief

A common experience that follows a codependent relationship breakup is grieving the loss of the other person. Indeed, the realization that you don't have access to them anymore can feel as though you are mourning the death of a loved one.

In a way, you are mourning a death—the death of an extremely addictive relationship. Similar to any addict who is going through withdrawal symptoms, you might fall physically sick, or feel depressed.

Being gentle and compassionate toward yourself is vital during this time. Breakups, for people with codependency issues, are extremely painful. This process is likely to make you experience a range of emotions and struggle to feel like yourself for some time. Be mindful of the way you speak to yourself, and how you make sense of what is happening.

Some of the harmful thoughts and emotions that you should attempt to avoid during this time include:

1. Blaming yourself for the breakup

Avoid the temptation to look at the negative outcome of the relationship as being your fault. You are not responsible for the other person's actions, state of mind, or decisions. You cannot fix or rescue them from their self-destructive behaviors, nor was it possible for you to "save" the relationships. While it is true that you are not completely innocent, be fair and level-headed when assessing the part you played in the relationship. Accept your mistakes and be generous to forgive yourself.

2. Feeling a sense of shame

Another emotion that you should avoid at all costs is feeling ashamed for staying in the relationship, or tolerating the harmful behaviors, for as long as you did. If you knew better, and maybe received the psychological tools many years earlier, perhaps you would have left the relationship sooner. Nonetheless, there is no purpose in thinking about what you should have done because you cannot change the past. Focus on the progress you are making right now. Celebrate the small efforts you are taking to heal from childhood traumas and past relationship mistakes. Cheer yourself on, and be the parent that you needed when you were a kid!

3. Believing that your future is hopeless

Beware of limiting beliefs that attempt to paint a negative outlook on the future. Beliefs such as "I will never find love again," or "I can't maintain healthy relationships" can make you feel anxious about starting over again and rebuilding your life. It is important to believe in your ability to unlearn trauma-informed behaviors and live the kind of positive and healthy lifestyle you desire. Continue to recite your positive affirmations, confronting limiting beliefs, and journal about difficult emotions that are uncomfortable to express in words. Constantly reaffirm your needs—especially your emotional needs—so you can take your power back and assume responsibility for your own happiness.

Avoiding blame, shame, and adopting a negative outlook on the future is only one way to cope with post-breakup grief. Another way is to find positive coping strategies to take your mind off the relationship. A few suggestions include:

- **Reach out to your friends and family.** Your social relationships are vital when healing from a painful breakup. Focus on the strong bonds with some of your close friends and family, particularly those relationships that feel emotionally safe. Share your thoughts and feelings, as well as aspects of your codependent relationship you are having a difficult time making peace with.
- **Prioritize your health.** Improve your overall moods by practicing healthy habits like getting proper sleep, eating healthy foods, and working out at least three times a week. Putting your health first can also boost your confidence and make you feel excited about this new chapter in your life.
- **Download a self-care app.** To keep yourself in a good headspace, incorporate self-care techniques into your daily routine. A powerful app that can show you is called Calm. The app allows you to focus on a number of self-care goals, like improving sleep, reducing stress and anxiety, or improving focus—to name a few—and keep track of your progress and milestones.
- **Create a post-break up music playlist.** Music has the ability to reduce stress and enhance positive moods. Get your phone out and create a one-of-a-kind post-breakup playlist. Keep the theme upbeat and motivational, so you can forget about the breakup blues.
- **Allow yourself to cry, yell, and scream.** Part of the process of

healing and recovering from a breakup is being able to process and let go of strong emotions. Create a safe space to express heavy emotions and feel the sense of loss. You don't need to be strong or keep it together during your recovery. It is okay to mourn, and continue mourning until you feel ready to embrace your new life.

Ending ties with a codependent relative, friend, or significant other is painful. Even though your relationship had become toxic, there was still a great deal of love there that caused you to have faith in things getting better. At the end, you decided to choose a happy and healthy life, instead of a life based on false hope. This decision wasn't easy, but it marks the beginning of a brand-new life, living under brand-new terms.

Celebrate This New Chapter

> *"We must be willing to get rid of the life we've planned, so as to have the life that is waiting for us. The old skin has to be shed before the new one can come."*
>
> — JOSEPH CAMPBELL

What Are You Looking Forward To?

It is tempting to reminisce about the past when you are beginning a new journey. As painful as the past chapter of your life was, it felt familiar. Now that you are on a different path, you may feel unprepared and anxious about the future.

However, perspective is everything when you are seeking to have a fresh start!

Decide, right now, what your future is going to look like. Are you going to be miserable? Go back to old patterns of behavior? Attract the same quality of men and women that you have been attracting in the past?

Your answer should be a big and bold "NO!"

If you are adamant that this next chapter of your life is not going to look or feel like the last one, then you must change your mentality. When you think differently, you move differently, and as a result, attract different things.

The best way to change your mentality is to set aspirational goals that become the new focus of your life. These goals paint a picture of the quality of life you intend on creating for yourself. It doesn't matter what others might think about your goals. All that matters is that they align with your values and make your life feel meaningful.

There are five steps that you can practice to set aspirational goals that give you something to look forward to:

Step 1: Make a Decision

For once and for all—decide on what you want and why you want it. Be absolutely clear about the intention behind your goal because that is what will keep you going on the journey. Ensure that the goal is a reflection of your desire, and not something that was inspired by someone else. A trick to figuring out if you have found the right goal is to ask yourself: *Would I regret not achieving this goal?*

Take some time to think about your goal and write it down below:

Step 2: Break Down Your Goal

This step is extremely crucial to making sure your goal doesn't overwhelm you. Break down your goal into smaller tasks that can be done on a daily, weekly, and monthly basis. Each task should be simple, easy to practice, and written as an instruction. Note that the less time-consuming and complicated your tasks, the less resistance you will feel to commit.

Use the table below to break down your goal and divide it into daily, weekly, and monthly tasks.

Daily Tasks	Weekly Tasks	Monthly Tasks

Step 3: Plan Your First Step

Now that you know what to focus on throughout the month, decide on your first step. Make sure that the first task is small enough to practice on any given day, with minimum resources required. After successfully completing it, plan your next small task.

Which task will break the ice and mark the beginning of this journey for you?

Step 4: Review Progress Regularly

Choose a day of the week or month that will become the "check-in" day. On that specific day, review the progress you have made for that period, as well as obstacles that you have encountered, so you can decide if a goal adjustment is necessary. The process of pursuing a goal should be challenging, but never demanding.

If you need to reduce the number of goal-related tasks completed monthly, feel free to do so! However, if you don't believe you are being challenged enough, find ways to increase the expectations for each task. For example, instead of working out for 15 minutes, twice per week, you can increase the intensity and workout for 30 minutes, three times per week.

Step 5: Celebrate Your Wins

Make it a point to acknowledge small and big wins. Take a moment to reflect on how far you have come, and what it took to achieve that victory. You can also express gratitude to the people you have played a role in helping you achieve the milestone. Celebrating your wins is what makes the journey worthwhile, so enjoy this small or big achievement!

Nurture Your Close Relationships

No matter how solid a relationship, when it isn't given the right amount of nurturing, it can start to fall apart. In this new chapter of your life, make a decision to prioritize close relationships with friends and family, so you can be rewarded with deep and satisfying connections.

The good news is that since you already have established close relationships, you won't need to start from scratch and get to know your loved ones. However, you may need to practice healthy habits that promote stronger and more fulfilling relationships. Below are five ways to nurture close relationships:

1. Listen with curiosity

Listening is a sign of respect and kindness. It also shows the other person that you care about what they are saying, which makes them feel seen and accepted. When listening, focus attentively on what the other person is saying. Tell yourself that nothing else matters besides what you are hearing. Pause before speaking, and process what you have heard. Truly appreciate their perspective and challenge yourself to learn something new!

2. Be intentional about spending quality time

Connections are maintained through spending quality time together. This doesn't need to be face-to-face interactions; they can also be online catch-ups through video chat or group messaging. If you tend to forget about your loved ones when your schedule gets busy, block out time in your calendar for uninterrupted quality time. Depending on each relationship, how you spend quality time will look different. Some of the suggestions you can consider are:

- coffee dates
- weekly date nights
- family picnics
- going on vacation together
- watching a movie together
- meeting for mentor-mentee appointments

When spending quality time with loved ones, be fully present. Put your devices away (or on silent) and put away as many distractions as possible. It is important for them to feel as though they have your undivided attention, and you have theirs.

3. Notice positive things and express gratitude

It is normal to start taking loved ones for granted because of how comfortable you are in the relationship. However, if you are not careful, you can start to neglect their core needs. Everybody desires to be recognized for their positive contributions—including your loved ones. Take the time to notice something good about them, each time you get together, and show appreciation.

Think about someone who has played an important part in your codependency recovery. It could be a cousin, friend, or colleague, who has always been there to listen and offer advice. Write a gratitude letter to them, mentioning how thankful you are for their support.

Your close relationships make up the core of your support system. These are the people who keep you grounded, offer emotional support, and help you through difficult times. Never miss an opportunity to show them how much significance they hold in your life.

How to Manage the First Healthy Romantic Relationship

An unhealthy relationship can change your perspective on love and closeness. You may doubt that it is possible to build friendships or romantic relationships that feel healthy and supportive. Well, the truth is that there are millions of good people out there, who are capable of meeting you halfway and consciously building healthy relationships with you.

When meeting someone new, you have an opportunity to start off with a solid and healthy foundation. How you approach the relationship—and the values and boundaries you communicate—will set the tone for what kind of dynamic both of you will create. It is therefore critical to decide, ahead of time, what kind of romantic relationship you want moving forward, as well as what standards you will enforce.

The first step in deciding what kind of romantic relationship you want is being clear and resolute about the kind of relationship you DON'T want. Create a list of unacceptable behaviors that are immediate dealbreakers or turn-offs. Examples of unacceptable behaviors include:

- yelling
- playing victim
- physical attacks
- name-calling
- silent treatment
- excessive jealousy
- not being supportive
- threatening to leave
- gaslighting
- controlling

Now that you know what you don't want, consider some of the standards that you will enforce. Remember that standards are not wishes, they are needs that make you feel safe, respected, loved, and supported in your romantic relationships. When these standards are not met, you may suffer emotional distress, like feeling anxious, neglected, or taken for granted.

Below is an example of some of the standards you can set and communicate in your new romantic relationships:

- I must feel attracted to the person.
- I must respect the person.
- I must feel safe around the person.
- I must feel wanted by the person.
- I must feel comfortable expressing my needs.
- I must feel safe sharing my thoughts and feelings.
- The person must believe in equality in a relationship.
- The person must show willingness to respect my boundaries.
- The person must respect my time with friends and family.
- The person must have separate hobbies and interests from mine.
- The person must be a positive influence in my life.

Take another look at your list and identify five non-negotiable standards. These are the standards that are mandatory in order to continue getting to know someone. Be mindful of these standards whenever you meet new people.

Rewrite Your Life Story

In Chapter 7, we spoke a little about negative life stories that produce limiting beliefs. But in this final section, we are going to take a closer look at these negative life stories and put a positive spin on them—one story at a time.

Just to recap, life stories are created after going through various experiences and drawing life lessons from them. Depending on how you perceived those experiences back then, you created empowering or disempowering stories.

It is important to identify life stories that are disempowering, so that you can reflect on those past experiences again and reframe them positively. Being able to look back on your life and find the goodness in everything that you have been through can be the kind of encouragement you need to face current challenges.

Below are five practical ways to rewrite disempowering life stories and regain control of your life. But before you go into them, write down your current life story below:

1. Challenge negativity bias

Negativity bias is the process of focusing on the negative aspects of a situation and overlooking or downplaying the positive aspects. Human brains are wired to do this naturally, so you will need to make a deliberate attempt to catch yourself when a life story starts to sound too negative.

Rewrite your life story and challenge yourself to find the silver lining of that situation, something positive that you can appreciate.

2. Change roles

Consider which movie "role" you play in your own story. For instance, are you the supporting actor or the main actor? Do you take orders from someone, or do you give orders? If your current story portrays you as anything other than the main actor, switch roles.

Rewrite your life story to highlight your strengths, victories, and talents. Read the new narrative and notice how you feel. Do you feel like a hero?

If not, take another look to see if you have cast yourself in the right role.

3. Allow opportunity for change

Rewrite your life story to allow opportunities for change. If your previous story made your life outcomes seem final, adjust them to allow for positive improvements in the future. For example, you can change "I wasted my youth making bad choices" to "I spent my youth learning what I didn't want in life, so I can live my adult years as I wish."

4. Create a new theme

What is the current theme of your life story? Does it motivate you to continue working on personal growth? Or does it feel discouraging? Look at your story from a fresh angle. See the possibilities where you once saw limitations. Create a new theme that inspires positive action and a continued effort to heal from past experiences.

5. Create a happy ending to defeat the villain

Often in movies, the villain is the character that is attempting to sabotage the hero. In your life, various people or self-destructive behaviors have played the role of villain. For many years, it seemed as though the villain was winning, but recently (when you began your codependency recovery journey), the hero remembered their own strength!

Change the ending of your life story to reflect the better position you are in right now. Show a change in how you present the villain; from being an undefeatable monster to an enemy that you have overcome!

Strengthen Your Relationship With the Divine

If you are spiritually inclined, or are at least curious to learn more about spirituality, you can make an effort to strengthen your relationship with the Divine. Spirituality is about embracing the fullness of life and allowing yourself to be guided. People have different views regarding who or what guides them, but for the purpose of this section, we will call that energy or entity, Divine.

The benefit of connecting to the Divine, especially after coming out of a codependent relationship, is to understand the meaning of life, and which direction you seek to take. Since the Divine represents infinite wisdom, it has the ability to guide you toward people, places, and opportunities that are aligned to your values, beliefs, and talents.

Growing up, you may have often felt a lack of guidance, particularly from the people who you trusted the most to provide a sense of security. For example, not being able to approach your parents about important conversations related to things like identity, puberty, sex and intimacy, or pursuing life goals, caused you to rely on your peers or the media to search for knowledge.

Looking back, you may agree that if you had proper guidance, perhaps you wouldn't have felt so alone, confused, or unprepared for life. Even though you cannot redo the past, it is possible to receive the guidance you have always longed for, by connecting to your higher power. The kind of guidance you are able to receive from the Divine can assist you with:

- Processing and releasing past trauma.
- Healing unhealthy attachments.
- Silencing the voice of the ego, so you can receive divine inspiration.
- Making important life transitions that can be terrifying.
- Healing the inner child and learning healthier patterns of relating to others.
- Living a life that is aligned to your values and beliefs.

Your ability to grow spiritually and connect to the Divine depends on your level of openness to change. The closer you get to the all-knowing, all-powerful entity, the more self-awareness you will gain. You will feel empowered to confront unhealthy habits and beliefs with compassion, and redefine who you are, what you desire most out of life, and the kinds of relationships you seek to build.

If you are ready to take this spiritual journey and connect to your higher power, below are a few spiritual practices you can try:

- **Practice silent meditation**

The moment you open your eyes, before getting out of bed, take five minutes to practice a silent meditation. The only thing you need to do is lie down on your back, close your eyes, and breathe. Allow the silence and gentle bringing to raise your consciousness and help you connect to a deeper part of yourself. If there are any inspired thoughts that come to your mind during this time, make a mental note, then write them down in a notebook afterward.

- **Practice manifesting Divine energy**

The Divine is an energy or entity that doesn't have a shape or form. However, on an energetic level, you can sense the presence of the Divine. It can feel like witnessing someone you love walk inside a room and brighten up the place with their smile. The warm, nurturing, and strong energy you feel whenever you are doing something you love, helping others, or witnessing a work of art is a sign that you have manifested Divine energy. Spend more time practicing activities that manifest that warm, nurturing, and strong energy within you. Find at least one hobby that provides this opportunity for you.

- **Be mindful of how you are being guided**

Tapping into your gut instinct, or intuition, can help you notice the various ways the Divine guides you. The form of guidance can be very specific, such as seeing images or symbols, hearing distinct sounds, having vivid dreams, or having miracle encounters with strangers. Look for the synchronicities, or patterns, between the guidance you receive and the real-life events or challenges you are faced with. Moreover, learn to take notes of signs that you believe have a deeper meaning.

- **Be available for guidance**

It is difficult to connect with the Divine when your mind has wandered to the past or future. Since Divine energy embodies pure consciousness, it is always available in the present moment. In order to connect to the Divine, you must also be present and focus on what is happening right now, right here. Practicing grounding techniques or meditation can help you cultivate presence and reduce mind-wandering.

- **Practice gratitude**

Divine energy is abundant energy. This means that when you trust in your higher power to take care of you, you can rest assured that goodness will find you, and every problem will have a solution or positive outcome. Therefore, cultivate an environment in your life where you are constantly thankful for what you have, or the experiences you are going through (even the challenging ones). Visualize every obstacle or opportunity working out favorably for you.

This new chapter of your life is going to be extraordinary. What will make it extraordinary are the positive actions that you will take to live a life that you never imagined was possible. Mourn the loss of the old you, along with relationships that had to be cut off. Show gratitude for those painful times that have taught you how to stand up for yourself and regain control over your life. Everything happens for a reason. Believe that the reason is always favorable to you!

Conclusion

> *"Holding on is believing that there's only a past; letting go is knowing that there's a future."*
>
> — DAPHNE ROSE KINGMA

The moment you realize that a relationship has become toxic, you are presented with an ultimatum: save the relationship or save yourself.

As someone living with codependency issues, who has been conditioned since childhood to put others' needs first, your initial choice may be to save the relationship. After all, who else can take care of others better than you? But after going through this book and learning about the value of self-care and enforcing boundaries to protect your needs, you may end up saving yourself.

It is important to take a moment and recognize how much of a big deal it is to finally come to a place where you can choose yourself. Many years ago, the thought of putting yourself first could have made you feel selfish.

Throughout your life, your focus has been on rescuing other people from their own personal dramas. The role of being a giver was forced upon you, before you were old enough to choose. Perhaps you were raised by a workaholic, alcoholic, or mentally ill parent, who relied on you to mature quickly and take care of the household in their absence, or provide emotional support for their needs.

As a result, the subconscious message you learned was that it was unacceptable to share your thoughts and express your longing for affection. What many people don't understand about putting others first is that it can make you feel invisible. There is only so much time, money, and energy you can give to others, before you start feeling drained and resentful for not getting the same effort and support given to you.

The road to codependency recovery is marked by the four stages that you will need to go through: abstinence, awareness, acceptance, and action. These four stages will support you in recognizing and healing unhealthy attachments, reaffirming your needs, and building safe relationships where you are able to express who you are without fear of rejection or judgment. During recovery, you are able to confront limiting beliefs, poor boundaries, and obsessive tendencies that make it difficult to form healthy and stable relationships with others.

Your openness to learning new information about yourself is what makes recovery possible. Unless you are able to challenge the current status quo in your life, you may struggle to adopt healthier patterns of behavior. Continue to lead with curiosity, and reflect on tough questions that get you to think about the "why" and the "how": *Why do I behave this way? How can I address it?*

To recap, here are the nine chapters (and strategies) presented in this book:

1. Define Codependency
2. Understand the Risk Factors
3. Recognize How Codependency Looks in Different Relationships
4. End the Terror of Obsessive Thinking
5. Put Yourself First and Set Boundaries
6. Learn the Art of Assertive Communication
7. Improve Your Relationship With Fear
8. Decide to Stay or Leave
9. Celebrate This New Chapter

The knowledge gained from these nine chapters is enough to support you on this amazing recovery journey. Feel free to flip through the pages of this book, whenever you need a reminder of who you are and the incredible life you deserve.

IV

Set Boundaries and Change Your Life Today

Life-Changing Strategies to Set Healthy Boundaries in Relationships, Start Saying No and Be Assertive

Introduction

"You are not required to set yourself on fire to keep others warm."

— UNKNOWN

Pouring From an Empty Cup

I was raised in what many refer to as a dysfunctional home environment. My mother and biological father went separate ways when I was one year old, and so I was raised by my mother and stepfather.

As young as I was, I felt responsible to take care of my parents and do whatever I could to make them happy since they both battled with mental health issues. My mother was diagnosed with bipolar disorder and my stepfather suffered from depression. Sadly, when I was seven years old, my stepfather lost his battle with depression and committed suicide.

From that moment onward, I told myself that my mother's well-being would become my priority. An enormous amount of guilt came over me for being the "lucky one" who didn't seem to be fighting inner demons. I felt that the only way not to feel as guilty was to sacrifice my time, energy, and well-being at the expense of taking care of others.

By the time I hit my teenage years, I was burned out and suffering from depression. The irony is that I didn't think I needed anyone to take care of me. I had convinced myself that my feelings and life experiences weren't as urgent as my family members'. I kept pouring into other people's cups, until eventually, I ran dry.

Finally, I had reached my breaking point and knew deep down that something had to change.

If you're reading this book, you might experience or know someone who experiences difficulties setting boundaries in relationships. Your story might look and sound different from mine, but we have one thing in common: We've both struggled to say 'no' at some point in our lives. For some reason, we grew up thinking that saying no to others might jeopardize the relationship or cause them to reject us. Since we couldn't risk losing them, we decided to hide or deny our own needs and desires.

As a qualified developmental psychologist, I often use my own life story as an analogy for what a lack of boundaries during early childhood leads to. In general, babies are able to start learning rules when they reach the 12-month milestone, and by four years old, the child can start learning about limits, choices, and consequences.

However, when a child is raised in a dysfunctional home environment where one or both parents are not emotionally available to enforce healthy discipline, reward good behavior, and offer positive reinforcement, the child grows up feeling unprepared to face the world. They may not have the proper mental and emotional tools to cultivate a healthy self-esteem and build mutually beneficial and safe relationships.

This book is dedicated to the grown-ups that were robbed of those early childhood lessons about setting boundaries and filling your own cup first. You will learn how to identify your emotional triggers and poor coping strategies that have been making it difficult to set healthy limits with others. You will also learn how to challenge that inner critic that feeds you fear-based beliefs about yourself and others, which causes you to feel afraid to stand up for yourself.

It took me many years to reach a point where I felt comfortable with being disliked, overlooked, or misunderstood. But the truth is, I would have never healed from my people-pleasing ways if I didn't get started on my journey. You can think of this book as the beginning of your own healing journey, too. You have the opportunity to work through deep insecurities that have been holding you back from living a fulfilling life, and redefine how you wish to live!

Are you ready to set boundaries and ultimately change your life for the better? If so, keep reading.

Living Within Boundaries

"Daring to set boundaries is about having the courage to love ourselves even when we risk disappointing others."

— BRENE BROWN

This chapter talks about:

- The benefits of setting healthy boundaries
- The difference between loose, rigid, and healthy boundaries
- Six types of boundaries to set in different areas of your life

Putting Up a Door, Not a Wall

The subject of setting boundaries is always a difficult one. Many of us grew up believing that boundaries were an aggressive way to keep others at bay. We saw setting boundaries as being the same as putting up walls, and since we didn't want to isolate ourselves from others, we thought that these walls were unnecessary.

Adults who experience a difficult time setting boundaries typically grew up in households where expressing a sense of self or having the freedom to voice ideas or concerns was shunned. Some parents may have explicitly said, "Your opinions, thoughts, and feelings don't matter," and others may have implicitly suggested it through their behaviors.

For these adults, creating limits with others or saying the word 'no' was therefore treated as an exception, not the norm. Unless they were severely under pressure, under-resourced, or exhausted to the point of barely moving their bodies, their answer would always be 'yes' and they would tolerate whatever attitudes or behaviors others decided to express toward them.

I used to be a kid afraid of disappointing others. This was partly due to my highly sensitive nature, where instead of checking in with myself first, I would become so engulfed in the other person's suffering or need and make it my mission to ease their burden. However, it was also due to the fact that I had never seen healthy boundaries modeled in front of me as a child.

My parents found it difficult to draw a line separating who they were—and the suffering they were dealing with—from who their children were. As a result, they often transferred their stress, anxiety, and trauma onto us as kids, and because we didn't know better, we felt responsible for our parents' mental, physical, and emotional well-being. Furthermore, since the lines between parent and child were blurred, we didn't know which behaviors were acceptable and unacceptable. This meant that we accepted poor behaviors like disrespect, name-calling, gaslighting, and manipulation, because to us, this was how we related to our parents.

Under these circumstances, you can imagine just how difficult setting boundaries would be. Essentially, it would mean compromising the relationship my siblings and I had with our parents. After all, if we related to each other in an unhealthy way, setting boundaries would significantly change the dynamics of those relationships.

The inability to set boundaries caught up to me during my adolescent years. The dysfunctional parent-child relationship I had grown up with was repeating itself in other relationships too. Once again, the line separating myself and the other individual was non-existent, and this meant their frustrations or emotional needs were being transferred to me. It was an exhausting feeling knowing that the well-being of my friends and family rested on my shoulders, and that if I didn't rescue them from their troubles, I would be the one to blame.

My understanding of what boundaries were had been warped since childhood. I knew that I had to adjust how I perceived boundaries so that I could take care of myself better. While pursuing my psychology degree in college, I was exposed to what boundaries actually are. Instead of this high wall that keeps people at a distance, I learned that boundaries are a door that regulates access to my time, space, energy, and resources.

Imagine that you were given $1 million to build your dream home. You started by laying the foundation, then built two stories, and finally added all of the fixtures and trimmings to complete your home. But after the money had been spent and the day of moving in had arrived, you realized that there wasn't a front door. As beautiful as your home was, it was under a significant security risk because anyone could enter the house during the day or in the evening and violate your privacy.

Let's assume you managed to raise enough money to buy a door. Great. Now you at least have better security. However, the house door won't be open 24/7. In fact, there will be times when it's inappropriate to have guests because you aren't home or are enjoying quality time with your family. The door is therefore a form of communication to let others know when you are available and when you are unavailable.

Boundaries serve as a door into your life. It doesn't matter how strong your core values are or how much work you have put into your personal development—if you don't have healthy boundaries, your sense of peace and emotional safety is at risk. Anyone, whether it be a friend, family member, or colleague, can have unlimited access to your time, energy, resources, and space. But even if you have boundaries (you at least have a door), when they are weak or too flexible, people can often violate them and continue to act as they please and mistreat you.

If you would never live in a $1 million home without a front door, then why would you continue building relationships without any healthy boundaries? Your sense of emotional safety should be top priority, more than the need to please others. Just like you wouldn't leave your front door open 24/7, you also don't need to be available to others 24/7. It's okay, and even necessary, to be unavailable sometimes because there are urgent tasks, needs, and goals you have to work on before making time for others.

The Benefit of Setting Healthy Boundaries

Every human being has a public self and a private self. The public self is the aspect of an individual that others get to interact with. This may include their personality, behaviors, and attitudes. Generally speaking, the public self is shaped by the individual's environment, relationship expectations, social responsibility, and how others might see them. Thus, the public self is likely to change based on external factors.

However, there's also the private self, which is the aspect of an individual that is hidden from others. It consists of their internal values, beliefs, thoughts, and emotions. The private self is a lot harder to express openly than the public self because to do so requires a great deal of vulnerability. Plus, since the private self is not determined by others' standards, expressing this aspect of self can go against social, relationship, or environmental expectations.

Boundaries are set up to protect the private self, not necessarily the public self. They can teach you how to recognize your internal needs, beliefs, and desires, and then establish boundaries to honor these important parts of who you are. When you step out in public and interact with others, boundaries ensure that you don't reach a point where you compromise your private self. Thus, your social interactions, whether at work or at home, become less stressful and more fulfilling.

There are numerous benefits for setting boundaries. Below are some of the most compelling reasons why you need healthier boundaries:

- **Boundaries help to express who you are to others.** People can learn a lot from you by the type of boundaries you set in your life. They can learn about your likes and dislikes and behavior you deem as acceptable or unacceptable.
- **Boundaries help you draw lines between yourself and others.** Within intimate relationships, it's common to become enmeshed with those you love. You and the other person behave as though you're one entity instead of two unique human beings. Boundaries protect your individuality and make it easier to identify where your needs end and where the other person's start.
- **Boundaries help you decide how you wish to be treated by others.** It can be surprising for some adults to learn that they don't need to accept any kind of difference from others. By setting boundaries, they get to redefine their relationships and ensure that their interactions with others align with their core values.
- **Boundaries help you live a life that empowers you.** When you set boundaries, your needs take center stage in your life. This doesn't mean you become selfish, but instead live in such a way that improves your overall health and well-being.
- **Boundaries give you more control over your life.** You cannot control how others act toward you, but when you set boundaries, you can control how you respond to bad treatment. Boundaries pull you out of a state of victimhood or people-pleasing and help you become

a better version of yourself.

What I have found in my practice is that many people understand what boundaries are (at least at a basic level) and are familiar with the benefits of setting boundaries. However, what they often lack is the ability to tell the difference between weak, rigid, and healthy boundaries.

Weak vs Rigid vs Healthy Boundaries

We all have boundaries. If we didn't, we wouldn't have survived through some of the atrocities in our lives. Every human being has the capacity to stay away from perceived danger, avoid making bad choices, and find ways to alleviate suffering. Having these abilities is essentially what boundaries are all about. But having said that, not everybody has healthy boundaries.

Indeed, if you study the people around you or reflect on your own life, you'll realize that some boundaries don't offer as much protection or freedom as others. For example, you might get upset when you're mistreated and feel within you that a boundary has been crossed. However, due to having a weak boundary, you're unable to stand up for yourself and do something about it. On the opposite end of the spectrum, you might notice the mistreatment but, due to having a rigid boundary, you end up cutting off the individual from your life completely rather than having a discussion about the matter.

The point I'm trying to make here is that we shouldn't assume that just because we have boundaries that they're necessarily healthy. Weak boundaries look different from rigid boundaries, and rigid boundaries are not the same as healthy boundaries. To help you understand the difference, below are a few signs of weak, rigid, and healthy boundaries.

Signs of Weak Boundaries

Weak boundaries are generally those that don't offer sufficient protection. While you might be able to express your limitations, you may struggle to follow through with the appropriate action. Moreover, if you receive pushback, you're more willing to adjust your boundaries rather than hold the other person accountable. Here are a few signs you may have weak boundaries:

- **Your calendar is often fully booked because you agree to take on more tasks than you can manage.** At work or at home, you're typically the one who assumes the most responsibility because you're unable to set limits. You may find yourself saying yes to tasks or gatherings you don't want to commit to.
- **When you are disrespected, you would rather keep silent or air out your grievance with a third party.** Having to confront someone who has mistreated you is an uncomfortable experience, thus you try to avoid it as much as possible.
- **Being rejected by others is one of your greatest fears.** Even though you desire to be respected by those closest to you, being accepted by them is more important to you. This means that you make a lot of personal sacrifices and compromises to stay in other people's good books rather than allow them to get to know who you truly are.
- **You internalize other people's thoughts and emotions.** It's difficult for you to separate your thoughts and emotions from another person's. For example, when someone is upset at you, you might assume you're responsible for making them feel that way instead of allowing them to take ownership of their emotions.

Signs of Rigid Boundaries

Rigid boundaries are on the opposite end of the spectrum. Instead of being too accommodating of others, you create boundaries that shut others out or severely punish them for boundary violations. Rigid boundaries tend to be a sign of anxious or avoidant attachment in relationships, where you prefer to create distance between yourself and others to protect yourself from getting hurt. While this distance makes you feel somewhat safe, it can be isolating and makes it harder to build healthy and mutually beneficial relationships. Below are a few signs that you may have rigid boundaries:

- **You are quick to block or cut people out of your life.** When you have been disrespected by others, you tend to take extreme measures to ensure the offense doesn't occur again. Rather than discuss the matter or allow the other person to apologize or explain themselves, you make an assumption that leads to blocking or cutting them out of your life.
- **You have strict rules about what you are willing to do and won't make any compromises.** The good news is that you're able to articulate what you like and dislike, however you often find it difficult to bend your rules so that you can accommodate people who might think or desire something different from you.
- **It takes a lot for you to trust others in close relationships.** Most of your relationships remain shallow because you have a difficult time opening up to others. Due to this, you might attract people who are happy to talk about themselves constantly and won't bother getting to know you or ask how you're doing. These lopsided relationships might feel safe, but they are unfulfilling in the long run.
- **You are highly sensitive to criticism.** Since your guard is always up, you often feel personally attacked when others share thoughts or feelings that are unfavorable. In your head it sounds like they're ripping you apart, but this isn't the case. As a result of being sensitive

to criticism, you may prefer to be around people who are agreeable rather than those who are likely to challenge you.

Signs of Healthy Boundaries

Ideally, we should all aim to set healthy boundaries. These normally fall somewhere between weak and rigid boundaries. You will know when you have set healthy boundaries because you won't feel vulnerable to disrespect, but won't be hyper-sensitive to it either. In other words, healthy boundaries allow you to set a standard for your life while recognizing that those around you have standards too, and in order to maintain healthy relationships, there must be mutual respect.

What differentiates healthy boundaries from weak boundaries is that you make clear and assertive limits. In contrast, what differentiates healthy boundaries from rigid boundaries is that they're flexible and can be adjusted when it's safe to do so. Therefore, what you end up with are boundaries that protect you from being mistreated by others, but also give you enough room to compromise in exceptional circumstances. Below are a few signs that you may have healthy boundaries:

- **You are able to separate your thoughts and emotions from others.** You are aware of your own physical, mental, and emotional needs and are able to express them whenever you need to. This means that you can easily identify thoughts and emotions that you disagree with or that might be projected onto you by others. For example, you can acknowledge that you aren't responsible for another person's emotional outburst.
- **You can articulate how you desire to be treated.** Since you're aware of what feels good and what doesn't, you can verbalize how you want to be treated. This might be as simple as saying no, or as elaborate as telling others what you need, what you are willing to accept (or not accept), and how they can show you support.

- **You are comfortable making choices that protect your interests.** There are times when you must make choices that don't benefit others, but protect your own interests. For example, you might decline an invitation to attend a social gathering because you're tired and would much rather have an early night. Even though you may feel guilty for not attending, you aren't worried about what others might think about your choice.
- **You are able to discuss your boundaries with others and hold them accountable.** The people closest to you are aware of your boundaries because you're open about discussing them. During conversations, or when a boundary has been crossed, you have the confidence to communicate your boundaries and request changed behavior. When your boundaries are repeatedly violated, you're also not afraid to enforce appropriate consequences.

Seven Types of Boundaries in Relationships

Healthy boundaries can be broken down into different categories to protect you in different aspects of your life. For example, you might desire to set limits when it comes to your personal space, privacy, or finances. Knowing what type of boundaries you need in your personal or work relationships will help you clearly communicate how you wish to be treated (as well as the consequences for boundary violations). Below are seven types of boundaries to consider:

Physical Boundaries

Your physical boundaries protect your need for privacy, personal space, and physical touch. It's always a good idea to let others know if their presence in your home, display of affection, or nosey behavior is making you feel uncomfortable. When communicating your physical boundaries, you might say:

- "I'm not in the mood for company tonight. Can we meet up tomorrow?"
- "I don't do hugs, but I can do a high five."
- "I'm not comfortable with you going through my phone."
- "May you please ask if I'm home before arriving at my house next time?"

Physical boundary violations will make you feel unsafe to be around a person. In extreme cases, these violations can lead to physical, sexual, or emotional abuse.

Emotional Boundaries

You have a range of emotions that deserve to be acknowledged and respected by those you're in relationships with. It isn't right for you to feel scared, judged, or embarrassed for expressing how you feel. Equally so, you shouldn't feel responsible for carrying another person's emotional baggage. Thus, emotional boundaries create clear limits when it comes to sharing feelings and resolving emotional situations. When communicating emotional boundaries, you might say:

- "When you yell at me during arguments, I feel disrespected."
- "I'm sorry that you're having a tough time. Since I'm not an expert, I can't speak much on the matter, but know that I'm here if you need someone to listen."
- "I'm not in the right frame of mind to have this discussion. Do you think we can have it another time?"
- "I prefer processing my feelings alone, but thank you for offering support. I truly appreciate it."

When your emotional boundaries are violated, you will feel judged, criticized, or misunderstood. If someone is emotionally dumping their frustrations onto you, it's possible to feel drained around that person or uncomfortable with the sensitive information you're being told. Other people, particularly those who are manipulative, might even make you feel guilty for expressing your emotional needs or take your kindness for granted.

Time Boundaries

How you decide to spend your time and who you decide to spend your time with is your personal choice. Time is a precious commodity because we can never earn it back; once it's been spent, it's gone. Therefore, if you value your time or perhaps live a busy lifestyle, you may want to set time boundaries with others so that you have more control over how you spend your time. Your time boundaries might sound like:

- "I won't be able to make it to the meeting tomorrow morning."
- "I only have 15 minutes to spare. What's up?"
- "I feel disrespected when you arrive to our appointments late. Next time I'll leave if you don't show up after 10 minutes of our agreed time."
- "I would be happy to assist you with this project. I charge an hourly rate of $50."

Time boundaries are violated when colleagues aren't punctual to meetings, when you aren't adequately compensated for your work, when friends cancel at the last minute on dates, or when a phone call with a friend drags on longer than you had agreed on.

Sexual Boundaries

Your sexual boundaries refer to your expectations when it comes to sexual intimacy, such as what type of sexual intimacy you're comfortable with, how often you prefer to engage in sex, your preferences when it comes to privacy, and so on. Sexual boundaries can sound like:

- "I'm not ready to be intimate with you at this stage."
- "I prefer it when you touch me like that."
- "I don't have sex without a condom."
- "I don't feel like having sex right now. Can we try later?"

It's extremely important for all parties to reach a mutual agreement on what kind of sex they would like to have. When consent is not given, or limits are not respected, a sexual boundary is violated.

Intellectual Boundaries

Similar to how you ought to feel safe sharing your feelings, you should also feel safe sharing your ideas and beliefs within a relationship. Since every human being is unique, there will be occasions where you enter into disagreements. This is natural and not something to feel bad about. In the heat of the moment, when you're engaging in a healthy debate or discussion with somebody, intellectual boundaries ensure that you're able to speak without fear of being shut down or dismissed. Your intellectual boundaries may sound like:

- "Let us agree to disagree."
- "You may not agree with me, but I don't tolerate name-calling."
- "I don't feel comfortable engaging in this topic any further."
- "I have the right to share my opinions too."

Intellectual boundaries are violated when your thoughts or beliefs are shunned or criticized. You might feel put down or invalidated. Remember that you can always end a conversation and walk away when you believe the discussion is unproductive or harmful.

Material Boundaries

Other great types of boundaries to have are material boundaries. These protect your material possessions, such as your money, home, car, or clothing from being exploited by others. It's important to be clear about what you're willing to share and what you prefer to keep to yourself. Moreover, you can communicate to others how you expect your material possessions to be treated. Your material boundaries may sound like:

- "If you want to use my car, may you please put gas inside it?"
- "I would love to help, but I only have $20 on me right now. Is this okay?"
- "Please ask for my permission before taking clothing out of my closet."
- "I'm happy to host the event at my house, but can you help me clean up afterward?"

When your material possessions are vandalized, stolen, or compromised by other people, your material boundaries are violated. You need to also be careful of those who use possessions like money to manipulate or control you.

Privacy Boundaries

Finally, privacy boundaries separate public and private information. When you share private information with someone, you might enforce certain rules about how they can safeguard your information. Privacy boundaries also govern who has access to your space, technological devices, social media accounts, work documents, passwords, cell number, and other materials that might contain sensitive information. Your privacy boundaries may sound like:

- "Please don't share what I'm about to tell you with anyone else."
- "I'm not comfortable being tagged on social media without my

permission."
- "You don't have the right to access my emails."
- "Please don't mention my name or company in the article."

Privacy boundaries can also govern how much personal data you share with others or on social media. Make sure you read the privacy policies on your favorite apps or social networks to understand how your data is handled and protected.

Chapter Takeaways

- Boundaries regulate the amount of access people have to your time, energy, space, and resources.
- When you set boundaries in relationships, your needs, values, and expectations are considered during every interaction.
- Healthy boundaries are clear and specific about limits, but depending on the situation, they can be loosened to accommodate others.

Childhood Attachments and Boundaries

"The only people who get upset about you setting boundaries are the ones who were benefiting from you having none."

— UNKNOWN

This chapter talks about:

- What makes a family 'dysfunctional' and how this dynamic can affect boundary-setting
- The three types of childhood attachment styles and how they manifest in adult relationships
- The effects of trauma on boundary-setting and what you can do to create a sense of safety

What Makes a Family Dysfunctional?

In an ideal world, each family is built on solid values, principles, and traditions that inform how family members relate to one another and protect the mental and emotional well-being of parents and children. The mutual trust and intimacy shared by both parents helps them identify themselves as the adults who are responsible for modeling healthy behaviors in front of their children.

Knowing that they are the adults and that there are certain experiences they cannot share with their children, such as their sexual intimacy or personal troubles, parents set boundaries to limit exposure to their private lives. However, a special bond is formed between parents and children that allows parents to protect, show affection, and teach their children the difference between acceptable and unacceptable behavior. Therefore, in the broader context, parents set boundaries for their children as a way to provide guidance, discipline, and teach them how to be responsible adults.

The unfortunate truth is that not every family is built this way. For instance, there are parents who are unable to identify themselves as the adults who are responsible for guiding their children. Instead, they might see themselves as being the ones who need to be taken care of. There are also parents who, due to their own childhood traumas and experiences, are unable to nurture their children or provide emotional validation—or they might be overly protective to the extent of smothering their children. Some single parents may even fail to keep sensitive information private and might depend on their children for emotional support.

These kinds of dynamics create what we call dysfunctional families. According to the APA, a dysfunctional family is one where relationships and communication between members is impaired, making it difficult for members to freely express themselves or feel close to each other (APA Dictionary of Psychology, 2022). One of the hallmarks of a dysfunctional family is the lack of clear and healthy boundaries.

In an ideal situation, healthy boundaries assist parents and children in defining their roles, setting expectations, and building trust. A lack of healthy boundaries blurs the roles that each family member plays and leads to issues like codependency, abuse, and emotional neglect. When parents are unable to model good behaviors or create structure for their children, it leaves the children feeling vulnerable. They might feel afraid to speak up for themselves, assert their own values or beliefs, or create their own identity apart from their parents.

Let's consider a common scenario of a lack of boundaries within a family: Imagine a child growing up with a parent who's a functioning alcoholic. When they aren't drinking, they're able to take on the role of adult in the relationship, become emotionally available for their child, and enforce healthy discipline. However, when they're intoxicated, the parent reverts to the role of being a child and cannot make logical decisions on behalf of the family.

The child grows up having to constantly switch between being a child (when their parent is sober) and being the adult in the relationship (when their parent is intoxicated). The child may have to take on adult responsibilities like cooking, cleaning, and paying bills, or even start working from an early age to cover for the negligence of their parent. Moreover, the child might also learn that it's unsafe to express their own needs or say no to their parent out of fear of receiving backlash or causing more conflict at home. Thus, the burden of taking care of the family falls on the child's shoulders, and they feel hopeless about doing anything about it.

You might be wondering how different this family dynamic would look if there were healthy boundaries. Well, first and foremost, if the family above had healthy boundaries, the parent would be more responsible regarding their lifestyle choices, particularly those that might violate the sense of security of their child. For example, consuming alcohol is not a bad thing, but when it starts to interfere with the ability to relate with others in a healthy way, there must be personal boundaries put in place. For example, the parent might restrict their alcohol consumption, especially when they're drinking around their child. This would ensure that their behavior is consistent and the child never has to step outside of their role.

Secondly, healthy boundaries between the parent and child could improve how both parties communicate with each other. The parent might speak freely about the kinds of behaviors they expect from their child, and the child might also feel comfortable expressing areas in their life where they need support. With words of affirmation and appropriate physical touch, both parent and child could affirm their love and appreciation for each other, and through this kind of relationship the family unit can be strengthened.

Being Close vs Being Enmeshed

In some families, dysfunction can be disguised as closeness. On the outside, the family appears to be affectionate, protective, and supportive of each family member, but if you look closer at the dynamic, you'll see that the boundaries between members have been blurred.

Families who are enmeshed don't encourage independence or autonomy. The parents who create this dynamic raise their children to depend on their instructions and put the needs and interests of the family above their own. In most cases, one or both parents have a desire to control the actions and future outcomes of their children by impressing their personal beliefs onto them.

When enmeshment occurs, boundaries become blurred. A controlling parent, for example, might violate the privacy of their child, make their child feel guilty for keeping certain information private, or encourage their child to go into career fields or pursue achievements that would reflect positively on the family. In other words, instead of developing a healthy sense of self, the child ends up becoming the image of what the family represents.

It's also difficult for a child raised in an enmeshed family to form relationships outside of their family. They might be discouraged from staying alone or spending too much time away from the family. When they do attempt to create their own separate life, they're often met with criticism or made to feel guilty, as though they were deserting their family. A parent with financial means may cut off their child financially for making decisions that aren't in the best interests of the family.

The difference between being close and being enmeshed is that a close family doesn't pressure its members to look within the family unit for satisfaction, support, and other emotional needs that could be found through external relationships. Children are free to express their individuality, cultivate meaningful relationships outside of the family, and make decisions about their own life. In contrast, with an enmeshed family, there isn't enough space given to each member to discover their sense of self and gain independence. Children often grow up with low self-esteem and being afraid to take risks or do anything that may upset their parents.

Since it's difficult to identify enmeshment when you're living in it, here are a few common signs of enmeshment in families:

- **Loyalty is overly emphasized.** People who aren't part of the family are often treated as "outsiders" and are not to be trusted. Parents might advise their children to stay away from certain social scenes or people, or to keep family secrets hidden from others.
- **Blurred family roles.** Parents might act more like their children's best friends rather than parental figures. This allows them to have more intimate access into their children's lives, but it also causes parents to overshare adult issues with their children.
- **Lack of privacy.** There's little concern for privacy within the family. For example, parents can arrive at their children's houses unannounced, call whatever time they want, or be overly opinionated about their children's personal relationships.
- **Feeling guilty when saying no.** Since solidifying a sense of self is

frowned upon, children grow up having a difficult time expressing their needs and saying no. They may go along with their parents' wishes to avoid confrontation or tension.

- **Easily hurt when bids for affection are not received.** What reinforces enmeshment in families is the abundance of reassurance and affection that is given. This becomes somewhat addictive, and when a parent or child doesn't respond to bids for affection positively, the other family member may feel hurt or betrayed.

It's important to remember that enmeshed families also have a dysfunctional dynamic. Just because they're close doesn't mean that boundaries are respected and each family member's mental and emotional well-being is supported.

Attachment Styles in Adult Relationships

The nature of your family dynamic as a child affects how you relate with others in your adult relationships. One of the commonly cited theories that explains this is the attachment theory, discovered by psychiatrist John Bowlby and psychologist Mary Ainsworth (Robinson et al., 2021). The theory suggests that the bond you develop with your parents during childhood ends up becoming how you show up in other relationships and respond to intimacy.

There are four attachment styles that characterize the type of behaviors you might display in relationships, depending on your unique parent-child bond. By identifying which attachment style most represents your childhood, you can gain insight on the kinds of challenges you face in relationships, which can include the fear of setting boundaries or setting boundaries that are too loose or too rigid. Below is an outline of each attachment style and the type of boundary problems you may experience.

Secure Attachment Style

When you have a secure attachment style, you're able to open up to others and feel safe in intimate relationships. You have the ability to manage conflict well and take ownership of your mistakes or hold others accountable for theirs. Even though you're still learning about yourself, you're comfortable expressing your needs, thoughts, and feelings with others.

If you identify with this attachment style, it's likely that your parents were emotionally available for parenting when you were a child. For instance, they might have picked you up when you were crying, offered positive reinforcement, and created a safe home environment without being overly protective. This allowed you to grow up feeling supported and confident enough to make decisions, learn from your mistakes, and take healthy risks.

Due to your upbringing, you're aware of what healthy boundaries look like and you aren't afraid to enforce them when necessary. In general, you trust people and can be vulnerable when you feel safe in a relationship. However, your level of emotional intelligence can work against you if you aren't careful. For example, you might be overly concerned about the needs of others at the expense of your own well-being. Or since you're able to empathize with people, you might think it's your responsibility to fix them. Remember to respond to your needs first so you have the capacity to take care of others.

Anxious-Preoccupied Attachment Style

People with an anxious-preoccupied attachment style are typically needy in relationships. They tend to seek reassurance constantly, and may feel uncertain when they don't receive it. One of the main reasons for the constant seeking of reassurance is that they have a low self-esteem. They worry that they aren't good enough to be loved or take care of others.

If you identify with this attachment style, you were likely raised by hot and cold parents. One minute you were smothered with affection, and the next minute you were given the cold shoulder. This made you grow up feeling anxious about forming relationships with others and deep down fearing the possibility of being abandoned. In your adult relationships, you may crave intimacy with others, but your trust issues get in the way. When you do eventually open up to others, you tend to fixate on the relationship or become overly dependent on the other person.

The type of boundary issues you may experience involve space. For you, being apart from friends and family for too long feels unbearable. When an intimate partner doesn't want to spend every minute of the day with you, you might feel offended. Moreover, you may find it difficult to truly express who you are with others because you fear being rejected. As a result, you might take on different personas depending on who you're around and have trouble saying no to others.

Avoidant-Dismissive Attachment Style

Think of people who display the avoidant-dismissive attachment style as being the polar opposite of those who identify as anxious-preoccupied. While the latter desires an extreme amount of closeness—and may even compromise their own needs to feel safe in a relationship—the former runs away or rejects any form of closeness. In fact, avoidant-dismissive people are so afraid of intimacy that they deliberately keep relationships on the surface.

If you identify with this attachment style, you were likely raised by parents who were emotionally unavailable or who abandoned you during childhood. Your needs for nurturing and affection were not met, and thus as an adult, you're uncomfortable with closeness. Part of your strategy to self-soothe was to build a wall around your emotions so that no one could hurt you. In adult relationships, you tend to be independent to a fault, not relying on others for assistance. You may even avoid people who are too emotional because you see them as being volatile and weak.

You're likely to have boundaries because these are what help you feel secure. However, unlike those with a secure attachment who cultivate healthy and flexible boundaries, your boundaries may lean toward being rigid. For example, you may be intolerant of other people's mistakes and take extreme measures to show your disapproval. Furthermore, due to your emotional unavailability, you may be responsible for violating other people's boundaries, such as keeping secrets, being promiscuous, or manipulating your way to getting out of trouble.

Disorganized Attachment Style

In most cases, people who develop disorganized attachment are survivors of childhood abuse and neglect. For them, the world is seen to be a dangerous place, and the only way to protect themselves is to emotionally shut down or withdraw from cultivating meaningful relationships. Think of this attachment style as the heightened form of avoidant-dismissive attachment.

If you've developed this attachment style, you've probably found it difficult to manage stressful situations like conflict, failure, and loss. Since you haven't learned the appropriate coping strategies, everyday life situations feel unsafe or overwhelming. Furthermore, without the necessary skills to build nurturing relationships, you're likely to repeat abusive patterns that were modeled in front of you as a child.

The type of boundary issues you might deal with revolve around your sense of safety. You might find it tough to ask others for what you need, and as a result are often unsatisfied with the quality of your relationships.

Opening yourself to others may also be something you fear due to past negative experiences. Thus, as a way to hold onto others, you may seek to control or manipulate them. Even though you desire a sense of security in your relationships, you're also afraid of getting hurt again. What's even more saddening is that without the proper tools to process your trauma, you're vulnerable to substance abuse, obsession, and addiction.

How Does Trauma Affect Boundaries?

There are some adults who were exposed to childhood trauma and, as a result of their experiences, were unable to learn how to set healthy boundaries. We can define trauma as a painful event or experience that threatens your sense of physical and psychological safety. For instance, after going through a traumatic experience, you might be afraid of certain people or environments, or you can lose your ability to stand up for yourself.

Even if you weren't directly impacted by the trauma, meaning the painful event didn't affect you personally, you can still grow up with secondary trauma. For example, a child witnessing domestic violence can grow up feeling traumatized and being afraid of certain people or environments, even though they were not directly abused.

It's also important to realize that trauma is an umbrella term to describe various types of abuse, loss, and personal injury. When we speak of childhood trauma, we almost always mention the different kinds of abuse, but other forms of trauma may include:

- witnessing or being personally affected by a natural disaster
- experiencing emotional neglect
- being bullied or harassed
- facing financial insecurity
- witnessing a parent lose their source of income

- being raised by a mentally ill or addicted parent
- experiencing the death of a loved one
- having learning or behavioral difficulties
- being hospitalized with a serious illness

The effects of trauma can last a few months or could take years to resolve. Early therapeutic intervention can prevent PTSD and other trauma-related conditions. When medical assistance is not received, traumatic symptoms like flashbacks, nightmares, anxiety, avoidant behavior, emotional outbursts, or depressed moods can continue into adulthood.

One of the signs of unresolved trauma in adulthood is difficulty in setting healthy boundaries. Since you were never able to rebuild your shuttered belief system, process the grief, or learn how to create your own sense of safety, your boundaries are typically loose. This may attract manipulators who prey on your vulnerability and inflict even more emotional damage.

Below are a few signs that you may have loose boundaries as a result of living with trauma:

- **You are an oversharer.** People who are oversharers tend to seek validation from others. This may be due to early childhood abandonment, where you felt like your parents' love needed to be earned. In adult relationships, oversharing could be your way of forcing a connection with others and trying to win over their love.
- **You often feel taken for granted.** You believe that others are constantly looking for ways to exploit you. This feeling may be due to your inability to say no or enforce consequences when boundaries have been violated. You somehow wish that people could read your mind and know when you have reached your limits.
- **You are attracted to people who don't respect your boundaries.** When you're living with unresolved trauma, it's common to recreate

abusive relationships from the past. By doing this, you subconsciously hope to finally heal whatever part of you that was wounded as a child. Unfortunately, the cycle of abuse ends up repeating itself, and you're left with more emotional damage to process.

- **You are afraid to stand up for yourself.** Some types of trauma, particularly emotional abuse, can cause you to lose your sense of identity and independence. You may feel powerless to stand up for yourself when you have been mistreated, or fear the consequences of voicing your opinions.
- **You tend to feel anxious or stressed in social interactions.** When you're living with unresolved trauma, a part of you is still vulnerable to getting hurt. Social interactions can become terrifying because they present many opportunities for you to be triggered by someone or something. Moreover, since you don't have clear and firm boundaries, you fear being put in uncomfortable social situations.

Setting healthy boundaries can be the first step to healing from trauma. They can slowly help you regain structure, routine, and a sense of safety in your life, which can empower you to address other emotional issues. It's important for you to feel like you're in control of your time, energy, space, and resources, and to close the door for abusers and manipulators. Here are just a few ways you can get started on establishing healthy boundaries:

- **Be aware of your wants and needs.** It's common for trauma survivors to create a sense of safety by putting other people's needs first. However, this can cause them to neglect their own needs. Each day, take a five-minute break to check in with yourself and ask the question: "What do I need right now?"
- **Identify your tolerance levels.** Every person has a tolerance level. Finding yours can help you draw a boundary as soon as you feel uncomfortable or burned out. To figure out your tolerance level, think about a few relationship scenarios with friends and family that make you feel comfortable and some that make you uncomfortable.

- **Practice voicing your boundaries.** While it's good to write down your boundaries, eventually you'll need to communicate them to others rather than assume they know your limits. Looking into a mirror, express your boundaries in different ways, using different facial expressions, body language, and tone and pitch.
- **Get clear on your non-negotiables.** Part of healing from trauma is giving yourself certainty that certain violations that occurred in the past will not happen again. For example, if you were emotionally abused in a past relationship, your non-negotiable might be name-calling. Think about some of the painful violations that threatened your sense of safety and create a list of non-negotiables. Create boundaries around these non-negotiables and ensure your loved ones are informed about them.
- **Don't be afraid of having different boundaries.** Your trauma impacted your life in a very unique way. As a result of overcoming painful experiences, you have a unique set of wants and needs. Realize that what is acceptable for someone else may not be acceptable for you, and that your friends and family may not always understand why you need a certain boundary put in place, but that doesn't mean you're wrong or that your boundary shouldn't exist.

Healing from childhood trauma is a journey all on its own, but having healthy boundaries put in place can make the journey feel a lot more comfortable. Essentially, when you heal from trauma, you're teaching your mind and body how to cultivate mutually beneficial and safe relationships again. Healthy boundaries can make it easier for you to articulate your thoughts and feelings around personal space, emotional needs, and expectations from others.

So far, you've learned the benefits of setting healthy boundaries, as well as the common reason behind a lack of boundaries in adult relationships. In the following chapter, you will discover what boundary violations look like and how to be assertive when holding others accountable.

Chapter Takeaways

- Growing up in a dysfunctional family can make it difficult to set and enforce healthy boundaries later in life. Instead, you're more likely to reenact the harmful relationship behaviors you learned—or saw as acceptable—when you were a child.
- Tight-knit families can create a nurturing and supportive environment for all members. However, when the closeness turns into enmeshment, boundaries become blurred and each member's rights and freedoms are stifled.
- Learning about your particular attachment style can help you identify specific boundary problems that you may be dealing with. For example, you might be overly needy of others and lower your standards in the process (anxious-preoccupied attachment) or you might be skeptical of others and find reasons to push them away with strict boundaries (avoidant-dismissive attachment).
- Depending on your childhood, you may be living with unresolved trauma. Setting healthy boundaries is the first step to regaining your sense of physical and psychological safety and learning how to communicate your needs.

What Boundary Violations Look Like

"The difference between successful people and really successful people is that really successful people say 'no' to almost everything."

— WARREN BUFFETT

This chapter talks about:

- what constitutes a boundary violation
- how to set and enforce appropriate consequences
- how to set boundaries with toxic friends and family

How to Tell When Your Boundaries Have Been Violated

Are you able to tell when someone has crossed the line with you? If so, how? Setting boundaries is winning half the battle. Enforcing these boundaries and making sure others are held accountable for boundary violations is the other half of the battle.

Celebrities are public figures whose boundaries are constantly violated. If it isn't one of their celebrity friends exposing their secrets, it's the paparazzi violating their personal space. While talking to *People* magazine in 2017, Oprah Winfrey accidentally announced her costar Mindy Kaling's pregnancy to the whole world. She told reporters that she was stunned when Kaling broke the news that she was five months pregnant.

Later on, Kaling admitted in a TV interview that Winfrey announced the news to the media. However, she didn't seem too bothered about it because of the status that Winfrey has. She said, "If anyone is going to announce big news about your private life, Oprah Winfrey is the person. You can't complain that much about it, and you also can't be like, 'Hey, Oprah, zip it,' because she's almost like a religious figure" (Price, 2017).

Imagine that it was one of her non-famous friends announcing a secret to the press—would that be considered a boundary violation?

Another celebrity that has experienced boundary violations is Jennifer Lawrence. Around 2014, the actress's nude photos were stolen from her personal device and leaked on the internet by some hacker who managed to get access to her iCloud account. But as if that wasn't enough of a violation, she has also been the subject of harassment by paparazzi.

In an interview, she expressed the emotional impact of being followed around by paparazzi all of the time: "I knew the paparazzi were going to be a reality in my life," she said, "but I didn't know that I would feel anxiety every time I open my front door, or that being chased by 10 men you don't know, or being surrounded, feels invasive and makes me feel scared and gets my adrenaline going every day" (Solove, 2014).

Just as Lawrence explained, having your boundary violated can make you feel anxious. It's similar to hearing a robber crack a window and forcefully enter your house. Boundaries are the imaginary lines you draw between yourself and others, thus when they're crossed you can feel deeply unsettled.

Due to the fact that no boundary is the same, boundary violations can look different for each individual. It's therefore up to each person to identify the criteria for a violation. Examples of internal boundary violations include:

- someone makes you feel worthless
- being yelled at or called names
- being told a lie or having a secret concealed from you
- receiving unsolicited advice
- feeling judged or criticized
- feeling controlled or manipulated

In contrast, external boundary violations may include:

- someone standing too close to you without your permission
- being touched without your consent
- having someone look through your belongings
- not being allowed to enjoy your privacy
- being pressured to smoke if you are a non-smoker

It's normally easier to tell when someone violates a physical boundary because they make you feel unsafe. For example, an unwanted touch can send shivers down your spine and cause you to feel vulnerable. Since these are not positive signs, you'll immediately recognize that a boundary has been violated.

However, you may have a difficult time deciphering when an emotional boundary has been violated because the signs are less obvious. For instance, if someone interrupts you while you're speaking, could this be a boundary violation or not? If your answer is "yes and no" then it proves just how tough it is to spot emotional boundary violations. Below are five signs that can help you identify emotional boundary violations when you're unsure:

- **You find ways of justifying someone's bad behavior.** While you're aware that what someone is doing or how they're treating you isn't right, you make up excuses for their behavior. The common excuse is "That's just who they are." If the person is battling with health issues, you may justify their behavior as a symptom of their condition.

- **You blame yourself for someone else's actions.** Instead of reacting appropriately to the offense by setting a boundary or issuing a consequence, you internalize the offense and see it as your fault. You might say to yourself, "If I didn't come home late, my husband wouldn't be insulting me."
- **You feel ashamed for calling the person out on their behavior.** You may feel like you're making a big deal out of nothing, or that you're causing more trouble in your relationship by communicating your boundaries or letting someone know when they have violated a boundary. For example, you may feel ashamed of telling your partner that you need time alone because you don't want them to think you're checking out of the relationship.
- **You tend to second-guess your decisions.** After you have made up your mind about a boundary, you tend to backtrack on your decision when someone challenges it. For example, you tell your mother how excited you are to apply for a new job, and at first she seems happy for you. However, as the conversation continues, she challenges you about your readiness and competence for the position, which makes you second-guess the decision to apply for the job.
- **You feel uncomfortable around someone but don't know why.** You may feel uneasy when you're around someone who's violating an emotional boundary, but can't quite put your finger on what it is that makes you uneasy. Oftentimes, the person could be passive-aggressive or a master manipulator who covers their tracks and makes it difficult to hold them accountable.
- **Your opinions are disregarded.** When a mental or emotional boundary is violated, you tend to feel like your voice doesn't matter in the relationship. Whether you express your opinions or not, the other person will not acknowledge them. This can leave you feeling

powerless to express your needs or hold the other person accountable for violating your boundaries.

Effective Ways to Respond to Boundary Violations

It isn't fair to expect others to understand or know how to adhere to your boundaries. Some boundary violations happen because those closest to you or those you work with aren't able to express the kind of respect, support, or consideration you need. However, that doesn't mean they should walk away scot-free after they have mistreated you.

The point here is that good-intentioned people can cross your boundaries too. When they do, it isn't always done to deliberately hurt you. But even when this is the case, good-intentioned people must be held accountable for violating your boundaries.

It's true that the people you love and respect the most are the hardest to confront about boundary violations. You might feel like doing so could jeopardize your relationship or make them treat you differently moving forward. However, think about the consequences of not holding them accountable. How much worse will your relationship get if a line isn't drawn? In general, the earlier you respond to a boundary violation, the better it will be for your relationship. This is because when both of you know where you stand with each other, you can deepen your level of trust and find the relationship mutually beneficial.

Depending on how safe you feel in the relationship, there are three ways you can approach boundary violators:

- **When You Feel Safe in the Relationship**

If you have already established healthy communication in the relationship and are comfortable expressing your thoughts and feelings, you can schedule time to sit down and speak to the boundary violator about your issue. If it's a violation that needs to be addressed urgently, like being cut off while you're speaking, then it's best to pull the person aside and express your concerns. However, if it's a violation that's deeply personal and might require some time to process, it can help to write down your feelings and think about what you want to say before approaching them.

When you have the conversation, remember to use "I" statements, such as "I feel" and "I need." Doing this helps the violator listen to you without feeling attacked or judged. Plus, when you use "I" you're showing the other person that you take full ownership of how you're feeling. For example, you might say "I feel disrespected when you cut me off while I'm speaking. Please be more mindful of your behavior next time."

- **When Your Relationship Might Not Feel Safe**

What challenges a relationship's sense of safety is the repetitive violation of boundaries. For instance, after you have made it known to a friend that you don't appreciate a certain behavior, they continue to do it anyway. What becomes obvious in these relationships is that the boundary violator is not willing to listen and respond to your needs. Perhaps they preferred it when you didn't have any boundaries, and now that you're setting boundaries, they're doing everything in their power to resist the change.

Once again, this resistance shouldn't stop you from addressing the boundary violations. If the violator isn't willing to speak to you about it, you can consider speaking to a therapist or trusted friend about your concerns. In some cases, a third party can advise you on ways to communicate better with the boundary violator, but if the violator is set on not respecting your boundaries, then any kind of intervention won't be successful. The bitter truth that's sometimes difficult to hear is that if somebody doesn't respect you, they won't respect your boundaries. Thus, this type of relationship will never feel safe because you aren't receiving the respect you deserve.

You may consider creating some distance so that they aren't close enough to hurt you. For example, you can ban someone who violates your personal space (like making a mess in your house or stealing your belongings, etc.) from coming to your house. Or you can stop giving out an invite to a friend who constantly has excuses for not attending your events or always arrives too late.

- **When You Know Your Relationship Isn't Safe**

Abusive relationships do not feel safe at all. The abuser has no sense of empathy for your needs and certainly won't respect your boundaries. Over the years, they have become comfortable disregarding your feelings, making you feel worthless, and turning the tables around when you confront them. Therefore, addressing boundary violations with abusers is no use. If you're not willing to stand for disrespect anymore, you can consider cutting off all communication with them and walking away from the relationship.

Of course, the more entangled your emotions are in the relationship, the harder it will be to leave. For example, if the violator is a boss at work you can look for a new job, but if the violator is a family member or romantic partner, leaving the relationship could feel wrong. Your support system will play a big role in helping you gather the strength to walk away from the relationship. If you don't have a support system, perhaps you can start creating one right now by finding a relatable and friendly therapist.

Addressing boundary violations with loved ones is about being clear on what respectful and healthy behavior looks like and trusting your gut instinct when deciding on the best ways to handle the situation. Some people may simply need to hear you articulating the boundary again in order for them to be on the same page. Others may not respect your boundaries no matter how many times you communicate them. Remember that your standards were never designed to accommodate the needs of your friends, family, and colleagues. They were put in place to protect your needs so that you feel safe in your relationships.

Of course, you can't force anyone to respect your boundaries, but you can enforce consequences when your boundaries are violated.

How to Create Effective Consequences for Boundary Violations

Believe it or not, many healthy boundaries that people set do not have consequences attached to them. This is because we operate under the assumption that those closest to us will honor our boundaries. However, as we have discovered, even good-intentioned people can violate boundaries.

Consequences are not a bad thing. They aren't a form of punishment that you issue whenever somebody disrespects you. All they're supposed to do is teach a lesson of cause and effect—with every action there's an equal reaction. For example, when a family member continues to enter your bedroom without permission, you might start locking your room when you're away. Your reaction is a consequence of their action. It's your way of showing the family member that entering your room without permission is unacceptable.

Contrary to popular belief, anger or the silent treatment are not consequences. They are emotional responses to a boundary violation. The reason why they can't serve as consequences is because they don't teach the violator a lesson of cause and effect. Using the same example as above, if you got angry each time your family member entered your bedroom without permission, would they learn a lesson? Your anger would be an inconvenience, not a reason for them to change their behavior.

Therefore, strong emotions should not be used as consequences for broken boundaries.

The best consequences are not punitive, but corrective. Their objective is to teach the violator how to honor your space, time, energy, and resources. Each time they violate one of your boundaries, they get an opportunity to be reminded of what you expect. Thus, as you start creating consequences, remember that your aim is to teach a lesson in a respectful way and not to hurt or humiliate the violator.

In his book *Boundaries With Teens*, author and psychologist Dr. John Townsend presented five principles for setting effective consequences (Townsend, 2022). These principles can help you set consequences that teach a lesson and help violators understand your needs better. The five principles include:

1. Take Away the Desirable

Think of something the violator enjoys access to or depends on when it comes to you. Remove or limit access to that thing and place conditions. For example, if your friend gets into the habit of arriving late on your dates, you can cut down on the amount of times you meet up during the month or limit the amount of time you have to spend with them. You might say, "I only have an hour to spend with you. If you arrive late, then we'll have less time to catch up."

2. Let Natural Consequences Take Over

Since every cause has an effect, every bad behavior will have a negative consequence. What's great is the universe has a way of issuing consequences without you having to orchestrate anything. For example, if your romantic partner cheats on you, it could naturally be the end of the relationship. Or if your friend shares personal information about you, it will lead to distrust. The only thing natural consequences require from you is to not get involved by justifying the violator's bad behaviors.

3. Make the Consequence Significant

In order to be effective, a consequence must be significant to the other person. In other words, it should be strong enough to make them pause and reflect on their behaviors. They must be able to understand the impact of their actions and what they could possibly stand to lose if their actions don't change. A coworker who makes embarrassing comments about you in front of others might understand the impact of their behavior if you don't show any response—completely ignore what they have said and continue to engage with others. This would make enough of an impact for them to question their harmful actions.

4. Find the Most Lenient Consequence That Works

Once again, consequences are not supposed to feel like punishments, nor are they meant to cause harm to your relationships. If possible, you should create consequences that are lenient while appropriately matching the violation. For example, if you're disrespected by a colleague, giving them the silent treatment would be too lenient and may even lead to more disrespect. But limiting your communication to only work-related matters is an appropriate consequence that teaches them the value of respect. Remember that your goal is to correct bad behavior, not crucify someone for it.

5. Praise Positive Changes

After you have issued a consequence, keep your eyes open and watch out for changed behavior. It's important that the violator feels supported and loved throughout the process of submitting to your consequence. In most cases, having to go along with your consequences can make them feel ashamed or embarrassed, so be sensitive not to rub it in their face or make jokes showing you're in a superior position. For example, when you notice your partner is no longer raising their voice during arguments, mention how positive it makes you feel and thank them for respecting your communication boundary.

As you can see, consequences were never supposed to damage relationships; all they were meant to do is hold those you love accountable for their actions. Nevertheless, it's still possible that you're in relationships with people who undermine your consequences and refuse to be held accountable. For this reason, you might need to consider alternative options.

Setting Boundaries With Toxic People

Have you ever thought about what makes a relationship toxic? The truth is that any relationship that makes you feel worse rather than better about yourself can become toxic. While no relationship is perfect, and it's common to have disagreements with people, a relationship should never threaten your physical and psychological well-being.

Only you can determine if the bad traits or behaviors of a person outweighs their positive traits and behaviors. For example, one person may not have an issue with being called a curse word, while another person may feel demeaned when they're called a curse word. Nonetheless, when any behavior shifts from being innocent to being used as an attack, it can become toxic. Below are hidden signs that you might be involved in a toxic relationship:

- You invest more into the relationship than you're getting out of it.
- You constantly feel like your needs aren't being met.
- Your self-esteem has lowered since entering the relationship.
- You feel tired, anxious, or depressed after spending time with the

individual.

- You notice yourself thinking or speaking negatively around the individual.
- Being around the individual brings out the worst side of you (E.g. you tend to gossip, judge others, or complain about life when you're with them.)
- You're afraid to express your true thoughts and feelings when you're around them.
- You spend a lot of time worrying if they're happy or being sensitive to their needs.

Toxic people can also come in all different shapes and sizes. What makes one person toxic might be different to what makes another person toxic. Learning about the different characteristics of toxic behavior can help you identify friends, family, and colleagues with toxic traits. Below are five types of toxic people:

- **The coworker who belittles you.** This person will make sarcastic remarks, implying that your thoughts or feelings are insignificant. They might make jokes at your expense or find ways to demean you in front of others. When confronting them about their behavior, they may say "I'm only kidding."
- **The parent with a bad temper.** Being around this person could make you feel on edge. You're never sure when they might erupt and have an emotional outburst. They're sensitive to criticism and don't like being questioned about their actions. When they feel under pressure, they'll lash out in rage.
- **The guilt-tripping partner.** This person feels safe when they have control in the relationship. One of the tactics they use to feel in control is to guilt-trip you. They often make you feel bad for not doing what they want you to do. When guilt-tripping doesn't work, they may accuse you of not being a loving or considerate partner.
- **The overreacting sibling.** When you attempt to confront this per-

son about their boundary violations, they become overly emotional and make it difficult to hold them accountable. You might end up comforting them and forget the main purpose of your discussion. Another variation of this toxic trait is turning the tables around and making their bad behavior seem like it's your fault.

- **The overdependent friend.** This person is so passive to the extent that they rely on you to take care of them and make most of the decisions on their behalf. It can feel like you're caring for a small child who can't think for themselves, and this can be emotionally draining. When you can't be there for them, you may feel guilty or anxious because you worry that something bad will happen to them.

Setting boundaries with a toxic person can be challenging because they have developed a habit of disregarding your needs and expectations in the relationship. However, that doesn't mean that they shouldn't face similar consequences as other good-intentioned boundary violators. When you have enforced consequences with a toxic person and they continue to violate your boundaries, there are few options available to you.

- **Decide whether the boundary is negotiable.** If the boundary being crossed isn't as important as some that are being respected, then you can consider making a compromise. However, remember that you're compromising with someone who isn't able to empathize with you, so being too lenient may come at the cost of your well-being. If the boundary repeatedly being crossed is non-negotiable, this could be a deal breaker in your relationship.
- **Get into the habit of writing down the violations.** Toxic people tend to twist the truth and use all sorts of manipulation to get you to doubt your own conception of reality. Write down every boundary violation, the consequence that was issued, and the response to your consequence. Having a record can help you when confronting the toxic person about their mistreatment, as well as when you're trying to weigh the pros and cons of the relationship.

- **Practice loving detachment.** When you lovingly detach from someone, you allow natural consequences to take over. Instead of trying to fix them, you accept them for who they are and maintain a healthy distance. This could include blocking their number on your cell phone, moving out of the apartment you share, declining invites to meet up, and so on. The relationship may fizzle out on its own, or the person may return ready to respect your boundaries.
- **If the relationship has become too volatile to maintain, go no-contact.** When you go no-contact, your primary concern is your mental, emotional, and physical health. Sometimes, maintaining certain relationships can start to make you sick, lose motivation, or feel hopeless. Going no-contact gives you time to prioritize your well-being, address your own psychological issues, and reassess the value of the relationship.
- **Get support from a third party.** When you're in a toxic relationship, you can feel isolated from everyone else. It's important to reach out to people who can give you unbiased advice about your situation so you have the confidence to stand up for yourself. If you don't feel safe talking to friends and family, look for a friendly therapist who can support you on this journey.

When setting boundaries and holding toxic people accountable to them, remind yourself that you have a choice in the matter. Just because you have known someone for many years or have built a close bond with them doesn't mean that you need to put up with abusive or manipulative behavior.

Choosing to continue to work on a toxic relationship requires two willing participants. If you're the only person who's committed to working on the relationship, then you won't see the kind of positive change you seek. Plus, since it's impossible to force someone to respect your boundaries, getting a toxic person to respond to your needs and help you feel safe in the relationship won't work.

It's possible that you're not ready to distance yourself from the toxic person, and this decision is okay too. Remember, you have choices! Instead of going no-contact, you might decide to limit access or detach emotionally. Rely on your gut instinct to tell you which option is best for you at this particular time.

Chapter Takeaways

- It's easier to detect physical boundary violations, such as feeling uncomfortable when someone touches your body. However, emotional boundary violations may not be so easy to spot.
- The best way to figure out if your emotional boundaries have been violated is to check if you're making excuses for mistreatment, whether you feel guilty for confronting the person or if your opinions are disregarded.
- Communicating boundary violations will require a different approach depending on how safe you feel in the relationship. If you feel comfortable voicing your concerns, all it could take is a meaningful one-on-one conversation. But if you don't feel safe at all, you can consider turning to a mediator for support.
- When creating consequences, ensure that they match the offense and are designed to teach the violator a lesson rather than punish them for breaking your boundary. After submitting to the consequence, the violator is meant to understand the impact of their actions and what they could lose if they don't correct their behavior.
- Toxic people may not respond well to consequences. Instead, they could use the confrontation as an opportunity to blame their behavior on your actions. You don't need to feel hopeless when setting boundaries with toxic people. Simply weigh your options and make a decision that protects your well-being. Once again, your support system will play a huge role in helping you safely walk away from a toxic relationship.

How to Communicate Boundaries Without Fear

"I set boundaries not to offend you but to respect myself."

— UNKNOWN

This chapter talks about:

- How to overcome the fear of what others might think of you
- How to define a healthy relationship according to your vision
- Phrases to use when communicating your boundaries assertively

The Fear of What Others Think

Have you ever been in a meeting and asked a question or shared your opinion, only for everybody present to stare at you like there was ketchup on your face? How did you feel at that moment?

We can't pretend that we aren't subconsciously hoping that the people around us like who we are. In fact, it's part of our human psychology to be concerned about what others might think about us. During the caveman days, our ancestors depended on groups, also known as tribes, in order to survive. Being part of a tribe was the security each individual needed to feel a sense of belonging.

Even though we don't operate in tribes anymore, there's still the natural human urge to form groups with others. We need a healthy dose of social validation to know that we're safe and valued. As we witnessed during the pandemic, being in complete isolation from others brought about anxiety and loneliness. Therefore, to some extent, we can't escape the need for relationships in our lives.

With all this said, when the need for relationships causes us to compromise on other physical, mental, and emotional needs, it becomes unhealthy. For example, when doing favors for others causes you to get behind on your work commitments, lose sleep, or put your goals on hold, then the cost becomes too high. Your generosity stops becoming a virtue, but rather a quality that makes you vulnerable to being taken for granted. When we are so focused on others that we make their thoughts and feelings more of a priority than our own, we risk satisfying other needs in our lives.

Caring about what other people think of us isn't bad, but living with the fear of what others might think can be harmful. For example, at work we might care about our reputation because it's important in building healthy work relationships. However, being afraid that our fellow coworkers don't like us can be a destructive thought. This is because it prevents us from taking necessary action and freely expressing who we are. We're always somewhat scared that we might step on someone's toes and make them upset.

The fear of what others might think can also make setting boundaries difficult. Since boundaries communicate our limits, we might be afraid that others may reject, ridicule, or judge us for drawing a separation between us and them. This often leads to loose boundaries that are too lenient and make us vulnerable to users and abusers.

It can be confusing to tell the difference between a healthy concern about how others perceive you and actually being afraid of what they might think (particularly if their perception is negative). Below are some of the common signs that you fear what others might think of you:

- When met with disapproval, you quickly change your stance and passively agree with the other person.
- If somebody comments about not liking something about you, you obsess about their comment until you start to see fault in yourself too.
- You prefer to let others make decisions for you, especially in a group setting where there may be a conflict of opinions.
- You are reluctant to express discomfort because you don't want to make the other person uncomfortable.
- You tend to beat yourself up when you make mistakes.
- You lose sleep over a disagreement with a friend or family member.
- You tend to apologize even when you're not in the wrong, just so you can clear the air.

If any of these signs have resonated with you, then it's a good idea to look for ways to not be so dependent on external validation. The following section will provide you with strategies on how to do it.

Strategies to Eliminate the Fear of What Others Think

Setting boundaries will continue to be a struggle until you overcome the fear of what others think. Recognizing that you're living with this issue is the first step. The second step involves practicing the following strategies:

- **Take People Off the Pedestal**

The first strategy is to remove anyone you have placed on a pedestal in your life. While it's normal to admire people, it's harmful to think that just because people are smart, beautiful, or successful that they're superior to you. Having skills, virtues, and talents doesn't make someone better than you, it simply means that they were able to cultivate their strengths. You have the same power to cultivate your strengths, thus there is nothing necessarily magical or supernatural about what they have done.

Start to see people for who they are, not who you have depicted them to be. Similar to you, every person you will encounter has strengths and weaknesses. They also have a complicated past and everyday work, health, and relationship struggles. Nobody you meet is perfect, nor can they achieve perfection. Therefore, when you observe people, have a sober evaluation of who they are and realize that you may have more in common than you think.

- **Accept That Not Everybody Will Like You**

If everyone had the same heart as your grandmother, perhaps they would think you were the best person in the world! But not everyone shares the same perspective as your grandmother. There are many reasons why some people won't like you—and most of them have nothing to do with you. In general, whether a person likes you or not has a lot to do with their formulated opinions (emphasis on 'their').

If you look at what informs a person's opinions, you'll find many factors that once again have little to do with you. For example, a person's opinion could be based on their upbringing, trauma, beliefs, emotions, desires, fears, and a whole bunch of other things. When a person rejects, criticizes, or judges you, all of these factors are triggered within them. Thus, it's impossible to connect with every person you meet or get them to understand your needs or where you're coming from.

- **Remind Yourself That Hurt People Hurt People**

It's unfair to expect someone who's dealing with emotional pain to treat you better than they treat themselves. Hurt people hurt people. This doesn't make their actions right or absolve them of any responsibility. However, it means that you can't expect them to empathize with you. Until they have gone through their healing process, they might always judge you negatively. Therefore, what they think of you isn't necessarily true, it's simply a reflection of their own pain.

- **Recognize the Voice of the Inner Critic**

There are times when you may think that someone dislikes you, but the truth is that you're projecting your own insecurities. The voice of the inner critic can sometimes sound like somebody else's thoughts and feelings, when in actuality they're your own thoughts and feelings. Be mindful of the internal dialogue you're having with yourself on a daily basis and how that might affect how you perceive yourself and others.

If you have a low self-esteem due to all of the past experiences you have endured, seek support from a therapist and slowly work toward having a positive self-perception. You can also consider cultivating deeper self-esteem by getting started with mirror work (refer to Chapter 5). When you can view yourself in a more positive light, it can become easier to tell the difference between your thoughts and what others believe about you.

- **Hold Off on Judging Others**

Another common reason that you might think others are judging you is because you're so used to judging others. In other words, you end up attracting the quality of thoughts you're constantly sending out. When you think negatively about others, you'll assume they're thinking negatively about you. However, if you were to think positively about others, you would assume they're thinking positively about you, too. The same applies to whom you call an enemy: An enemy is only an enemy because you have made them so. If you start to have a neutral or positive perception about them, they stop becoming an enemy. Thus, if you want to eliminate the fear of what others might think, practice thinking good thoughts about them and interpreting their actions in a positive way.

Craft Your Ideal Relationships

You may be able to set healthy boundaries in your current relationships, but if these relationships continue to feel unsafe, your boundaries may not work. In order to feel empowered in your relationships, safety is incredibly important, and moving forward, this characteristic might be something you look for in the relationships you form.

Healthy people who have good intentions will never put you down for setting boundaries. This is because they understand that relationships involve two unique people who have unique needs. Healthy people also understand the value of mutual respect and compromise. Instead of seeking to always get their way, they're considerate about your needs and feelings.

As you prepare to live a healthier lifestyle where your relationships feel safe and your needs are respected, it's worth thinking about the kind of relationships you desire. What do you want in a romantic partner, best friend, or boss? How do you want to feel when communicating with them? What kinds of values do you want to see shining forth? If you have grown up in a dysfunctional environment, you may not know what healthy relationships look or feel like. You may even think that you don't deserve to have relationships where you are honored, adored, and listened to.

I'm here to encourage you that healthy relationships exist, and that you deserve to have many of them in your life. You're not asking for too much when you say that you want to be around kind, honest, affectionate, generous, and friendly people. When it comes to romantic relationships, you're not asking for too much when you mention a list of qualities you need from your partner. In fact, relationship experts have found that there are qualities in a relationship that are more important than love, such as (Newsome, 2016):

- the ability to trust each other
- having a foundation of mutual respect
- feeling safe to express your thoughts and feelings
- having more happy experiences than hurtful experiences
- becoming good friends and leaning on each other
- maintaining your sense of self and having separate hobbies and interests
- showing commitment by actively making the relationship better
- regularly updating each other about your needs and boundaries

As you can see, love is never enough when it comes to building healthy relationships. Take a moment and think about your existing relationships in different areas of your life. Reflect on the current state of these relationships and what qualities are missing in order for you to feel satisfied. Write down a list of these qualities—you'll need them when you complete your relationship vision statement.

How to Create a Relationship Vision Statement

The concept of a relationship vision statement may seem strange, however, just like companies establish a vision statement, so can you when crafting your ideal relationships.

A relationship vision statement gives you the opportunity to think about the quality of interactions you desire based on your needs, beliefs, values, and past experiences. Unless the people you're in relationships with have a similar vision, you'll often have disagreements or communication issues.

Starting off new relationships with a vision can set you up to succeed. But this doesn't mean that your existing relationships can't benefit from a vision either. Of course, both you and the other individual must agree that your relationship needs a fresh start and work together to form a new vision. If it's only you who desires a fresh start, this exercise won't be useful.

Below are the steps on how you can create a relationship vision statement together with the person you're in a relationship with:

Step 1: Write Down 'We' Statements

On separate pieces of paper, write down statements about the kind of relationship you want. Start each statement with the word 'we,' like "We enjoy spending quality time together." Ensure that each statement is written in the present tense, as though it's how your relationship is operating right now. Write down 5–10 statements, and when you're done, read them aloud to each other.

Step 2: Discuss and Consolidate Your Lists

Take turns discussing each statement in more depth to truly understand the expectation. You're welcome to raise questions and challenge the expectations in a respectful way. For example, you might say, "I hear that you'd like us to spend more time together, but what happens when I'm busy throughout the week?" Remember, challenging isn't the same as judging. You challenge by validating what the other person is saying and sharing your ideas, thoughts, or concerns to trigger a deeper conversation and compromise.

After you have discussed each statement, decide on which vision statements you agree on and would like to work on together. Not every statement on your list or theirs will make the final list. This is okay. The final list should only consist of vision statements that hold true and feel meaningful for both of you.

Step 3: Hold Each Other Accountable

Your final list should be treated as a working document, meaning that you're both constantly editing, adding, and removing statements according to your relationship's needs. Make copies of the list so that you can both access it regularly and hold yourselves and each other accountable. For example, if your friend raises their voice at you during a conversation, you can remind them of your vision statement that states "We will speak to each other with respect." This is how you can ensure your relationship reflects ideals that both of you share.

If you need inspiration on what relationship vision statements look like, below are a few examples to consider:

- We are free to share any thought or feeling without being judged.
- We spend at least one weekend in the month together.
- We speak highly of each other to friends and family.
- We avoid making jokes about each other's feelings.
- We compliment each other often.
- We tell each other the truth even if it's painful.
- We explore new activities together.
- We have sex at least once a week.
- We respect each other's need for privacy.
- We support each other's goals.

Communicating Boundaries Assertively

Getting over the hurdle of what others think will give you the necessary confidence to ask for what you need. This doesn't mean that your boundaries will always be well received, but it does mean that you'll be able to draw limits with others. A great communication skill that will improve how you articulate boundaries is assertiveness.

To be assertive is to stand up for yourself and what you believe in.

Assertive communication, therefore, is a style of communication where you make confident statements while showing respect to others. It shouldn't be confused with arrogance, since an arrogant speaker is self-absorbed and will not listen or empathize with the other person.

Assertive communication is also not defensive, nor is it aggressive. You don't need to raise your voice or intimidate others to get them to listen. In fact, aggressive communication is more likely to cause the other person to shut down or walk away, which prevents you from getting what you need.

Assertiveness is important when communicating boundaries because it sends a clear and direct message. Unlike passive communication, where the listener is confused about what you're actually saying, assertive communication gets down to the nitty-gritties and states boundaries boldly. For example, instead of saying to a friend, "Oh, so you're ignoring me now?" which is a question that's hiding a deeper meaning, you can plainly say, "I don't feel seen or loved when you give me the silent treatment. If you're not prepared to talk, I'll leave."

What's the difference between these two statements? The first one is indirect and somewhat sarcastic. It's likely to aggravate your friend rather than allow them to see how their behavior is impacting you. The second statement focuses on your experience rather than theirs, and sets a boundary followed by a consequence.

Now practice saying both statements to yourself and notice the difference in tone. The first statement doesn't allow you to convey as much clarity and confidence as the second one. And this is why assertive communication will always work when communicating boundaries.

Constructing assertive statements isn't as difficult as it seems. There's a simple formula that you can follow whenever you desire to convey messages assertively:

- **Think about what you want to say and write it down.** Don't skip this step because it'll help you map out your thoughts and ensure you're being as clear as possible. Sometimes when you have a million thoughts running through your mind, it becomes tough to know exactly what boundary has been violated and the appropriate consequence to issue.
- **Tune into your feelings.** Assertive communication places the spotlight on your experiences. For example, instead of saying "You make me feel," you would say "I feel." Check in with yourself and figure out what emotions were triggered when your boundary was violated. Write these emotions down on paper too, starting with "I feel" or "I felt."
- **Mentally prepare yourself to enforce the consequence.** After demonstrating confidence in communicating your boundary, you must be willing to follow through with the consequence if the other person isn't willing to listen. Think about what you'll do if the other person is uncooperative. Have at least three different options that you can revert to at that very moment.

So far, you understand what assertive communication is and how to construct assertive statements. Now we'll get a little bit more specific and look at five elements that your statements need in order to qualify as assertive.

- **Clearly Describe the Transgression/Behavior**

It's important for the other person to understand what they might have done to offend you. Remember, even good-intentioned people can violate boundaries, so we can't assume that everyone who violates our boundaries means any harm. By explaining what has happened, you give them an opportunity to reflect on their behavior and see where they might have gone wrong.

Here's an example of describing the transgression/behavior:

> *"When you interrupt me while I'm speaking..."*

- **Be Honest About the Emotional Impact**

The next component is displaying vulnerability by sharing your feelings. This will probably feel awkward if you aren't used to expressing your emotions, but it explains why the boundary violation means so much to you. If the relationship doesn't feel psychologically safe, you may not feel comfortable opening up about your emotions. This is okay, and you shouldn't feel guilty for not trusting another person with your emotions. Simply remove this component from your statement.

Here's an example of conveying the emotional impact:

> "I feel frustrated."

- **Share Your Thoughts**

It's common for a boundary violation to make you draw assumptions or perceive the violator in a certain way. Once again, it's important for the other person to know what thoughts are running through your mind when they violate your boundaries. This gives them an opportunity to step inside your shoes and imagine what you're experiencing. When sharing your thoughts, be respectful and considerate of their emotions too. While it's good to get everything off your chest, it's never good to make another person feel small, insulted, or ashamed.

Here's an example of sharing your thoughts:

> *"It makes me think that you don't care about my opinions."*

- **Suggest an Alternative Behavior**

The goal of communicating boundaries isn't to punish the other person, but to teach them about how they can respond to your needs better. Therefore, a crucial component of your statement is the alternative behavior. Instead of their current behavior, think about how they can act differently (within reason, of course). The alternative behavior must be realistic and simple enough for the other person to follow.

Here's an example of suggesting an alternative behavior:

> *"I would appreciate it if you waited for me to complete my train of thought before you speak."*

- **Clearly Define the Consequences**

Lastly, end your assertive statement by defining the consequences. In other words, if the other person doesn't make the effort to follow the alternative behavior, what will you do in response? Remember to choose a consequence that matches the violation and is effective while also being a teachable moment.

Here's an example of a definitive consequence:

> *"If you continue interrupting me while I speak, I'll disengage from the conversation."*

Now, let's combine all five components to see how communicating boundaries assertively looks and sounds like:

"When you interrupt me while I'm speaking (1), I feel frustrated (2). It makes me think that you don't care about my opinions (3). I would appreciate it if you waited for me to complete my train of thought before you speak (4). If you continue interrupting me while I speak, I'll disengage from the conversation (5)."

Practice saying this paragraph in the mirror. Repeat it over and over again until you feel a sense of confidence take over your body. This is the kind of confidence you need when approaching someone who has violated your boundary.

Phrases to Help You Communicate Boldly

Communicating boundaries won't come naturally at the beginning, but with much practice, you'll learn how to articulate yourself better. To end off the chapter, I'll present to you phrases that can become your template when communicating boundaries.

To start off with, here are sentence openers that you can use to initiate a conversation about your boundaries:

- "I would like to bring something to your attention."
- "May I please make a request from you?"
- "I would like to revisit the incident that took place yesterday."
- "I have taken the time to think about your request."
- "Is this a good time for us to have a heartfelt conversation?"

There are also specific phrases that you can use when setting certain kinds of boundaries. For example, you can use the following phrases when disagreeing with someone in a respectful way:

- "I disagree with your approach to this situation."
- "I'm not willing to change my mind about this matter."

- "I hear what you're saying. However, that hasn't been my experience."
- "Your ideas are fascinating. However, I'm not sure how they would work in practice."
- "Let's agree to disagree on this subject."

There will be times when you'll need to make it clear that the answer is a firm 'no.' Here are a few phrases to help you state your position confidently:

- "I don't have the time to take on more projects."
- "I know my original response was yes, but after looking at my schedule, I can't commit to any more tasks."
- "I can't answer your call right now. Please send a text."
- "I would be happy to help you, but my hourly rate is $100."
- "I can't see you this weekend. Let's reschedule for another time."

In certain situations, you'll be put on the spot and forced to set a boundary at that moment. An example would be someone asking you a question that you're unprepared to answer. Here are some phrases that can help you set boundaries right there and then:

- "I'm uncomfortable answering that question."
- "Give me some time to have a look through my emails and I'll get back to you."
- "I'm not in the position to share that information with you."
- "I'm not in a good place to have this conversation right now."
- "I'm not an expert on that topic, but I'll find someone who is."

Every now and again, you'll encounter people who are negative and seek to bring you down. They may be your friends, family, customers, or strangers you meet in public. Here are some of the ways you can set boundaries and protect your mental and emotional well-being:

- "Please excuse me while I take five minutes to recollect myself."
- "I'm feeling overwhelmed by this conversation. I would like us to change topics and come back to this subject later."
- "What you have shared with me is a lot to take in. Please give me a few days to process this information and I'll get back to you."
- "I feel misunderstood and I don't think we'll get very far with this topic. Let's agree to disagree."
- "I don't appreciate being spoken to like that. You can disagree with me, but insulting me is unacceptable."
- "I would like us to find a middle ground, but if you aren't prepared to compromise, I'm willing to walk away."

Sometimes, you'll want to convey the emotional impact that a boundary violation has on you. Here are some of the ways you can describe your emotional experience:

- "I feel afraid to be honest with you."
- "I don't feel like my needs are being considered."
- "I feel shut out when you emotionally withdraw from me."
- "I feel undermined when you tease me in front of our friends."
- "I feel betrayed when you share my secrets with your family members."
- "I don't feel comfortable opening up to you about that situation right now."

Finally, there will be times when good-intentioned people give you unsolicited advice. Instead of putting them down, you can set a clear boundary and redirect the conversation to something else. Here are a few phrases to help you:

- "I think we're getting distracted. Let's focus on the task at hand."
- "I value your friendship, but this is a family matter."
- "Thank you for those encouraging words. I'll go home and think about it."

- "That may have been the case in your situation, but my situation is different."
- "Let me talk to my partner first and then I'll get back to you."
- "I understand that you have more experience, but allow me to do it my way."

Chapter Takeaways

- Caring about what others think of you isn't necessarily a bad thing. However, when you become fearful of criticism or judgment, it can hold you back from making decisions that could improve your quality of life.
- Realize that not everybody will like you or have enough empathy to accept you as you are. Their dislike of you has more to do with their personal experiences, biases, and assumptions than who you are as a person.
- You can protect yourself from one-sided or unsupportive relationships by creating relationship vision statements with your friends and family and holding each other accountable to that shared vision.
- When communicating boundaries, assertiveness is key. It gives you the confidence to stand up for yourself while being mindful of others. The five components that make boundary statements assertive are: describing the transgression, describing the emotional impact, sharing your thoughts, suggesting an alternative behavior, and defining the consequence.

What Self-Love Has to Do With It

"Loving yourself does not mean being self-absorbed or narcissistic, or disregarding others. Rather it means welcoming yourself as the most honored guest in your own heart, a guest worthy of respect, a lovable companion."

— MARGO ANAND

This chapter talks about:

- The emotional impact of not being shown love as a child
- How to identify old relationship patterns so you can stop attracting toxic people
- The true meaning of self-love and steps on how to get started with mirror work

Robbed of the Affection You Needed

Love is an emotion that's essential for your survival. It isn't optional, nor is it a privilege that only some people get. When you're robbed of love, you become physically, mentally, and emotionally sick. The lack of love, especially in the lives of children, is serious enough to cause trauma.

Love is more than hugs and kisses. It's about feeling safe and accepted.

Think back to some of your earliest childhood memories and connect to your emotional experiences. Reflect on how your parents made you feel in their presence and absence, or how you felt living in that household environment. If what you felt back then was fear, confusion, stress, or unworthiness, then it means your parent-child relationship or the household environment lacked love.

If you want to dig deeper, you can even think about nonverbal cues that your parents showed that signaled being emotionally unavailable. A few of these might have been avoiding eye contact when you spoke, being short-tempered, failing to soothe you when you were distressed, invalidating your feelings, and so on.

The lack of love in childhood may have affected you in several ways, but one of them was in how you built your sense of self; who you believe you are and what you believe you deserve. Being raised by emotionally unavailable parents meant that you weren't able to see yourself correctly. You interpreted the coldness or neglect as a consequence for being a certain way. Instead of viewing your parents' behaviors as a sign of their own dysfunction or mental health issues, you internalized the mistreatment and saw it as a reflection of who you are.

An example of this would be a daughter who was raised by a narcissistic mother, but is too young to see her mother's self-absorbed and controlling behavior as a sign of her own psychological state of mind. She internalizes her mother's daily criticism and gaslighting as a sign that she needs to change something about herself. "Perhaps if I just shut up and agreed to what mom says," she thinks, "then she'll be pleased with me." Desperate to receive her mother's unconditional love, she internalizes the criticism and seeks to correct "flaws" in her own character. Of course, the worse her mother's behavior gets, the more flaws she believes need to be corrected in herself.

Maybe you have a similar experience of questioning your character as a result of internalizing your parents' suffering. Due to being young and not having a sense of boundaries, you internalized the negative energy and dysfunction in your environment and developed a warped sense of self. You may have even concluded that you're unlovable or that you don't like affection, only because you were robbed of unconditional love.

You might be wondering what all of this has to do with setting boundaries. The lack of love during childhood creates patterns later on in life. These patterns can manifest in different ways, although they all resemble the dysfunctional parent-child relationship. For instance, not being shown love as a child can make you desperate for love as an adult, which often means compromising your own standards just to please others. You're so desperate for others to validate you to the extent that their thoughts and opinions about you matter more than what you believe about yourself.

Another pattern that could manifest is pushing people away because you don't trust that they can protect you and give you the kind of love you need. You may even adopt the belief that love is dangerous (if you were abused by someone you trusted) or that love is painful (if you were betrayed). These beliefs cause you to place barriers between yourself and others, making it extremely difficult to connect or build intimacy.

These patterns continue to unfold in your adult relationships until you recognize them and make different choices. One of the first choices you will need to make is to stop looking at love from a negative perspective and start embracing the idea that healthy love exists, and you deserve to experience it!

How to Stop Attracting Toxic People

A quote that I read a while back said, "You stop attracting certain people when you heal the part of you that once needed them." (Tygielski, 2017) It may sound strange to think that a part of you is drawn to people who disrespect your boundaries or prove to be unreliable or emotionally unavailable after knowing them for some time. However, if you understand the fact that your adult relationships follow patterns you learned from childhood, it becomes a lot easier to accept why you're constantly attracting one toxic person after the next.

Another uncomfortable truth to hear is that due to not receiving sufficient nurturing and affection as a child, opening yourself up to healthy and loving relationships feels terrifying. In other words, having someone treat you with respect, be attuned to your needs, and respect your boundaries can make you suspicious, and you might unintentionally find ways of sabotaging that healthy relationship.

Responding negatively to love is a sign of childhood trauma that must be addressed before you can cultivate healthy relationships. This behavior prevents you from making genuine connections with good-intentioned people. In fact, when a stable and secure person notices how detached you are from your feelings or how defensive you get when they attempt to get close, they will often walk away from the relationship. A toxic person, on the other hand, will notice the same negative behaviors and feel safe in your company because they respond to love in the same unhealthy way.

To process and overcome your negative views about love, it's important to understand what causes you to react to love in that manner. Below are the three main reasons you may find it difficult to accept genuine love:

- **Being genuinely loved makes you feel anxious because it threatens your defense mechanisms.** To protect yourself from emotional distress, you learned defense mechanisms, like pulling away, acting indifferent, or getting angry. Healthy love challenges these defense mechanisms and leaves you feeling vulnerable.

- **Being genuinely loved triggers feelings of disappointment from the past.** When someone comes into your life and desires to love you without asking for anything in return, this can bring up pain from the past, particularly relationships where you felt like you had to earn the other person's love. You may feel afraid of experiencing the same disappointment all over again.
- **Being genuinely loved causes you to question who you are.** Since your sense of self was built on internalized negative beliefs and experiences, being in a loving relationship can feel confusing because it challenges who you grew up thinking you were. All of a sudden, you're forced to question your feelings of inadequacy and other insecurities that aren't being mirrored back to you in this healthy relationship.

Since you're a creature of habit like any other human being and rely on learned patterns, defenses, and habits to protect yourself, you're more likely to recreate the relationship you had with your parents growing up in your adult relationships. Even when you have the opportunity to meet wonderful people who are willing to respect your boundaries, you will subconsciously seek to maintain a sense of pseudo-safety by sabotaging the healthy relationship. For example, if you sense that someone admires you, it might cause you to create distance or find a way to cause conflict. Or you might find a way to provoke the other person so that they recreate the same dynamic you experienced with your parents.

What's most interesting is that you may not even realize that you're pushing good people away and attracting toxic people toward you. Remember, all of this tends to happen on a subconscious level. To end the cycle of dysfunctional relationships and start cultivating healthy relationships, you'll need to learn how to identify your self-sabotaging behaviors.

Recognize the Old Relationship Patterns

Have you ever wondered why someone would treat two people differently? To the first person they're polite and agreeable, but to the second person they're obnoxious and self-centered. It isn't because they have two different personalities, but instead that each person places a different demand on them.

When you don't have any boundaries to protect your physical, mental, and emotional well-being, you give those around you the license to treat you however they want to. Instead of placing a demand on them, like being very clear on your intolerance of disrespect, you accept whatever treatment given. Someone else who might have more solid boundaries might correct people whenever they step out of line, which influences how those around them act.

If you're tired of being surrounded by negative people, manipulators, or those who are emotionally unavailable, it's time to look at yourself in the mirror and ask a sobering question: *What demands have I placed on those around me?* If you haven't placed any demands, don't be surprised when your boundaries are frequently violated. The truth about toxic people is that they can only get away with as much as you allow them to. When you decide to stop participating in their dysfunctional patterns, they won't have an opportunity to take advantage of you.

The kind of treatment you were accustomed to receiving as a child is the kind of treatment you expect—and sometimes seek—in others. This creates a toxic cycle where your adult relationships reinforce behaviors that were acceptable or normal growing up. Earlier on, in Chapter 2, we discussed the four attachment styles. If you're still unclear about your attachment style, please go over that chapter again. Learning your attachment style gives you insight on patterns that you must break in order to stop sabotaging yourself in relationships.

It's also crucial to be honest with yourself during this time about your ideas of love. Reflect on what your relationship with your parents taught you about love. If you didn't have healthy love modeled in front of you as a child, you'll tend to have a negative or limited understanding of love. Breaking old relationship patterns involves challenging these ideas about love by holding them loosely and being open to change your mind. You can undo these patterns by simply acknowledging that unconditional love isn't supposed to hurt.

A scripture in the Holy Bible describes what unconditional love is supposed to look and feel like (*New International Version*, 2011/1984, 1 Corinthians 13:4-7):

> Love is patient, love is kind. It does not envy, it does not boast, it is not proud. It does not dishonor others, it is not self-seeking, it is not easily angered, it keeps no record of wrongs. Love does not delight in evil but rejoices with the truth. It always protects, always trusts, always hopes, always perseveres.

What Is Self-Love?

Learning how to love yourself when you weren't shown affection or given positive reinforcement as a child can be really difficult. It requires more than just spoiling yourself with new clothes or gadgets, going to the gym, or wearing makeup. Self-love is about making up for the emotional needs you hadn't received as a child and reparenting yourself. In other words, making it your responsibility to care for your physical, mental, and emotional well-being.

Self-love can be defined as showing up for yourself. You can do this in three different ways: forgiving, accepting, and respecting who you are. Let's look at each of these components in more detail.

- **Self-Forgiveness: Hold Yourself Accountable for Self-Inflicted Pain**

When thinking about forgiveness, you might think about forgiving others for the hurt they have caused you. But how often do you think about the hurt you allowed against yourself? What about the many times you betrayed yourself by accepting the bare minimum from people, allowing others to walk all over you, or making decisions that sabotaged your sense of safety?

The reason self-forgiveness is crucial to cultivating self-love is because before you can love yourself, you have to be honest about the role you have played in your own suffering. This doesn't excuse wrongdoers for what they have done to hurt you, but it also doesn't allow you to walk away scot-free. You must be able to sit down with yourself and take responsibility for pain that was self-inflicted. Setting loose boundaries, for example, is self-inflicted pain because when you fail to stand up for yourself, you can't hold others accountable for their mistreatment.

Take a moment right now and think about some of the ways you have inflicted pain upon yourself by not protecting your physical, mental, and emotional well-being as well as you should have. Please note that reflecting on your own shortcomings is not a form of judgment or thinking poorly of yourself. Instead, it's a way for you to confront injustices that you have permitted in your life with honesty and transparency. You are not a bad person for having these shortcomings, and they certainly don't define who you are. However, if you desire to deepen self-love, you should be able to have tough conversations with yourself about unacceptable behaviors you exhibit that are unloving.

- **Acceptance: Be Content With Who You Are**

The moment you come to terms with your own acts of deception, you can move forward and learn to accept yourself as you are. Acceptance is an important part of cultivating self-love because you make peace with the person you see in the mirror. Yes, that individual is flawed and may even be holding on to a lot of pain from the past, but take a closer look at them and you'll see a survivor.

Every human being has a story, and if you were to learn about their story, you would understand something about life: Bad things happen to good people too. Just because your life story didn't unfold like a fairytale doesn't mean you were destined to live an unfulfilling life. Certainly, there are many past events that you wish didn't happen or that you wish you could change, but even those painful events played a role in shaping who you are today.

Accepting who you are is about putting down your mental weapons and ending the inner war that has continued for so many years. Instead of finding fault in yourself, you embrace your weaknesses and admit to your own dysfunctional behaviors. You recognize that you have limitations and sometimes these limitations get in your way. This level of honesty with yourself makes it possible to feel comfortable in your own skin. When you're comfortable in your own skin, you can start to appreciate your life and become more sympathetic to your own needs.

- **Respect: Treat Yourself Like a VIP**

When you love something, like a gadget, piece of clothing, or jewelry, you're extremely careful about how you take care of it. You might place it in an isolated area, so that no one else has access to it, or put terms and conditions about how others can use it. The same applies when you love another person, like a close friend or sibling. You're protective over them and care deeply about their well-being. If they're upset, you get upset too because you have a lot of compassion for them.

Self-love is compassion and consideration directed inwards. Because you think highly of yourself, you're protective about your mental and emotional well-being. When you detect discomfort (whether physical or emotional), you respond immediately and restore your sense of wholeness. The reason you think highly of yourself and go to such great lengths to show yourself compassion is because you respect the person that you are.

Self-respect is the confidence you have in yourself that causes you to behave with dignity. Just like a precious piece of jewelry, you limit the access people have to you, especially to your private life. Moreover, you set standards regarding how others treat you and hold them accountable whenever they don't meet your standards. You don't have to be rich, classy, or famous to treat yourself with self-respect. All you need to do is recognize that you're worthy of love and good treatment from yourself and others.

One of the barriers that prevent you from deepening the love you have for yourself is the fear of what others might think. In this context, you may be afraid that others will think you're being selfish for treating yourself like a VIP, setting healthy boundaries, and honoring your needs. Or maybe your fear stems from growing up in a family where self-love was seen as indulgent, whereas self-sacrifice was seen as noble. Whatever the case may be, it's important to challenge the idea that self-love is wrong.

If you remember the last time you were on a plane, the air host or hostess gave you and other passengers flight safety precautions. One of those precautions had to do with the loss of cabin pressure. They stated that in the event of the loss of cabin pressure, you were responsible for putting an oxygen mask over yourself before assisting other passengers. Now, would you classify this precaution as selfish or indulgent? Absolutely not.

It's a safety procedure that can potentially keep you alive.

The same can be said about practicing self-love. Setting standards for how others treat you and putting your needs first are habits that protect your well-being and keep you healthy. When your needs are taken care of, you're able to invest more time and energy in taking care of others. Self-love makes it possible for you to build healthy relationships because you can sincerely love and accept who you are, which means that you won't demand love and acceptance from others.

Speaking about self-compassion, Professor Kristin Neff writes, "Self-compassion involves treating yourself with the same kindness, concern, and support you'd show to a good friend. When faced with difficult life struggles or confronting personal mistakes, failures, and inadequacies, self-compassion responds with kindness rather than harsh self-judgment, recognizing that imperfection is part of the shared human experience" (Neff & Dahm, 2015).

It's not wrong to give yourself the same love and respect you give to others. Yes, this might cause others to feel uncomfortable around you, however, realize that the discomfort they feel has more to do with their own emotional wounds. Misery loves company, and when you no longer think low of yourself, there will be friends and family you can't seem to get along with anymore. You'll need to choose between continuing on your healing journey (even if it means ending unhealthy relationships) or giving in to the social pressure.

If you're interested in deepening the love you have for yourself, be prepared to work for it! It won't be an easy journey, but in the end it will be worth it. One of the techniques that can help you cultivate self-love is mirror work. The following section will explain the technique in more detail.

Step-by-Step Process to Practice Mirror Work

Mirror work is a technique that literally gets you face-to-face with your own image. It's a simple yet incredibly powerful way of coming to terms with who you are and loving the person you see staring back at you in the mirror.

The technique was created by motivational teacher Louise Hay. She found that looking at yourself in the mirror can help you get in touch with your inner self. The purpose of mirror work is to build a stronger relationship with yourself and, over time, cultivate self-love and a healthy self-esteem.

Even though all you need is a mirror, this technique can feel overwhelming. The reflection you see in the mirror can bring up many memories, strong emotions, or negative thoughts you have about yourself. You may feel embarrassed about how you look, unsettled by the eye contact, or angry at yourself for past mistakes and regrets. In her book, *Mirror Work,* Louise Hay explains why staring at a mirror can be unpleasant. She writes, "The mirror reflects back to you the feelings you have about yourself. It makes you immediately aware of where you are resisting and where you are open and flowing" (Hay, 2016).

In other words, looking at yourself in the mirror forces you to be vulnerable. It gives you no room to hide what you think or how you feel about yourself. Of course, this also creates an opportunity to strengthen the relationship you have with yourself by confronting the 'ugly' truth that you have concealed for so many years.

There isn't a rigid set of rules you need to follow when practicing mirror work. However, there are five steps that can help you get the best out of your practice. The five steps are as follows:

Step 1: Show Commitment

It's possible to stare at yourself in front of a mirror and not get anything out of it. What makes mirror work powerful isn't looking at the mirror, but rather opening yourself up emotionally so that you can connect to your soul. Commit yourself to the experience of soul-searching and embracing every aspect of who you are. No, it won't feel comfortable all the time, however, it will bring up thoughts and emotions you have stored deep in your subconscious mind.

So, how can you show commitment? Dedicate a minimum of two minutes a day looking into a mirror and practicing one of the exercises that will be mentioned in the following steps.

Step 2: Create a List of Personalized Affirmations

One of the exercises you can practice while staring at a mirror is reciting positive affirmations. Simply put, positive affirmations are statements written in the present tense that affirm positive qualities, strengths, and beliefs about who you are. What makes positive affirmations powerful is that they create positive suggestions in your mind. Over time, these suggestions inform how you think about yourself and others. For example, if you're battling with negative self-talk, positive affirmations can counteract those thoughts and slowly change the quality of your internal dialogue.

While you can find thousands of positive affirmations online, it's recommended to create personalized affirmations that target aspects of yourself that you would like to improve. For example, you can create an affirmation based on how you desire to feel about yourself, such as: "I am at peace with myself." Note that the affirmation is positive and written in the present tense. You may also wish to affirm something that you hope to one day display, such as: "I am confident in expressing my needs."

If affirming certain qualities about yourself feels too difficult, choose milder qualities. The point is not to fake something that you don't feel comfortable with yet. For example, staring at yourself in a mirror and saying "I love you" may be difficult to do at this stage. But you can think of a milder affirmation that feels more believable, such as "I accept you for who you are."

You can also refer to this list of positive affirmations when affirming your strengths, desires, and beliefs:

- I am growing.
- Life is getting better for me.
- I am a survivor.
- I am unstoppable.
- I wake up motivated.
- My life is constantly unfolding.
- I am a walking, breathing, talking miracle.
- I inspire everyone who I encounter.
- I am driven to pursue my dreams.
- I am free from the bondage of fear.
- I am healing every day.

Step 3: Validate Your Emotions

It's common to become emotional during the practice of mirror work. You may not even understand where the emotion is coming from. For example, after reciting an affirmation, it may trigger deep sadness or anger. The affirmation only serves as a channel to give you access to deeper parts of your subconscious. Thus, when you speak certain words, they trigger past memories or traumas that haven't yet been healed.

Don't be afraid of your emotions. They are a good indication that the mirror is doing its job! You're supposed to cry, get angry, laugh, or feel embarrassed, because these emotions must be released in order to process pain. When you feel an emotion bubbling up within you, invite it to come forward and spend a few minutes with you. You can speak directly to the emotion and say, "I can feel you, anger. It's okay to come forward." When your emotion reveals itself, allow it to have its moment. Don't hold back how you feel or what comes naturally to you at that moment. Validate the emotion as though you were comforting your younger self. Say to yourself, "I get it. I'm here for you."

Step 4: Ground Yourself in Your Body

Mirror work can get extremely intense, particularly if traumatic wounds have resurfaced. In this place of vulnerability, it's important to show yourself compassion and remain present in your body. Ideally, you want to offer positive reassurance while avoiding being caught up in the memory and drifting to the past. One of the ways to remain present in your body is to ground yourself through gentle touch.

Touch awakens your senses and keeps you connected to the moment. It's also a great way to self-soothe and reduce feelings of being exposed or ashamed. While staring at the mirror, give yourself a warm hug, stroke your arms, place your hand over your heart, touch your face, or any other loving touch that can make you feel safe. While touching yourself, you can even repeat, "You are not alone. You will get through this."

Step 5: Document the Experience

After you have completed your practice, take a few minutes to journal about your experience. Write down what came up, what triggered it, and the emotional experience that followed. If there was something new that you learned about yourself, or any epiphanies you had, write these down too. As time goes on, you'll be able to track your healing process by reading your journal and looking at how far you have come.

While mirror work is centered around the relationship you have with yourself, in the long run it can also improve the relationship you have with others. By gaining more awareness of who you are and learning to love the person you see in the mirror, your connections with others become stronger and more meaningful too!

Chapter Takeaways

- You're prone to repeating relationship patterns you learned growing up in your adult relationships. If you didn't receive the affection you needed, the possibility of opening yourself up to love as an adult can be scary.
- Desiring healthy relationships doesn't necessarily mean you'll attract secure and well-adjusted people, especially if you're holding on to old defense mechanisms, like shutting down or creating distance between yourself and others.
- Cultivating healthy relationships is a process that begins with you; you need to first get to know yourself and accept your strengths and weaknesses before you can open yourself to others.
- Attracting loving relationships becomes easier when you have first developed self-love and can stand up for yourself. Self-love isn't selfish or indulgent, but rather a necessary habit to protect your overall well-being. It's only after you have poured into your own cup that you can pour into others'.

Discovering Your Core Values and Raising Your Standards

"It is not until you change your identity to match your life blueprint that you will understand why everything in the past never worked."

— SHANNON L. ALDER

This chapter talks about:

- How your beliefs shape your life experiences
- How to identify your core values
- How raising your standards helps you become the best version of yourself

What Do You Believe In?

Whenever you meet a stranger, you get an opportunity to express who you are. Typically, without even knowing it, your attitudes and behaviors do most of the speaking on your behalf. Research has shown that people make their first impression of you based on nonverbal communication, like how you carry yourself and the energy you bring into a room.

You don't have to be a human behavioral scientist to spot an insecure person in a crowded room. They're the person who arrives late to make an entrance, struggles to make eye contact or engage in meaningful conversation, and shows signs of high agreeableness, like showing support for what everyone says but failing to offer their own insight. On the other side of the spectrum, they might reveal their insecurity by displaying domineering behavior (standing over people), cutting others off when speaking, and showing disinterest when they're not the center of attention.

The traits and behaviors you display to others say a lot about how you feel about yourself. When you think low of yourself, you tend to act in ways that reinforce your inferiority complex. Skills like setting healthy boundaries or communicating assertively may not have the intended effects on your relationships because on a deeper soul level, you're dealing with a sense of low self-worth.

This is why techniques like confronting your negative beliefs (turn to Chapter 9) are so important to practice on this healing journey. They allow you to take a good look at who you are and ask tough questions like, "What do I believe in?" What you believe in ends up becoming who you are. Your reality is merely a reflection of the quality of your thoughts about yourself and others. This is because your thoughts inform what you consider to be true about people, the world, and your past, as well as your future.

Consider a belief like, "I'm not worthy of love." The belief might be based on a series of past traumatic relationships that left you feeling betrayed and emotionally wounded. Believing that you're not worthy of love comes with an implication: You will subconsciously look for evidence—or create an environment—that reinforces what you believe is the truth. In other words, every experience you have will be seen and evaluated based on the filter that you are unworthy of love.

Imagine how this belief might affect your relationships with others. Regardless of how much love they show you and how often they express their appreciation or respect your boundaries, your mind will discount or overlook any kind of information that doesn't support your belief. Instead, it will work tirelessly to find evidence of the relationship being wrong or the person not being the right fit for you.

Therefore, if you desire to change the first impression that others have of you, or perhaps improve the quality of your relationships, then the first thing to do is assess the quality of your beliefs. What kind of negative suggestions are you constantly feeding yourself? When you meet people, what kind of interactions are you subconsciously expecting? You may not be able to control what happens to you, but you can control how you perceive situations and how they shape you. The power lies in your beliefs.

Core Values: The Center of Your Belief System

A belief system is a network of beliefs that help you make sense of life, understand how to show up in relationships, and distinguish between acceptable and unacceptable behaviors. Your experience of reality is also predicated on your belief system. In essence, what you like or dislike about yourself, your job, or other people is based on a network of beliefs with which you live by.

Not all beliefs that are part of your belief system stem from childhood. Some of them are a result of good or bad experiences you have had later on in life. Furthermore, not all of your beliefs will be based on moral or religious principles. You may have several that stem from your ideas about gender, sexuality, race, politics, health, education, or how society is structured.

What makes your belief system unique from others is how your beliefs are interconnected with each other (how they form a system). For example, believing that men are dangerous, women are undermined in the workplace, and that true love doesn't exist creates a unique belief system that informs how you interact with the world. Thus, when two strangers meet to form any type of relationship, they each bring along their unique belief systems. At times there are similarities between their systems, and other times there aren't any.

Two strangers who have unresolved childhood trauma may have belief systems that complement each other. As a result, they're able to relate to one another, even when what they're relating to would be considered toxic. For example, someone with an avoidant-dismissive attachment style who believes that love is painful might end up attracting someone with an anxious-preoccupied attachment style who doesn't believe they deserve to be loved. While these two people have slightly different belief systems, they're able to complement each other based on their perceptions about love.

What do belief systems have to do with setting healthy boundaries? The answer is simple. Setting healthy boundaries would be a breeze if you actually believed they were valuable or necessary. The fact that you don't have a lot of healthy boundaries means there are some beliefs that you hold that conflict with the act of setting healthy boundaries. One of those beliefs might be the sense that you need to prove yourself to others. Proving yourself to others means placing their needs above yours, hence the lack of healthy boundaries.

What also makes setting healthy boundaries difficult is the fact that, due to your history, you have never gotten the opportunity to think about or put into effect your core values. Core values are at the heart of your belief system. When you have solid core values, you're able to build a life that aligns with what matters to you most, which includes decisions about work, relationships, and the kinds of goals you pursue.

Core values also influence your sense of right and wrong. When setting boundaries, they dictate where your limits are. And since they're the foundation of your belief system, they predict what you believe about yourself and others. For instance, if you value time, then you'll likely believe in task efficiency, punctuality, and planning. Not knowing what your core values are means that your beliefs aren't anchored to what matters most in your life. Instead, they're subject to shift and change based on your life experiences. This results in constant mood swings, anxiety, and confusion whenever you're faced with difficult circumstances.

The best way to ensure that your healthy boundaries remain stable and consistent over time is to get clear about your core values. Figure out what matters to you most and live your life on that model. When you're clear about your core values, you'll notice that your belief system changes. The new beliefs you adopt will be aligned to the fundamental principles that you hold about life, health, goals, work, and relationships. In the following section, we'll think practically about how to identify core values.

Identify Your Core Values

You made dinner plans with a friend and both of you agreed to meet at 7 p.m. sharp. It's been 45 minutes, and they still haven't shown up. Are you waiting or leaving?

After a month of dating your partner, you find out that they lied about not having kids. Is this a deal breaker, or can it be resolved through a conversation?

Your boss just gave you a performance bonus. Do you put the money toward your retirement or start planning your upcoming vacation?

These questions represent some of the many decisions you make on a daily basis. Your decisions determine how you interact with the world and reflect what you value most in your work, family, health, and friendships. If you didn't have core values, making decisions would be overwhelming. It would be tough deciding which outcome is best for you because you wouldn't have a blueprint that you live by.

Furthermore, since life will always introduce you to different kinds of people and situations, having core values gives you a greater sense of control. In every relationship or situation, you can make decisions that are consistent with what you believe. This doesn't mean you can control the other person or manipulate a situation to work in your favor, but your values will help you set boundaries so that your interests are taken care of.

The following steps are designed to get you thinking about your core values. Get a pen and paper and go through each step at your own pace.

Step 1: Create a List of Values You Are Already Aware Of

The first step is to create a long list of values that you believe reflect what matters most to you. Try not to think too hard about these values, because later on you'll get the chance to narrow them down. If you can't think of values from the top of your mind, refer to the list below for inspiration:

- productivity
- family
- balance
- hard work
- acceptance
- respect
- beauty
- goal-oriented
- success
- accountability

- security
- growth
- ambition
- purpose
- generosity
- simplicity
- peace
- freedom
- kindness
- commitment
- honesty
- fun
- intelligence
- communication

Step 2: Extract Values From Your Past Experiences

Now that you have a long list of values to work with, go a bit deeper and think of past experiences (extreme highs or lows) that revealed some of your core values. Which values shone through during that joyful or painful time? Think of at least three experiences and add more values to your list.

Step 3: Complete a Self-Assessment

Next, turn to yourself and reflect on your personality, mannerisms, beliefs, and attitudes. Identify a few more values based on the following criteria:

- how you structure your daily routine
- the healthiest relationships in your life
- situations that make you angry
- situations that you complain about
- the ideal life you wish to live
- what it takes for you to feel accomplished

You can also take a trip down memory lane and think about what kind of child or teenager you were, how you spent most of your time, and the kinds of interactions that made you sad or happy. Write down values that are illustrated by some of these childhood memories.

Step 4: Create Groups and Highlight Central Themes

At this stage, you should have a list of over 20 values. Identify values that are related to each other and group them together. For example, success, ambition, and goal-oriented would fall under one group because they're similar. Do this for all of your values until you have a few groups.

For each group, select a theme that represents all of the values within it. For example, trust might be a theme that represents values like communication, honesty, and accountability. When you're done, every group should have a central theme.

Step 5: Create Your List of Core Values

The final step is to arrange your themes in order of priority, the number one spot being reserved for the most important theme. Here are a few questions to help you identify which themes take the highest priority (Don't forget that each theme represents a group of similar values.):

- Which themes are essential to your life?
- Which themes represent your authentic self?
- Which themes support the building of healthy relationships?
- Which themes support your deepest desires?

There's no limit to how long your list of core values should be. However, when your list is too long (i.e. having more than 10 core values), you'll easily forget what matters most to you, or you may struggle to incorporate all of them into your daily life. The sweet spot is having a list of 5–10 core values.

The bonus step is to create positive statements that can help you memorize each value. These are known as value statements. The most effective value statements include the following qualities:

- consist of inspiring words
- trigger positive emotions
- highlight your strengths
- designed to be meaningful, not perfect

Below is an example of how you write a value statement structured around your theme and associated values:

1. **Theme:** Love
2. **Associated values:** Compassion, acceptance, support
3. **Value statement:** Love is when someone shows compassion for my feelings, accepts me for who I am, and shows up when I need them most.

Now, go ahead and create value statements for your list of core values!

It's Time to Raise the Standard

Something magical happens when you realize what you value in life—you finally raise your standards!

A standard is an acceptable norm or average that sets a benchmark or expectation. If you had dreams of becoming a doctor, you would need to pursue a medicine degree that takes an average of six years to complete. This is the standard recommended by international institutions for qualifying as a doctor. If you had a goal of losing a few pounds of weight, you would need to reduce your calorie intake and increase physical activity. This standard formula is what your body responds favorably to.

Elon Musk, who's now ranked the richest person in the world, didn't accumulate his wealth and success by sheer luck. He created a standard of excellence that helped him design his daily routine and the amount of hours he would dedicate to his work. His day is organized in five-minute segments, and he's known to work at least 100 hours a week.

When he was establishing his company, Tesla, Musk was known to sleep on the production floor or in the conference room just so he could maximize the amount of productive hours (SCB, 2022). Of course, this kind of lifestyle isn't healthy. However, what's important to learn about Musk's approach to success is that he consistently practiced behaviors that were his personal benchmark and informed how he ran his businesses and structured his life.

A C student in high school achieves a C on their report card because they invest "C" amount of effort. In contrast, an A student achieves an A on their report card because they invest "A" amount of effort. When both students leave high school, they'll have access to different kinds of opportunities. The C student's options will be limited due to their minimal effort in high school, whereas the A student will have a variety of options to choose from.

This analogy can be applied to your life. If you set "C" standards regarding how others treat you, you'll get "C" treatment. But if you raise your standards and expect more from yourself and others, you'll receive better treatment. Low standards cause you to accept whatever others have to offer without creating a benchmark. This means that they can say or do anything to you or around you and there won't be any consequences for it. However, when you raise your standards, you create a new normal in your life and make it clear what you can and can't tolerate.

Raising your standards also means modeling the kind of behaviors you expect from others. People often learn how to treat you by watching how you treat yourself. For example, if you don't display any self-respect or self-control, people won't be afraid to walk all over you. Whether you're at work, amongst friends, or at home, it's important to be aware of how your attitudes and behaviors come across to others. Unfortunately, you're judged based on what others perceive about you, not your good intentions. As the police warning goes: Anything you do or say can and will be held against you!

Three Ways to Raise Your Standards

It only takes 30 seconds of first meeting you for someone to create a story about you, but seven positive interactions for you to make up for a bad first impression. Based on their perception about your standards (i.e. whether you're somebody with high or low standards) they'll adjust their behaviors and engage with you accordingly. Therefore, it's crucial to create a benchmark for yourself and display behaviors that represent who you are and what you stand for.

If you're tired of attracting the wrong kind of attention or treatment from people, perhaps it's time for you to raise your standards. The following three-step process will show you how:

- **Figure Out What You Want**

If you aren't clear about the way you want to be treated, then you won't be able to model those behaviors to others. Clarifying what you want will also make it easier to recognize boundary violations and other undesirable behaviors. Write down a list of at least 10 behaviors you would like to adopt. These are the behaviors that will create a benchmark for how others treat you. For example, if you want others to respect you, then you must practice self-respect (and believe you deserve to be respected).

- **Bridge the Gap**

Your standards should always reflect who you desire to be (your future self) so that you're inspired to evolve and become that person. If you assess your life right now, you'll find that there's a gap between your present and future self. Your present self is the person you are right now. This version of you also has standards, however, they're not a reflection of who you desire to be—the future self. Write a letter to your future self expressing how you would like others to see you. Describe scenarios at work, amongst your friends, and with family that would make you feel accepted and respected.

You can also bridge the gap, you can ask yourself sobering questions about your current standards and what needs to change in order to become a better person. Here are a few questions to start you off:

- What are three standards that are keeping you stuck in the past?
- What are three standards that reinforce the same unhealthy relationship patterns?
- What standards do you maintain at work? How might these standards be holding you back?
- What standards do you maintain about your health? How might these be compromising your physical well-being?
- What standards did you learn from other people (e.g. parents, coworkers, friends, ex-partners, etc.) that are negatively impacting your life?

The aim with bridging the gap is to assess areas where you can improve your standards. For example, you might find that you have great work and dating standards, but when it comes to your health and family, you need to raise your standards. Furthermore, while completing the self-assessment, you may find standards that are toxic and can no longer be maintained. Be honest about what you're not willing to tolerate anymore and why it's important for you to make these changes.

- **Find the Right Mentors**

Now that you're clear about what you want and understand what it will take to bridge the gap, the next step is to find great mentors. The beauty about standards is that you can always find a person who exemplifies what you desire to become or display. Think about role models like Michelle Obama, Serena Williams, or Warren Buffett. These individuals may be different, but what they have in common is that they're all living based on their highest standards—and it shows in their mindsets, characters, and professional lives.

Find a few people who exemplify the kind of standards you hope to develop. The purpose is not to idolize them, but to draw inspiration from their journeys. If you can't think of any celebrity figure, think about people who you have encountered in your life who left a positive impact on you. What was it about your parents, school teacher, or football coach that you admire and would like to embody?

When you have completed these three steps, it's time to take action by developing daily or weekly rituals. Rituals are simply behaviors carried out the same way, at the same time, which support the new standards you have set for yourself. To make your rituals effective, ensure they're small, easy to follow, and don't require a lot of time and money. For example, waking up at 6:30 a.m. and meditating for 10 minutes is a great way to cultivate inner peace.

Challenge yourself to explore different rituals until you find those that accommodate your lifestyle and help you become a better person.

Chapter Takeaways

- People treat you as well as you treat yourself. Whenever you're engaging with people, be aware of how others might perceive you. Consider how your attitudes and behaviors come across, and make the best first impression!
- Your belief system is a network of beliefs that help you interpret the world. If your beliefs are negative, your behaviors will be negative too. It's only when you start challenging your beliefs that you can change how you act, think, or show up in the world.
- At the heart of your belief system are your core values. These are the ideas or principles that matter most to you. When you make decisions based on your core values, you're able to live a life that's consistent with what you believe.
- Discovering your core values helps you create personal standards or benchmarks in various aspects of your life. These standards teach others how to relate to you and how much respect to show you. However, the most important part about setting personal standards is that you get to adopt new behaviors that help you become the best version of yourself.

Boundaries in Relationships

"Evaluating the benefits and drawbacks of any relationship is your responsibility. You do not have to passively accept what is brought to you. You can choose."

— DEBORAH DAY

This chapter talks about:

- How to maintain your individuality in relationships by going through the process of individuation
- How to start a conversation about boundaries with friends, romantic partners, and family members

Embrace the Process of Individuation

Tanya and Zach decided to go for couple's therapy after two years of being together. Both of them felt ready for marriage, except they kept on getting into the same kinds of struggles for power.

Zach was an assertive, straight-talking man in his mid 30s who was raised in a liberal household, where mutual respect lay the foundation for his relationships with his parents. He grew up with a love for accounting and with the support of his parents, he climbed the corporate ladder and became one of the youngest directors at his company.

What made him fall in love with Tanya was her kind and agreeable nature—but these traits also became what sparked many arguments. "Whenever I ask her to make a decision," Zach told the therapist, "she always goes with what I like instead of making her own choices."

Tanya was a typical people-pleaser who felt uncomfortable speaking up for herself. She was raised by strict parents who restricted many of her freedoms and kept a close watch on everything she did. From an early age, she learned that being agreeable was the best way to relate to her parents and get along with others. When she met Zach, this relationship pattern played out once again, but unfortunately it created more tension than harmony in their relationship.

Observing their relationship, the therapist realized that most of their conflict was due to their patterns of individuation. Psychoanalyst Carl Jung discovered the concept of individuation, which is the process of forming a separate identity from others and realizing who you are. This is an ongoing process that begins from infancy and continues into adulthood, and is most noticeable in how people relate with one another.

One of the signs of individuation is developing a separate identity from your friends and family. In other words, you seek to find out what your strengths and weaknesses are, what kind of personality you have, and what you desire out of life. During this process of exploration, you may discover hidden aspects of your identity that weren't revealed as a child. As you can imagine, going on this journey takes a lot of courage because what you might learn about yourself could change the nature of your relationships.

Parents are typically responsible for helping their children along the process of individuation in order to prepare them for life as an independent adult. However, not all parents take their children through this journey, hence the dynamic between Tanya and Zach. Tanya's strict parents imposed their own beliefs and expectations on their daughter, which made self-realization impossible. Even in her adult life, Tanya struggled to develop an independent identity from her romantic partners because she was never encouraged to.

On the other hand, Zach's parents raised him to have a healthy sense of autonomy from a young age. They created an environment where he felt safe to voice his opinions and make important decisions for his life, such as deciding to pursue a career in finance. Knowing that he was supported by his parents gave Zach the self-confidence to discover who he was and build a stable life for himself.

Since relationships are a necessary part of growing up and living a fulfilling life, it's important to undergo the process of individuation to form a separate identity from others. Perhaps you grew up in a family similar to Tanya's, where you weren't encouraged to find your voice, communicate your needs, and express your individuality. Not having the support of your parents in discovering who you are meant that you depended on others for validation: At work this might show up as a lack of assertiveness, and in romantic relationships it might show up as passivity or neediness.

The good news is that it's never too late to continue the process of individuation and create an independent identity from your parents or people who you have deep emotional ties with.

Three Stages of Individuation

If you desire to become your own person and gain the confidence to think, feel, and behave in ways that are authentic to you, then it's important to go through the process of individuation. Depending on how restrictive your past relationships were, there may still be aspects of your identity that are tied to your parents' or ex-lovers' thoughts, beliefs, and values. You can redeem these aspects of your identity by following the three stages of individuation: declaring, separating, and reconnecting.

Declaring

The first stage is to declare your freedom from whomever your identity has been tied to for all these years. You can make this declaration to yourself by stating that you're severing the emotional ties that have kept you enmeshed with another person's ideas, thoughts, and feelings.

This stage can involve mirror work, where you look at yourself in the mirror and declare your freedom out loud. You can also write letters to yourself in a journal and explain the decision you're making and why you have chosen to cut emotional ties. It isn't necessary to share your declaration with the person you're emotionally separating from, although if you do, ensure that you don't overly explain yourself or get caught up in blackmail and other forms of manipulation.

Declaring your freedom might sound like this:

> *"I'm going through a process of making positive changes in my life and relationships. I take responsibility for not always standing up for myself, expressing my emotions, and protecting my boundaries. I have decided that in order to continue my personal evolution and maintain the health of this relationship, I have to become more independent and stand on my own. This doesn't mean I don't love you, however, I need to fight for myself and my own wishes more than I depend on others to carry me."*

Separating

The second stage of individuation is the actual separation. You can interpret this separation in two ways. First, it could be setting healthy boundaries with the other person so that you have the space to grow and explore who you are. Alternatively, if the relationship no longer feels safe, you can make a physical separation and request some time apart. Whether you decide to set healthy boundaries or create physical distance, it's important to disconnect emotionally—until you have created a life for yourself.

The purpose of separating isn't to hurt the person who you have been enmeshed with, but instead to get clear on who you are and take full responsibility for your life. It's also during this stage of separation that you're able to reflect on your relationship dynamic and identify harmful patterns of behavior like codependency, seeking validation, or using the other person to distract you from your feelings of loneliness.

In an article titled *How to Individuate,* author Jake Eagle recounts a story about a grown child who was finally ready to separate from their parents. Below is their story of how the process of separation occurred (Eagle, 2011):

> *"I haven't lived with my parents for years, but I called them every week. I always asked about them, but they never asked about me. Or, if they did, it was because they wanted to tell me what I should be doing in some area of my life. I got sick of it, so I told my parents that if they wanted to know how I was they should call me. I told them I was going to stop calling them for a while. And I did. And they never called me. This caused me to rethink my relationship with them. I struggled to accept that my parents didn't reach out to me, but only after experiencing this did I begin to understand myself much better. Someday I will reach out to my parents, but not until their response*

is less important to me."

Reconnecting

The last stage of individuation is reconnecting to those whom you separated from. Please note that in some cases, especially when the relationship was toxic or no longer felt safe, reconnecting may not be possible. However, you won't know for sure until you have gone through the first and second stage.

If the relationship is salvageable, it means that there's commitment from both parties to respect each other's autonomy. In other words, the person who felt subjected to must commit to respecting your boundaries and giving you the space to think for yourself and lead a separate life. Think of this as a new chapter in your relationship, where both of you get to relearn each other and operate under a new vision (refer to Chapter 4).

If coming to a mutual agreement is difficult (i.e. the other person refuses to cooperate or respect your new boundaries), then it may be necessary to take your relationship back to the separation stage. Reuniting with someone who isn't willing to change will recreate the same patterns of dependency that you don't desire anymore. There will also be some people whom you reconnect with but continue to maintain your distance from. These may be family members who you can't walk away from but also can't allow full access into your life.

This three-stage individuation process is generally directed toward your parents, because the parent-child relationship is the primary one that sets the tone for all other relationships in your life. If your parents are deceased, or maybe you're afraid of making the separation, then you'll most likely project the unresolved issues from your parent-child relationship onto your romantic relationships. For example, if your parents were emotionally unavailable, you may be emotionally needy in your romantic relationships.

The reason why it's so important to separate from your parents is to accept that how they raised you was the best they could do with what they knew at the time. Their parenting was in no way a reflection on who you are. The lack of unconditional love from your parents didn't make you unlovable or unworthy of receiving love. Therefore, since your parents' actions and behaviors had very little to do with you as a person, you don't need to reinforce those patterns in your adult relationships.

Communicating Boundaries With Friends

Friendships tend to change over time as the people who are part of the friendship evolve. The kind of friendship expectations you had when you were in high school are different from what you expect in your friendships at this stage of your life. Plus, from each friendship dynamic, you may desire something different. For example, there might be a friend you call whenever you want to socialize, and another friend you call whenever you want to have deep meaningful conversations. Both friendships are valuable in their own way because they respond to your friendship needs.

While each friendship may look different, there are standards that healthy friendships must uphold. These standards are:

- **Being emotionally available for each other.** Even though there are many things that fight for your attention, it's important to pay attention to how your friends are coping and what their needs are, and vice versa. Having concern for one another's well-being is what builds mutual connection.
- **Having a balance of give-and-take.** Reciprocity is essential to healthy friendships because it ensures that both people's needs are considered and taken care of. One-sided friendships often consist of one person who always gives and another who always takes. There

can be no harmony in these types of friendships due to one person who has overextended themselves.

- **Offering support during difficult times.** Life isn't always full of joyful moments, and as much as you can celebrate with your friends, you also want to count on them to hold your hand during tough times. Support might look different for each of your friendships. For example, you might approach some people for emotional support and others to teach you skills or share their knowledge. What matters is knowing that you can rely on your friends to carry you during moments of weakness, and vice versa.
- **Feeling safe to be vulnerable.** Healthy friendships offer a psychologically safe space where you can share your thoughts and emotions without feeling judged or exposed. Sharing personal information must be a mutual agreement and something that you both do freely in order to build a strong connection. The inability to be vulnerable could be an indicator of a lack of trust.
- **Maintaining a level of consistency.** Friendships are not static; they ebb and flow as time passes by. However, healthy friendships are built on values, traditions, and common practices that make them feel stable and reliable. For example, friends might agree to meet up at least once a month for a catchup or check up on each other over text once a week. These small practices are what keep friendships intact.

There will be moments when you're forced to set boundaries with friends. This isn't always a sign that your friendship is in trouble or that your friend is toxic. As we have mentioned in earlier chapters, even good-intentioned people sometimes violate our boundaries. There are many reasons why setting boundaries would be necessary. Some of those include:

- You're overwhelmed with personal responsibilities and don't have the bandwidth to be there for your friend.
- You have gone through a life transition and your priorities have

changed. You're no longer available to hang out like you used to or engage in the types of activities you and a friend used to enjoy.
- The friendship is one-sided and you often find yourself investing more time and energy into maintaining the friendship than your friend.
- You don't feel comfortable sharing personal information with your friend. This could be due to a number of reasons. For instance, the friendship may be new, trust could have been broken in the past, or perhaps your friend is secretive and doesn't share much about themselves.
- You struggle to keep up with your friend's expectations. As much as you desire to respond to their needs, you tend to feel overwhelmed by how much they expect from you. For example, having a friend who wants to hang out every weekend or expects you to help them make decisions about their own life.

Some boundary violations may be obvious, and others will require you to trust your gut instinct. You can also think about how the behavior committed made you feel. That could be a good indication of a boundary violation. When communicating your boundaries with friends, remember these important tips:

- **Be clear and straightforward.** Get to the point and explain what happened and how it made you feel. If possible, avoid making assumptions or accusations. Simply state the boundary that was crossed and a way forward that both of you can take.
- **Create an atmosphere for open dialogue.** After communicating your issue, give your friend an opportunity to speak and share what's on their mind. They may want to clarify any misunderstandings that have occurred. Seek to understand where they may have been coming from or how they may have been feeling at the time. Being able to talk freely about your experiences can strengthen your friendship.
- **Emphasize how much you value the friendship.** Communicating

your boundaries doesn't need to be a combative situation. After all, the aim isn't to damage your friendship, but to make it stronger. Before and after you define the consequences, express how committed you are to making the friendship work and how much you care about your friend.

Setting boundaries in friendships is all about communicating how your needs have changed and how you would like your friends to treat you moving forward. The aim is never to end a friendship, but to make your needs clearer. In romantic relationships, the type of boundaries you set looks a bit different, especially earlier on during the dating stage!

How to Talk About Boundaries During the Dating Stage

How would you respond if the man or woman you had only known for a week asked you to send nudes? Or what would you say if the man or woman you had recently started dating asked to borrow a large sum of money?

Setting boundaries in the early stages of dating can feel awkward because you're forced to communicate your limits with somebody you barely know. If you have a tendency to people-please, you might fear that setting boundaries so early may cause them to run away or have a negative perception about you.

The truth is that boundaries are a lifesaver when it comes to screening singles in the dating scene. They protect your interests and ensure that the people you eventually allow into your life understand how to treat you. Healthy boundaries aren't a mood killer. In fact, they can strengthen the attraction between you and your partner since both of your needs are being met. Plus, if you have experienced abusive relationships in the past, having boundaries in place protects you from re-traumatization.

Communicating boundaries with a romantic partner sounds and looks similar to how you would communicate boundaries with anyone else. Nevertheless, there are a few guidelines that will make approaching this situation less daunting:

- **Speak about your boundaries as soon as possible.** Ideally, you want to set the ground rules for your romantic relationship after the first few dates, when you begin to take the other person seriously. This doesn't have to be a formal conversation; it can be a topic that you bring up on a fun date. For instance, you might start the conversation by asking, "What's important for you in a relationship?"
- **Use "I" statements.** The purpose of dating is to get to know someone better. Therefore, it's normal to share your likes and dislikes. If your partner has violated one of your boundaries, there's a good chance that they weren't even aware of it. Use "I" statements to teach your partner what you like and dislike. You might say, "When you make last-minute plans, I don't feel considered."
- **Share your sexual boundaries before you engage in sex.** Good sex is all about consent. When there's no consent, the act becomes a sexual violation. Be clear ahead of time about your sexual boundaries. You may even want to have an open discussion about your sexual beliefs, like waiting until a relationship reaches a certain milestone before having sex or practicing safe sex by wearing condoms. Remember that both you and your partner can withdraw consent at any time, so check in with each other regularly to see if your sexual boundaries are being upheld.
- **Be clear about your non-negotiables.** It's normal to enter a new romantic relationship with non-negotiables, especially if you're living based on your core values. Your partner should know what you need in order to feel safe and honored in the relationship. In some cases your partner may not be willing to accept your non-negotiables, and this could make them walk away. Don't see this as a bad sign. It simply means that you weren't compatible in the first place.

- **Look out for yourself.** It's common for new lovers to become so besotted with each other that they forget to protect their own interests. For a relationship to make it past the honeymoon phase, both you and your partner must feel comfortable being yourselves and continuing to live separate lives, together. Neither of you should feel like you're compromising yourselves by staying in the relationship.

Your mindset during the dating process is another factor to consider. Be careful about the beliefs you hold about yourself, such as thinking you're not good enough to be treated a certain way. Your mindset will also affect your behaviors. If you think low of yourself, it will be evident in how you carry yourself on each date, as well as how loose your boundaries are. Remember, you teach people how to treat you through your behaviors. Act like a king or queen, and you will be treated like one!

Unlike bad dates, you can't walk away as easily from family. Nevertheless, your difficult family members must be held accountable for boundary violations just like any other relationship in your life.

Setting Clear Boundaries With Difficult Family Members

What makes setting boundaries with family so hard is the fact that these relationships hold so much value. For instance, as frustrated as you might be with your parent's selfish behavior or manipulative tactics, they will always be your parent. Many people end up excusing bad behavior from family members as a way of ignoring the boundary violation. However, doing this only leads to further hurt in the future.

Abuse or mistreatment of any kind is unacceptable, regardless of who the transgressor may be. It's important to get to the point where your mental, physical, and emotional well-being matter more than what others think or react toward you. Individuation is the first step to figuring out who you are and how you desire to be treated. When you think like an independent person with independent needs, you'll find it a lot easier to protect yourself against unfair or abusive behavior.

Once again, communicating your behaviors with difficult family members will follow the same process as other relationships. However, below are some guidelines that will help you set limits with family members without damaging your relationships:

- **Decide what's best for you.** Take a moment and think about what would make the relationship with a family member feel safe and fulfilling for you. Try not to think about them and their experience, but focus on your unmet needs. Write down a list of these needs, and for each one, set a boundary to protect it. Schedule a time to communicate these boundaries with your family member.
- **Prepare for pushback.** Depending on how long this particular family member has overlooked your needs, they may resist adhering to your boundaries. Don't be tempted to compromise or revert back to how your relationship used to be. Remain calm and level-headed, and repeat the same boundaries. If they violate your boundaries (perhaps to test how serious you are), enforce the appropriate consequence and explain once again why the boundary means so much to you.
- **Know what triggers you, and make the necessary preparations.** Triggers are words, behaviors, or attitudes that cause a negative emotional response. You may already know what triggers you about a family member's actions, however, to protect your state of mind you need to learn how to anticipate these triggers and the best ways to respond. For example, if you suspect that visiting your parents will be stressful, plan ahead of time how long you'll stay there, what topics you'll discuss (and those off the table), and an exit plan if the environment becomes toxic.
- **Practice saying no without explaining yourself.** It isn't always necessary to justify your decisions. It's okay to refuse to do something

and not have to feel guilty about it either. Your 'no' doesn't have to be aggressive to be clear. It just needs to sound certain and not as if there's a question mark at the end. Look into a mirror and practice the different ways of saying no. Hear yourself saying no with confidence and assertiveness. Notice what facial expressions or gestures work well when saying no. Play around with this until you feel comfortable saying no without explaining yourself.

- **Create a list of self-care rituals.** For some people, walking away from family isn't an option. This is usually the case when you're taking care of family members. While healthy boundaries will make the relationship feel a lot more stable, you'll need to practice self-care rituals as a way of disconnecting from others and prioritizing your needs. These may include going to the gym, picking up a hobby, journaling, or finding a support group.

Family relationships are complicated, but that doesn't mean that difficult family members aren't held accountable. Everyone who desires to be a part of your life, whether it be a friend or a family member, must be willing to treat you the way that you want to be treated.

Chapter Takeaways

- When you become an adult, you must complete the process of creating a separate identity from your parents. This prevents you from internalizing your parents' beliefs, behaviors, and traumas, and repeating them in new relationships.
- There are three stages of individuation: declaring, separating, and reconnecting. Declaring your freedom is a conscious choice to think of yourself as someone unique rather than a shadow of your parents. Separating is the painful but necessary stage of creating emotional or physical distance in order to begin the journey of self-discovery. Reconnecting occurs after you have built a solid sense of self and are willing to renegotiate the terms of the relationships.

- Communicating boundaries with friends, romantic partners, or family members is never an easy conversation. However, the sooner you get it done, the more stable and consistent these relationship will be. Always start the conversation with the intention to strengthen your bond, not tear it down. Listen as much as you speak, and be willing to stand up for yourself if necessary.

Boundaries at Work

"A boundary shows me where I end and someone else begins, leading me to a sense of ownership. Knowing what I am to own and take responsibility for gives me freedom."

— HENRY CLOUD

This chapter talks about:

- The importance of establishing healthy boundaries with coworkers
- Whether forming friendships at work is a good or bad thing
- How to communicate assertively in a workplace environment

Why Are Boundaries Necessary at Work?

Work relationships are unique in the sense that they aren't based on attraction or compatibility, but rather collaborating on shared goals. Boundaries with coworkers are useful to ensure that you're not taken for granted (doing more work than you ought to), as well as to work in harmony with others.

Many people fail to set boundaries at work because they assume that coworkers know how to behave respectfully and professionally. This assumption leads to poor communication, being overworked, and resentment amongst colleagues. Just like we can't assume our close friends know what we need, we also can't assume that the people we work with know how to treat us.

The benefits of setting boundaries at work are:

- **You earn the respect of your coworkers.** Having boundaries makes you feel a lot more comfortable sharing your thoughts and suggestions with others without the fear of being shut down or judged. Your boundaries can also teach others how to communicate with you respectfully, so that every interaction is constructive.
- **You set the standards of behavior.** People often test how far they can go with behaviors to see what you will and won't tolerate. By setting boundaries, you communicate clear expectations of what you will and won't tolerate, which ends up becoming how others approach and build relationships with you.
- **You get better at resolving conflict.** Unfortunately, conflict at work can't be ignored like conflict in a friendship or romantic relationship. It needs to be addressed immediately so that it doesn't hamper your workflow. Responding to boundary violations with decisive action reduces the back-and-forth and helps you reach a mutual understanding.
- **You can manage your coworkers' expectations.** There's no doubt that you're exceptional at your job, however, you have limits. For instance, working fast doesn't mean you can take on more workload. Your boundaries draw the line with coworkers and protect you from overcommitting yourself.

As beneficial as having boundaries at work is, there's still the fear of what coworkers might think. Tough conversations with people you aren't close to feel awkward, however, just imagine reporting to a manager or working on a team with a coworker who makes you feel small and undervalued. How would this affect your satisfaction at work?

To make the process of setting boundaries at work less overwhelming, the following section will provide you with examples of what your boundaries might look like.

Examples of Work Boundaries

Healthy work relationships start with healthy boundaries. Take a moment and think about how you desire to feel when you walk into the office in the morning or join a Zoom meeting. Now think about how you desire to feel when you're sharing your ideas or making a presentation. These emotions don't just happen. They come after countless attempts at teaching people how to treat you or how to behave around you. If you desire to feel safe, accepted, and valued at work, consider the kinds of boundaries you would need to establish for that to take place.

To get you started on setting work boundaries, there are three areas you can focus on: job responsibilities, interpersonal boundaries, and personal boundaries. Let's look at each area more closely.

Job Responsibility

Your job responsibilities are the duties that come with your specific role. Before you accept the job position, you agree to complete all of your job responsibilities. This is a boundary created by your manager. If you're unclear about what's expected from you, then you can't work to the best of your ability—and this might cause you to violate the boundary that had been set by your manager. To ensure that you're fulfilling your job responsibilities, answer the following questions:

- What tasks do you perform on a daily basis?
- How does your job contribute to the greater good of the company?
- Who do you report to?
- How is your performance measured?

- What are your current work goals?

Once you're settled in the role, you get to set your own boundaries around your job responsibilities. This means creating rules about the way you work and interact with others. Of course, these rules can't go against your company's policies or culture. They should be directed toward improving your work efficiency and achieving your work goals. Here are a few examples of boundaries you can create:

- asking coworkers not to call your phone after hours
- checking and responding to work emails during designated time slots
- declining meeting invitations that have nothing to do with your current work tasks
- saying no to projects until your schedule has cleared up
- approaching your manager when there's an issue you would like to discuss

Interpersonal Boundaries

Interpersonal boundaries are the limits you create with your manager and coworkers. These boundaries are typically centered around communication preferences, like how you would like coworkers to speak to you or resolve conflict. Examples of interpersonal boundaries at work include:

- the tone of voice others use when speaking to you
- the topics you're open to speak about and those off the table
- how to resolve conflict or work amicably when there's tension within the team
- limits about the sharing of personal or company information

Even if your work relationships are going well and you believe there's no need to set interpersonal boundaries, have a discussion with your coworkers about them. This will help you know how to respond if at any point you or your coworkers violate a boundary.

Personal Boundaries

Personal boundaries are those limits you set with yourself to maintain a healthy work-life balance. They protect you from overworking and ensure you invest your time and energy in other aspects of your life too. Examples of personal boundaries include:

- switching off your work phone when you're at home
- leaving your laptop in the office or in the car after work hours
- scheduling five-minute rest breaks throughout your work day
- taking days off and making sure you don't touch any work during that time
- decluttering your email mailbox after every quarter
- updating your resume every six months

Having these boundaries in place won't protect you from boundary violations. However, if you have read Chapter 3, then you have the necessary tools to set effective consequences and hold coworkers accountable. If you feel intimidated or harassed by a coworker, or maybe that your consequences aren't bringing about the desired change, then you should escalate the matter and allow a third party to intervene.

Can Coworkers Be Friends?

A question that many people grapple with is whether or not to be friends with their coworkers. For instance, what happens when you're placed in a team with someone whom you get along with, and even share many interests with? Is your relationship supposed to be kept strictly professional?

It's possible to meet someone at work and find yourselves instantly bonding. Perhaps you know each other, have mutual friends, or are drawn to each other's personalities. Feeling drawn to your coworkers isn't a bad thing. In fact, if you manage work relationships well, you can balance having both platonic and professional relationships at work. The secret, though, is to take things slow—slower than you would a first date!

The reason for taking things slow is simple: Neither of you are at work to make friends. You're there to accomplish shared goals and objectives. It's in your and their best interest to keep the working relationship at a superficial level until you have built respect for each other and understand one another's work standards and behaviors. After having plenty of professional interactions and going through different work situations together, you can assess if you'd like to get to know your coworker on a friendship level.

Below are more guidelines that will help you navigate the process of cultivating friendships at work:

- **Avoid misreading another person's intentions.** It's polite to smile and be cordial with others at work. Some company cultures may even encourage team bonding events and other social activities. This isn't an indication that you have something in common with your coworker beyond your work duties. Not everyone is open to making friends at work, specifically in competitive environments. Thus, don't be quick to assume that kindness is a sign of friendship.
- **Have as many face-to-face interactions at the beginning.** If you like somebody and would like to get to know them better, take the opportunity to speak to them at work. Avoid sharing personal information about yourself, including your private social media accounts, until you're certain that you trust the other person.
- **Know what (and what not) to talk about.** In some workplaces, employees get to spend a lot of time together. It could be during

brainstorming sessions, team projects, or happy hour. It's easy to forget where you are and who you're talking to when you spend many hours with the same people. However, until you're ready to open yourself up to a friendship, maintain your boundaries when it comes to sharing personal information. You'll know that you've overshared when you feel vulnerable or exposed.

- **When it comes to your boss, tread lightly.** The boss-employee relationship is more sensitive than the relationship between coworkers. This is because your boss is your boss. There's a greater level of consideration you need to have in how you present yourself because you want them to respect you and provide a fair evaluation about your work. Plus, you can still have fun and engage with your boss without being their friend.
- **Avoid forming cliques.** Knowing a lot of people at work and cultivating friendships is good. However, remind yourself that you're no longer in high school. You don't need to form cliques or alliances in the office—and you certainly shouldn't be using these friendships as an opportunity to gossip about or alienate other employees. If you find yourself in a routine of hanging out with the same employees at the same spot, break the routine and get to know other members of your team. You also shouldn't feel pressured to act a certain way just so you can relate to a group of employees. Be yourself and maintain your work standards.

Your coworkers can become some of your closest friends. With the right boundaries in place, you can even balance being personal and professional with one another. Nonetheless, you should be careful of work friendships that are one-sided or only feel like a friendship when certain conditions are met. A good rule of thumb is: If it feels forced, the feeling might not be mutual. If you're ever doubtful about where your relationship stands with a coworker, it's also not a bad idea to be upfront and ask them what their intentions are.

Assertiveness at Work

In Chapter 4, we discussed how to communicate boundaries assertively. From a work context, assertiveness goes much deeper than how you articulate yourself. The main benefit of being assertive at work is gaining the respect of your coworkers. Nevertheless, it's still not an easy skill to learn. If you observe many of your work relationships, you'll find very few people who can communicate assertively. Many of them might fall under the passive, passive-aggressive, or aggressive categories. Below are the common characteristics of these types of employees:

- **Passive coworker:** Internalizes their negative emotions to avoid confrontations or making other employees feel bad or guilty. Their conflict resolution strategy is to go with the flow, even when their needs are compromised. They might say, "I don't mind. Let's go with your idea."
- **Passive-aggressive coworker:** Internalizes their negative emotions, but finds subtle ways of releasing their built-up resentment without their true intentions being known. For example, they're notorious for committing acts of sabotage like missing deadlines or failing to show up to a meeting, and making up an excuse for why they "forgot" to follow through.
- **Aggressive coworker:** They'll express their negative emotions without thinking about the impact of their behavior on work relationships, or whether they're managing the situation in a professional way. When resolving conflict, the aggressive coworker tends to speak more than they listen, and they're likely to defend their position even when they discover they're in the wrong.

Assertive employees aren't necessarily born with the confidence to share their opinions and balance their needs and desires with those of others. In fact, it's possible that due to many boundary violations, the passive or passive-aggressive employee taught themselves how to speak up for themselves and be transparent in how they address issues. As much as all the other types of communicators want to be respected at work, it's only the assertive employee who earns true respect due to their direct and human approach to building relationships.

The assertive employee knows that if they want respect from others, they need to show respect too. Now, this is usually straightforward when there's no conflict amongst employees. When conflict ensues, mutual respect goes out of the window, and the assertive employee must find other ways to appeal to their disgruntled coworker and reach some kind of middle ground. The level of maturity that it takes to be calm and level-headed, even when you're not shown the same decency, is part of what makes an assertive employee respectable. They have a way of seeing the bigger picture, which is typically a win-win situation that dissolves the conflict.

If you would like to strengthen your assertive communication skills, there are a few habits that you can start practicing at work:

1. Express Your Opinions Boldly

Assertiveness is deepened when you find ways to validate yourself rather than seeking validation from others. You have to believe within yourself that you're qualified to perform your job and that you have a lot of value to offer your company. These beliefs must be something you know to be true, otherwise, expressing your opinions boldly will make you feel too self-conscious. Each type of communicator will express their opinions differently, but to be more assertive, focus on being direct while maintaining respect in your delivery.

2. Maintain Eye Contact

Eye contact is a nonverbal cue that displays assertiveness. It portrays confidence and helps you hold other people's attention. In many cultures, maintaining eye contact is also a form of respect, particularly to people who have a higher social ranking. If you work in a traditional environment, this may be a great way to show coworkers respect without using words. When looking into someone's eyes, be careful not to stare without blinking (this could be interpreted as a sign of aggressiveness).

3. Be the First to Admit When You Were Wrong

Part of strengthening your work relationships and earning others' trust is being able to admit when you were in the wrong. Don't allow your position at work to make it hard for you to apologize and make amends. Just as you're confident to stand up for what's right, it's important to show your coworkers that you can own up to your mistakes. If the entire team made a mistake, own your part instead of passing the blame.

4. Be Inclusive of Others

It's also important to make sure that those you work with feel seen and accepted. For example, when making decisions, make sure that everyone has added their input. Being accepting of others is a great way to model how you would like coworkers to treat you. Ideally, you also want to be seen and accepted in all matters relating to your work. When coworkers feel seen and accepted by you, they're more likely to behave according to your standards and show you the respect you deserve.

5. Be Quick to Forgive

Another great way to model a standard is when it comes to forgiveness. Tension often remains in a team or department long after the conflict has been resolved. This can negatively affect teamwork and the general mood in the atmosphere. If you want to work in a harmonious environment, create a standard by being quick to forgive others. Once the disagreement has been settled, be deliberate in keeping the lines of communication open. Make sure that no one feels alienated or ganged up on, and that the team is able to recover and get back to a healthy space.

You'll find that it's easier to be assertive with other assertive communicators at work. However, when you're dealing with a passive or aggressive communicator, you can lose control of your emotions. What often helps when interacting with non-assertive communicators is to prepare yourself for these encounters. At home, spend time rehearsing what passive and aggressive language sounds like so that you can pick up on a coworker's style of communication.

After you have identified a non-assertive communicator, take a moment to tune into your own emotions. Figure out how you're feeling and what you need at that moment. If you don't feel confident enough to engage in the conversation, you can set an immediate boundary. You might say, "I hear what you're saying, but I don't think I'm getting through to you. Can we reschedule this conversation for another time?" If you agree to engage, remember that a conversation includes back-and-forth. Be willing to listen and validate their experiences, and request the same decency in return.

It's also important to remember that some people might never understand where you're coming from despite your attempts to explain your position. It's okay to not win over every coworker or reach a point where you can squash conflict. You're only responsible for your actions and reactions, not how others act or react towards you. Having said all of this, below are a few tips on how to communicate with the passive, passive-aggressive, and aggressive coworker:

If you want to get through to an aggressive coworker, remember the following:

- **Acknowledge their feelings, even when they don't acknowledge yours.** Aggressive coworkers enter a conversation already having high walls. They're so sensitive to criticism or rejection that anything can send them into attack mode. Make them feel more calm by acknowledging how they feel and emphasizing that you're willing to listen and hopefully reach a win-win situation by the end of the conversation.
- **Take a moment to pause before responding to an emotional outburst.** It's important to calm yourself down and make sure you're feeling strong before responding to an outburst. Responding immediately might cause you to escalate your voice or say something you don't mean. If you start to feel like you're acting out of character, it's okay to draw a boundary immediately and walk away.
- **Be intentional about finding common ground.** You don't have to give an aggressive coworker what they're looking for, which is a fight. Go into the conversation being clear about your intentions of understanding where they're coming from and walking away having reached a settlement. It might also be necessary to repeat several times during the conversation that you desire to understand where they're coming from and come to a reasonable solution.

Speaking to passive and passive-aggressive coworkers requires a different strategy. Here are a few pointers that will help you get through to them:

- **Encourage them to share their opinions.** Both passive and passive-aggressive coworkers are afraid of being upfront about what they're thinking or feeling. You may need to encourage them to speak freely, especially if you notice that you've been speaking for a long time. You can also read their body language and point out that they're looking confused, uncomfortable, or like they want to say something.

- **Use nonverbal communication to show openness.** It takes a lot of reassurance for passive coworkers to warm up to others. When you're speaking, be mindful of your nonverbal cues, like your facial expressions or gestures. Communicate positive body language by nodding, smiling, making eye contact, and reacting when they make a joke or say something interesting.
- **Show that you accept them for who they are.** Passive and passive-aggressive coworkers are aware of how their lack of assertiveness makes them appear to others. They're also more alert to boundary violations because of their lack of self-defense skills. When communicating, show them respect by giving them an opportunity to speak and having the conversation at their own pace. Never push or insist on them doing something that makes them uncomfortable, like asking for their opinion in front of a group of people.

As you can tell, not everybody at work communicates in the same way. However, the advantage of being an assertive communicator is that you can place yourself in other coworkers' shoes and communicate in a style that makes them feel comfortable.

Chapter Takeaways

- Work relationships are unique because what brings you together isn't a mutual connection, but rather shared goals and objectives. Therefore, what matters most in these types of relationships isn't being emotionally validated, but being respected.
- It's important to create work standards around your job responsibilities, interpersonal boundaries, and personal boundaries. These will create expectations regarding how you work or structure your work

day, the acceptable and unacceptable forms of communication with coworkers, and healthy limits to create a good work-life balance.

- Even though forming friendships at work isn't wrong, be careful about how much you share about yourself during the early stages of getting to know coworkers. Ideally, you want to establish a professional relationship with other employees and iron out any boundary issues or expectations before you can invite each other into your personal lives.
- Assertiveness at work can help you earn the respect of your peers and model the kinds of behaviors you would like others to show you. Being assertive entering conversations with your guard down, being open to listen and admit mistakes, and being intentional about finding common ground.

Boundaries Around Social Media

"Don't say anything online that you wouldn't want plastered on a billboard with your face on it."

— ERIN BURY

This chapter talks about:

- Why online privacy should be a priority when sharing data online
- The benefits of creating social media boundaries for your mental health
- How oversharing can cost you your job, and how to avoid it at all costs

The Importance of Online Privacy

In Chapter 1, we discussed how you can set boundaries around your privacy. In this chapter, we'll explore the different ways that you can protect your privacy online. It can be difficult to explain online privacy, because technically no one else has access to your tech gadgets besides you. However, even when you have secure passwords and restricted access to your accounts, your digital footprint can still be traced. This means that people are always keeping tabs on you and your content, as well as your data.

Just because you share information online doesn't mean it should be accessible to everyone. Personal data is the term used to describe information that identifies an individual, which might include (but is not limited to) your cell phone number, home address, company address, banking information, etc. You have the right to keep this type of data private, or in some instances choose who you would like to share it with.

If you're somebody who naturally enjoys their privacy at home, then your online activity doesn't need to be any different. Psychological safety still applies in digital spaces, as it does in your relationships. For example, while networking on social media, you deserve to feel free to share your opinions without being trolled or bullied. Although, even when you do experience harassment of any kind, you have the right to enforce consequences. Of course, the boundaries and consequences you establish online will look different to those you establish in your relationships. However, the sense of safety and contentment you feel will be the same.

Take a moment to create a list of your favorite or go-to mobile apps and websites where you have a registered account. For each app or website, write down the type of personal data you have stored there. It could be your cell phone number, email address, banking details, home address, relationship status, educational history, credit profile, social security number, etc. Looking at your list, you can see just how important maintaining your privacy truly is. The more privacy you have, the easier it is to protect your identity online.

Your homework is to go down the list, log into every app or website, and check your privacy or security settings once again. Perhaps when you registered an account on that platform, you were unaware of the importance of your personal data. Now that you know what these platforms have access to, you can adjust your privacy permissions according to how much you're willing to share. It's also good to be on the lookout for privacy policy updates and to take time to read them so you can ensure there are no privacy violations.

How to Set Up Social Media Boundaries

Social media boundaries aren't necessarily created to keep people out—you can simply use the block button or restrict access to your social media accounts for that. Instead, the boundaries you establish around your social media usage are created to protect your mental health.

You have probably noticed how excessive social media consumption can take a toll on your mental health. However, this doesn't mean that social media is completely bad for you. There's no better way to stay connected with loved ones, build successful businesses, and stay updated on the latest world events than through social media. Nevertheless, if you don't create limits for yourself, then your use of social media becomes toxic. Below are some of the dangers of not having social media boundaries:

- **You can become addicted.** Social media can be addictive because of its effects on your mood. This partly has to do with the instant gratification you receive when you get a 'like' or scroll down an endless feed full of curated content.
- **It limits real life social behavior.** When you're so accustomed to online engagement, it can make real life encounters feel unnatural. Online relationships can also be superficial at times, since you never get to fully discover who the person on the other side of the screen is, or how they're truly feeling.
- **You tend to compare yourself to others.** What's considered a normal life online is often not a realistic goal that you can aim at. For example, in real life it takes more than six months to make millions of dollars, find a soulmate, or buy a dream home. Therefore, when you're wrapped up in the illusions fed by social media, you can start to resent your real life.
- **You become distracted from your daily tasks.** It's easy to lose track

of time when you're going through social media. Most platforms are designed to keep you engaged for as long as possible, which makes it difficult to log out once you're online. You can find yourself being easily distracted from your tasks, or performing tasks mindlessly because the real focus is on the content you're watching.

- **You find it difficult to fall asleep at night.** One of the causes of poor sleep is increased screen time before bed. Researchers have found that the blue light emitted from devices keeps your body awake and delays the natural process of sleep. Taking your devices with you to bed can also keep your mind running and make it harder for it to calm down.

So, what are the boundaries you can establish for yourself to monitor your social media usage and protect your mental health? Consider the following suggestions:

- **Technology-free Sundays:** Are Sundays your rest days? Good! This means that you don't need to be scrolling on your social media either. True rest is about being present and practicing self-care, not checking in on what's happening around the world.
- **Technology curfews:** During the week, you can also limit your social media usage by setting a curfew. For instance, after 8 p.m. you can close your laptop, switch off your TV, and put your phone on silent. Disengaging from technology at least an hour before bed will also improve the quality of your sleep!
- **Put your cell phone away when you're with other people:** Answering text messages, creating content, or responding to notifications can be considered rude when you're having a conversation with someone. Not only that, it can also make it harder to pay attention to what they're saying.
- **Conduct a friendship audit:** Go through the list of people you follow on each social media platform and do a purge! Look specifically for accounts that show harmful content and those that make you

feel bad about yourself. Ideally, you don't want to be exposed to any content that doesn't align with your core values or the type of lifestyle you live.

- **Put yourself on a timer:** Like any other task, add "check social media" on your calendar. Dedicate an amount of time to checking your social media, and once that time lapses, switch to another task.
- **Take time getting to know strangers:** Be mindful of the information you disclose to strangers online. It's never wise to share too much about yourself before meeting face-to-face and having a real life encounter. Get to know who they are offline before investing your time, money, and energy into the relationship.

Be Careful Not to Overshare

Oversharing can be defined as sharing inappropriate or compromising information online. On social media, it would be sharing content that might offend your followers, or that is too personal to share on public platforms (even if your social media accounts are private).

Yes, it's true that social media gives you the freedom to express your views, but what happens when these views re-trigger your trauma, create insecurities, or cost you your job? For example, in past decades, we have read many stories of professionals being fired over racist, homophobic, or violent social media posts. This is because HR departments are now taking social media activity into consideration during the hiring process. Not only can oversharing negatively impact your professional life, it can also lead to an increase in frustration and emotional posting (this is particularly true when you notice that your content is receiving traction).

The cycle often begins with an angry tweet or revealing post that gets a lot of likes or reposts. Perhaps you said something controversial, political, or shared a tragic story about your life. Seeing the positive reaction from the post creates a desire for more validation, until you find yourself desperate for constant attention and reassurance from others—even if it means baring your soul on a public platform.

Giving away so much information about yourself simply to satisfy the demands of others isn't safe, nor is it good for your mental health. You shouldn't feel like you owe others your personal life stories or that in order to be accepted, you need to expose sensitive details about your life. Social media connections can't compensate for real life connections, and sometimes oversharing can be a sign of lack of real support. This doesn't mean that you should delete your social media or limit your engagement. All it means is to be aware that your life shouldn't live on the internet.

Below are some of the tips to avoid oversharing on social media:

- **Decide which platforms are for personal and professional use.** Each social media platform has its own expectations when it comes to creating content. TikTok is great for creating short videos, Instagram is a place to share photos, and LinkedIn is where professionals meet to share knowledge. Ensure that the content you share is appropriate for the platform it's uploaded on.
- **Decide whether content is suitable as a post.** Not every idea or experience you have is shareable. There are some stories that are too sensitive to be broadcasted on a post, or may be taken out of context. Consider how the post will be received by others, how they might react, and if it offers enough value to share.
- **Avoid posting when you're emotional.** It's never wise to post when you're not in the right frame of mind. This may include when you're angry or under the influence of drugs or alcohol. What you post can be used against you, even if you didn't mean to hurt anyone. As a rule of thumb, write down what you intend on posting on a notepad and wait a few hours before making the decision to post it.
- **Be mindful of the groups and forums you're associated with.** Sometimes it's not what you say that gets you in hot water, but

the controversial people, groups, or forums you're associated with. Moreover, if you have your company logo on your profile and post content that's questionable, people can associate what you say with your company's reputation.

- **Do a Google search on yourself.** Type your name into Google and see what search results come up. If there's any information that can be used against you or discredits the person you are today, make sure you delete it. You can also adjust your privacy settings on websites you're subscribed to so that you can manage your online reputation.

In a world where content is in high demand, it can be tempting to become an open book and share intimate details about yourself. If sharing personal information is part of your job and you have built a following around it, then it's more than acceptable. However, many of us are associated with people, businesses, and organizations that expect us to safeguard their reputations through our social media usage. A good rule of thumb to use when checking if you should post something or not is asking yourself how well it will age. For example, in a year's time, will people still react positively to your post as they do now?

Chapter Takeaways

- Online privacy ensures that your identity and personal data is safe online. You can strengthen your online privacy by regularly checking and adjusting your privacy settings on apps and websites.
- Privacy is also crucial on social media, but even more important is protecting your mental health. Social media boundaries can help you set healthy social media limits so that you don't leave feeling drained or discouraged after spending time online.
- Social media boundaries can also protect you from being heavily influenced by unrealistic expectations or investing too much time in online relationships rather than maintaining real relationships.
- While it's good to express yourself on social media, be mindful of

how your posts can be perceived by others. The type of content you post should be appropriate for each platform, and create a positive reflection of who you are.

Extra Exercises to Set Boundaries

"Hold yourself back, or heal yourself back together. You decide."

— BRITTANY BURGUNDER

This chapter talks about:

- Boundary building exercises to boost your confidence

Recognizing Boundary Violations

It's important to notice when a boundary has been crossed so you can communicate the violation clearly. Have a look at the tables below and make a note for each boundary violation you resonate with.

Communication Boundaries	
Violation	**Notes**
Texting, calling, or emailing excessively.	
Responding to you sarcastically.	
Yelling or raising their voice at you.	
Interrupting while you're speaking.	
Ignoring or minimizing your feelings.	
Others:	

Physical Boundaries	
Violation	**Notes**
Trying to isolate you from friends or family.	
Touching your body without consent.	
Going through your belongings without your permission.	
Denying your privacy.	
Standing or talking too closely.	
Others:	

Emotional Boundaries	
Violation	**Notes**
Constantly coming to you with bad news.	
Relying on you too much for emotional support.	
Failing to keep promises.	
Using humor in a demeaning way.	
Changing the topic or refusing to address your hurt feelings.	
Others:	

Control Your Urges

When a boundary has been violated, you might be triggered to act without thinking clearly about your decision. The following exercise will help you slow down your thinking and process your urges rather than acting upon them.

- **What do you have an urge to do?**

- **What boundary violation has triggered this urge?**

- **If you decide to give in to this urge, what will be the negative consequences?**

- **If you decide to control your urge, what will be the positive consequences?**

- **What coping strategies can you turn to as a distraction from the urge?**

- **Is there anyone you can speak to about your urge?**

Confronting Your Negative Beliefs

Your belief system reflects stories that you have told yourself about who you are and how safe it is to interact with the world and others. By recognizing thoughts that are harmful, you can pause and replace the thought with one that aligns with the kind of world you desire to live in. Below are examples of thoughts and the types of beliefs they reinforce. In the third column, write down a healthy replacement for the thought.

Thought	**Belief**	**Replacement**
Nobody understands me.	Overgeneralization	
My parents ruined my childhood.	Blaming	
I'm stupid and weak. That's why others take advantage of me.	Assumption	
If I get married, only then will people respect me.	Does not follow	
I feel betrayed. This friendship is over.	Emotional reasoning	
I don't need friends. I'm okay spending time by myself.	Relative deprivation	
If I raise an issue with my boss, they'll fire me.	Aggression as an argument	
They'll either respect me, or I'll cut them out.	Black and white thinking	
I'm judged because I'm different.	Mind reading	

Journaling About Your Feelings

Find a quiet room in the house or office where you can spend 20 minutes. Write about something that has been on your mind that you haven't spoken about. Don't worry about grammar, spelling, or punctuation—simply allow the pen to move on paper. Describe the emotional impact of this issue and the toll it has taken on your well-being. It's normal to get emotional during this exercise. Write as much as you feel comfortable sharing, then look over what you have written at a later time.

Responding to Threatening Communication

When you're communicating with an aggressive person, perhaps a family member or coworker, and they make threatening remarks that aren't true, it's important to stop them and challenge their opinions with your truth. Your truth is based on the positive perceptions you hold about yourself (i.e. your belief system and core values). When challenging threatening messages, focus on providing positive evidence from past experiences or what you know to be true about yourself.

Consider each threatening message written below and provide counter-arguments that reflect your truth—the positive beliefs you hold about yourself. For example, if a friend said, "You wouldn't be able to do anything without me," you might respond, "The truth is I have a whole life outside of this friendship and my current goals are proof of that."

Threatening Message	**Challenge**
You will never amount to anything.	
You can't do anything right.	
That was such a stupid mistake.	
Do you listen with your ears?	
You need to fix the problem now, otherwise there will be consequences.	
Do you honestly think this is your best work?	
I think you're living in a fairytale. This is the real world.	
You need to try harder to impress me.	
I have never met someone so slow like you.	
Toughen up. Other people have it harder than you.	

Conclusion

Setting boundaries is one of those skills that's easy enough to explain, but difficult to put into practice. What makes boundaries tough to establish isn't necessarily that you don't know what you want, but instead that you're afraid of not getting what you need. You may be afraid of being turned down, ridiculed, or criticized for requesting others to respond to your needs.

It's possible that you didn't grow up in a household where there were any house rules, where adults behaved like adults, and where children were allowed to be children. As a result, you grew up without having a solid sense of self that could protect you from abusive or manipulative people you would meet as a young adult and well into your adult years.

The purpose of this book was to help you address that crippling fear and offer you the necessary tools to set healthy boundaries. However, even more than that, the strategies and exercises offered were designed to help you start believing more in yourself. The secret of communicating assertively, enforcing consequences, and knowing when to leave a relationship lies in having a high sense of self-worth. You need to believe without a doubt that you deserve feeling psychologically safe in relationships, voicing your opinions, and being shown the same respect you show others.

As you continue to practice setting boundaries, remind yourself that putting your needs first isn't selfish. It's an act of self-love. If you don't prioritize your needs, who will? Get comfortable with the process of setting standards with others and holding them accountable for their actions—yes, even those difficult family members or toxic coworkers. Setting boundaries will never stop being something that you do, because you're either meeting new people or discovering new needs from your relationships.

Therefore, make conversations about boundaries a common topic in your personal and professional relationships. Create an environment for open and honest communication about limits and expectations so that you leave very little room for misunderstandings. With time, you'll gain more confidence in standing up for yourself and teaching others how to relate to you.

Be patient with yourself; you'll start to notice your relationships becoming how you desire them to be. And if you're not able to rehabilitate a relationship, accept the situation and be willing to move on.

BONUS: Your Free Gift

I'm only offering these bonuses for FREE to my readers. This is a way of saying thanks for your purchase. In this gift, you will find a guide with extra tools to start your inner journey and a self-development course.

Healing your Inner Child First Guide

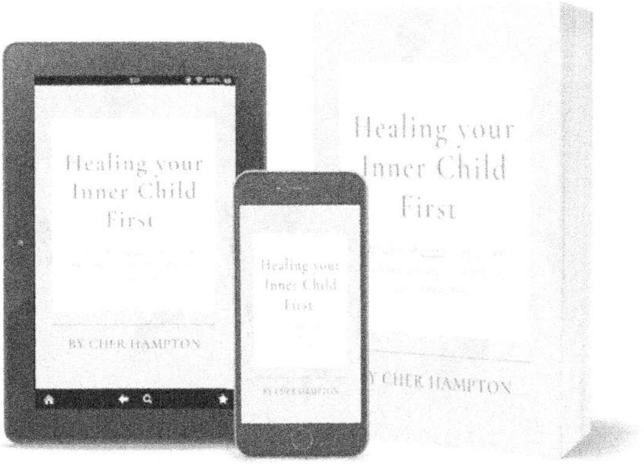

Inside this guide, you'll discover:

1. How to use Journaling in the Healing Process.
2. Questions to Remember Your Inner Child.
3. Space to Write Your Thoughts Down.

4. Questions to Better Understand Your Inner Child's Pain.
5. Motivational Things to Say to Your Inner Child.
6. Positive Affirmations + a 5-Step Method to Make Your Own.
7. An Extra Inner Child Meditation.
8. A Checklist.
9. And More...

The Personality Development Wisdom Course

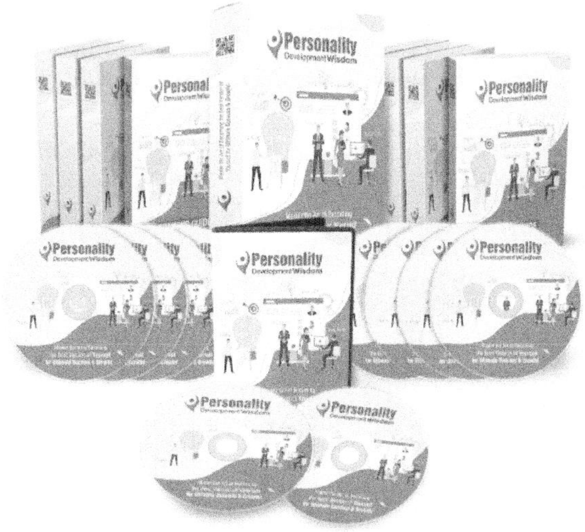

Inside this course, you will find:

1. Personality Development - An Overview
2. How to Transform Yourself into a Better Version
3. How To Improve Your Body Language
4. How to Boost Up Your Self-Confidence, Self-Esteem, and Motivation
5. Best Tips to Overcome Procrastination
6. The Power of Positive Thinking

7. How to Improve Your Workplace Wellness
8. How to Enhance Your Soft skill
9. Learn and Practice the Art of Work-Life Balance
10. How to Deal With Failures
11. How to Manage and Overcome Your Fears
12. Best Ways to Deal With Difficult People
13. Stress and Energy Management
14. How to Have a Productive Day
15. Bonus 1 - Cheat Sheet
16. Bonus 2 - Mind Map
17. Bonus 3 - Top Resource Report
18. Bonus 4 - 10 Extra Articles

To receive these extra **bonuses,** go to: https://booksforbetterlife.com/thrive-through-healing

Or scan the QR code:

Thank you!

I really appreciate you for purchasing my book!

You had the chance to pick a lot of other books, but you chose this one.

So, **thank you so much** for purchasing this book and reading it to the very last page! I hope that I was able to help you in your healing process, as my goal is to help as many people as possible!

Before you close the book, I want to ask for **a small favor**. Would you please consider ***leaving an honest review*** about the book? **This would be really helpful for me**, as I'm an independent author and posting reviews is the best and easiest way to support me.

The feedback you provide will help me so I can continue selling, improving, and writing books. **It will mean the world to me to hear from you!**

Go to this book on Amazon and scroll down (https://mybook.to/thrive-through-healing), or scan the QR code to leave a review:

Amazon US <—— ——> Amazon UK

Amazon CA <—— ——> Rest of the World

References

Ainsworth, M. D. S., & Bell, S. M. (1970). Attachment, exploration, and separation: Illustrated by the behavior of one-year-olds in a strange situation. *Child Development, 41*(1), 49–67. https://doi.org/10.2307/1127388

Amanda Palmer quote. (n.d.). Goodreads.

Amstel, B. (2019, June 9). *Individuation in therapy*. goodtherapy. https://www.goodtherapy.org/learn-about-therapy/issues/individuation

Anderson, K. (n.d.). *The stages of trauma and recovery.* Clarity Therapy NYC. https://www.claritytherapynyc.com/stages-of-trauma-and-recovery/.

APA Dictionary of Psychology. (2022). Dictionary apa. https://dictionary.apa.org/dysfunctional-family

APA. (2022). *Handout 27: 5 Steps of cognitive restructuring instructions.* American Psychological Association.

Bowlby, J. (1969). *Attachment and loss* (Vol. 1). Basic Books.

Brazelton, T. B., & Yogman, M. W. (1986). *Affective development in infancy* (pp. 95–124). Ablex Pub. Co.

Bretherton, I. (1992). The origins of attachment theory: John Bowlby and

Mary Ainsworth. *Developmental Psychology, 28*(5), 759–775. https://doi.org/10.1037/0012-1649.28.5.759

Chen, G. (2020, December 30). *How the arts benefit your children academically and behaviorally*. Public School Review.

Cherry, K. (2022, May 2). *What is attachment theory?* Verywell Mind. https://www.verywellmind.com/what-is-attachment-theory-2795337

Chopra, D. (2013, August 9). *How to communicate your emotional needs in relationships*. Chopra. https://chopra.com/articles/how-to-identify-and-express-your-needs-in-relationships

Christiansen, L. (2020, July 30). *What is an obsessive personality? Signs, symptoms and treatments*. Straight Talk Clinic. https://www.straighttalkcounseling.org/post/what-is-an-obsessive-personality-signs-symptoms-treatments-by-lauren-christiansen

Cotec, I. (2020). *Shadow work and healing the inner child (In 5 steps)*. HeroRise. https://www.herorise.us/shadow-work-and-the-inner-child/.

Diamond, D. (2008, June 7). *Essential secrets of psychotherapy: The inner child*. Psychology. https://www.psychologytoday.com/ca/blog/evil-deeds/200806/essential-secrets-psychotherapy-the-inner-child.

Delagran, L. (n.d.). *How to deal with fear and anxiety*. University of Minnesota. https://www.takingcharge.csh.umn.edu/how-deal-fear-and-anxiety.

Eagle, J. (2011, December 1). *How to individuate*. Live Conscious. https://liveconscious.com/2011/12/how-to-individuate-step-one/#:~:text=If%20you%20want%20to%20learn

Eagle, J. (2011, December 2). *How to individuate. Learn the second step in this 3-step process*. Live Conscious. https://liveconscious.com/2011/12/how-to-individuate-step-two/

Eanes, R. (2016, January 15). *Turning toward our children: Answering bids for connection*. The Gottman Institute.

Elizabeth Gilbert quote. (n.d.). Goodreads.

Estrada, J. (2019, October 30). *Reparenting therapy can help you heal your inner child—here's how*. Well+Good. https://www.wellandgood.com/reparenting-therapy/.

Firestone, L. (2022). *Freeing Yourself from childhood trauma*. PsychAlive. https://www.psychalive.org/freeing-yourself-from-childhood-trauma/.

Fredrickson, B. (2014). *The science of happiness, theory and practice*. Pursuit of Happiness. https://www.pursuit-of-happiness.org/history-of-happiness/barb-fredrickson.

Harvard Health Publishing. (2020, July 6). *Understanding the stress response*. Harvard Medical School.

Hay, L. L. (2016). *Mirror work : 21 Days to heal your life*. Hay House, Inc.

Hanh, T. (2022). *Body Scan*. Spirituality & Practice Resources for Spiritual Journeys. https://www.spiritualityandpractice.com/practices/practices/view/28468/body-scan.

Henry Cloud quote. (n.d.). Goodreads.

Howie, V. (2021, January 7). *Heal your sacral chakra inner child*. Chakra Boosters. https://www.chakraboosters.com/heal-sacral-chakra-inner-c

hild.

H Raven Rose quote. (n.d.). Goodreads.

Kabat-Zinn, J. (2003). Mindfulness-based interventions in context: Past, present, and future. *Clinical Psychology: Science and Practice, 10*(2), 144–156. https://doi.org/10.1093/clipsy.bpg016.

Jacobs Hendel, H. (2018, July 16). *Getting to know your three brains: Part 4 triggers*. Hilary Jacobs Hendel.

Kellend, M. (2015). "Carl Jung." In *Personality Theory in a Cultural Context*. Portland State University. https://pdx.pressbooks.pub/thebalanceofpersonality/chapter/chapter-5-carl-jung.

Khodabakhsh, M. (2012). Attachment styles as predictors of empathy in nursing students. *Journal of Medical Ethics and History of Medicine, 5.*

Lancer, D. (2022, July 2). *What is a trauma bond? What Is Codependency?* https://whatiscodependency.com/what-is-a-trauma-bond/

MasterClass. (2022, January 14). *Paradigm shift definition: 6 Examples of paradigm shifts*. MasterClass.

Meyerowitz, A. (2020, November 20). *Why we should embrace our inner child and 5 ways to do it.* Red. https://www.redonline.co.uk/health-self/self/a34725323/how-to-embrace-inner-child/.

Moulik, S. (2022, April 25). *Individuation process: Learn to master your "self" in 5 stages.* Change Your Mind Change Your Life. https://medium.com/change-your-mind/individuation-process-learn-to-master-your-self-in-5-stages-52ac89b19ce7

Munger, K. (n.d.). *How your attachment style impacts your stress response.* FuelEd.

Neff, K., & Dahm, K. (2015). *Self-Compassion: What it is, what it does, and how it relates to mindfulness.* In Springer. https://self-compassion.org/wp-content/uploads/publications/Mindfulness_and_SC_chapter_in_press.pdf

New International Version. (2011). Bible Gateway. https://www.biblegateway.com/passage/?search=1%20Corinthians%2013%3A4-7&version=NIV

Newsome, T. (2016, May 13). *Things more important than love in a relationship.* Bustle. https://www.bustle.com/articles/160467-11-things-that-are-more-important-than-love-in-a-relationship

Patrick Rothfuss quote. (n.d.). Goodreads.

Pandey, S. (2021, December 31). *Break the cycle of trauma: Re-parent your inner child.* The Bliss Key. https://www.theblisskey.com/post/break-the-cycle-of-trauma-re-parent-your-inner-child.

Price, L. (2017, October 13). *9 Times stars shamelessly spilled other celebs' secrets*. People. https://people.com/celebrity/stars-telling-other-stars-secrets/

Proyer, R. T., Gander, F., Bertenshaw, E. J., & Brauer, K. (2018). The positive relationships of playfulness with indicators of health, activity, and physical fitness. *Frontiers in Psychology,* 9. https://doi.org/10.3389/fpsyg.2018.01440.

Robinson, L., Smith, M., & Segal, J. (2018, November). *Emotional and psychological trauma*. HelpGuide. https://www.helpguide.org/articles/pt

sd-trauma/coping-with-emotional-and-psychological-trauma.htm.

Robinson, (2021, July). *Laughter is the best medicine.* HelpGuide. https://www.helpguide.org/articles/mental-health/laughter-is-the-best-medicine.htm.

Robinson, L., Segal, J., & Jaffe, J. (2021, February). *How attachment styles affect adult relationships.* HelpGuide. https://www.helpguide.org/articles/relationships-communication/attachment-and-adult-relationships.htm

Rowe Ward, P., & Ward, L. (2021, December 20). *Loving-kindness: healing your inner child.* Lion's Roar. https://www.lionsroar.com/loving-kindness-healing-your-inner-child/.

SCB. (2022). *Elon Musk's working style - Iron Man in the real world.* SCB. https://www.scb.co.th/en/personal-banking/stories/success-story/elon-musk-working-style.html?hash_primary=6772730A47BFEB83D5B792387B6168E4C32460AC#:~:text=Works%20like%20a%20mad%20man

Shelley Klammer quote. (n.d.). Goodreads.

Siegel, D. (n.d.). *Reflections on the mindful brain.* https://communityofmindfulparenting.com/documents/research/Siegel-Mindfulness.pdf.

Sinclair, J. (2021, July 12). *How mindful breathing can change your day (and your life).* BetterUp.

Sjöblom, M., Öhrling, K., Prellwitz, M., & Kostenius, C. (2016). Health throughout the lifespan: The phenomenon of the inner child reflected in events during childhood experienced by older persons. *International Journal of Qualitative Studies on Health and Well-Being, 11*(1), 1062-1071. https://doi.org/10.3402/qhw.v11.31486.

Snowise, K. (2015). *Authenticity: Are you embracing your true-self?* Thrive.How. https://thrive.how/authenticity-are-you-embracing-your-true-self/.

Solove, D. J. (2014, November 24). *Should celebrities have privacy? A response to Jennifer Lawrence*. TeachPrivacy. https://teachprivacy.com/celebrities-privacy-response-jennifer-lawrence/

Sorgen, C. (n.d.). *Bonding with baby before birth*. WebMD.

Stelter, G. (2016, December 18). *A beginner's guide to the 7 chakras and their meanings*. Healthline. https://www.healthline.com/health/fitness-exercise/ 7-chakras.

Tara Bianca (November 18, 2019). *The Flower of Heaven*.

Thoughtless Delineation. (2018, December 27). *Moving on from childhood trauma*. Medium. https://medium.com/thoughtless-delineation/moving-on-from-childhood-trauma-e222b9c7e28b.

Townsend, J. (2022, May 26). *How to determine the right consequences when setting boundaries.* Boundaries Books. https://www.boundariesbooks.com/blogs/boundaries-blog/how-to-determine-the-right-consequences-when-setting-boundaries

Tygielski, S. (2017, February 9). *You stop attracting certain people when you heal the part of you that once needed them.* Shelly Tygielski. https://www.shellytygielski.com/you-stop-attracting-certain-people-when-you-heal-the-part-of-you-that-once-needed-them/

Vironika Tugaleva quote. (n.d.). Goodreads.

Vishnu. (2015, May 29). *9 Ways to release your limiting beliefs so you can find love again*. Tiny Buddha.

Printed in Great Britain
by Amazon

35994619R00341